Further Praise for *Your Drug-Free Guide to Digestive Health*

I am very impressed by the thoroughness of this work. This book will be useful as a self-help book and for professionals. Here we have an excellent textbook and desktop reference to help them address aspects of treatment not covered by homeopathic philosophy and practice such as fields of nutrition, natural and environmental medicine. The homeopathic tips and advice are comprehensive yet easy to follow and are obviously based on in-depth experience and research. I am sure many people will benefit from the book. Well done! ~ Robin Logan RSHom (NA) FSHom, author of 'The Homeopathic Treatment of Eczema' and creator of '7 Cream' www.natural-skin-health.com

Your Drug Free Guide to Digestive Health masterfully negotiates the needs of both practitioner and patient. This book contains a treasure of reliable information delivered in a smart and easy to use format. Bravo Heather! ~ David Brule, Homeopath, Coordinator, Homeopathic Research Network of Canada, Riverdale Homeopathic Resources, www.rhronline.ca

I'm a 47 year old female who has struggled with irritable bowel syndrome (IBS) since I was 18. Over the years I have tried many herbal remedies, supplements and dietary changes in an effort to relieve my IBS symptoms. By following the protocol that homeopath Heather Caruso developed for me, I am completely IBS symptom free for the first time in 29 years! Her knowledge and genuine interest in helping me have changed my life. I know her book *Your Drug-Free Guide to Digestive Health* will provide others with the tools to change their lives, too. ~ Cathy Newton, Guelph, Ontario

As a primary health care practitioner I believe that Heather Caruso's book *Your Drug-Free Guide to Digestive Health* is an excellent reference for a growing number of people with digestive disorders. In addition, often times in practice we encounter people that will need that extra piece of advice, supplement or remedy. This book has made that an easy task. I highly recommend this book as reference in your practice.
~ Dr. Michelle Whitney, D.C., Ann Street Family Chiropractic, Guelph, Ontario

Reading Heather's book, *Your Drug Free Guide to Digestive Disorders*, broken down into an A-Z format makes us realize how much valuable help is out there for gastrointestinal problems. I wish that I had this book when my sons were little because children often have digestive issues. I could have used it alongside my Mendelson natural health bible. This book is a must for every home and healing office.
~ Lori Wilson B.A., M.S.W., author of Demystifying Medical Intuition and founder of Inner Access www.inneraccess101.com

Author's Acknowledgements

After having spent a year writing this book, I have many people to thank. Those friends who have helped me along the way such as Cathy Newton, Micheline Duhamel, Deborah Caruso and Susan Maclean are much appreciated. Thanks to those who have generously leant me a hand in writing this book simply because I asked. I am especially grateful to my husband for without his support I would not have done this project nor would I be a homeopath. Thanks to my mother for her support of my career decision and faith in me.

Disclaimer

Every effort has been made to ensure that the information in this book is whole and correct. However, neither the publisher nor the author has given professional advice to you, the individual reader. Any health book, including this one, is not a substitute for professional advice from your medical doctor. You are responsible for seeking professional advice from your medical doctor or homeopath.

As you may be aware, the natural remedies in this book are not a full picture of all of the herbs, supplements or homeopathic remedies available to treat every disorder. They are only the more commonly used ones. **If you have any serious disorder, you are strongly recommended to seek the help of your doctor or a qualified alternative health professional (such as a homeopath or naturopath).**

This book provides information about natural remedies for gastrointestinal illnesses. Neither the author nor the publisher assumes any responsibility for any loss, injury or damage arising from any information or suggestion in this book.

TABLE OF CONTENTS

INTRODUCTION

THE OBJECTIVE OF THIS BOOK

I decided to write this book because gastrointestinal (GI) disorders affect much of our population. According to *Forbes.com*, a recent survey of statistics on drug sales found that Nexium and Prevacid are the third and fourth most popular prescriptions in North America. Both these drugs treat heartburn and/or acid reflux. I saw a new television commercial of a man jumping for joy in his apartment hallway with a few different food delivery men. They were holding pizza, chicken wings, Chinese food and burgers. He was rejoicing because he could now eat all the junk food he wants without consequence. This was due to his new antacid medication. However, anyone with common sense knows that when you eat junk, there are consequences even if they are unseen. Pharmaceutical drugs do help to reduce some of the symptoms of gastrointestinal disease but they are often not a complete cure. There are harmful side effects with most drug therapy and they tend to only suppress the symptoms. Homeopathic and natural remedies offer a safe and natural cure without side effects. Many remedies can be used in conjunction with prescription drugs. This is beneficial because working together helps to reduce symptoms but a person's overall foundation of health is consistently and progressively strengthened using a natural approach. This can reduce the need and dosage of many prescription drugs, which in the long run is an excellent goal with no potentially harmful side effects.

In practice, I use natural remedies and diet to treat various disorders successfully. I see approximately one in four clients with digestive disorders. I am surprised at how easy it is to heal from these disorders naturally, yet many people do not choose this route. It is either due to a lack of knowledge or discipline. It should be everyone's priority to be healthy by making <u>positive</u> choices, not to just try to mask their symptoms. I have seen some of the tougher digestive disorders to treat, such as irritable bowel syndrome IBS), Crohn's disease and colitis abate using a completely natural approach. Surgery and aggressive drugs should and can be used as a last resort.

Homeopathy, natural supplements and diet are powerful tools for healing. Various homeopathic texts dating as far back as the late 1790s have documented full cures of various GI diseases. Homeopathy is not a new medicine. Many people think of it as a "New Age" type of healing. However, it has been around formally since 1790 and even noted in Hippocrates' times. It is based on a logical, systematic use of certain laws. It is a medical practice due as much respect as allopathic, meaning mainstream, medicine. Many medical doctors are becoming trained in homeopathy and seek natural health treatments for themselves and their families. These are exciting times for homeopathy.

Diet is often an obstacle to cure. Many medical doctors do not discuss diet with their patients. A lot of people believe that their diet is healthy. However, they have not had proper education regarding healthy food choices and how to properly combine foods for optimum nutrient digestion. Some people may eat the same food repeatedly or eat too much of one food group. Many people eat mostly fast or junk food. Education is crucial. Nights of suffering and doctor's visits can be easily prevented with a proper diet.

Although gastrointestinal conditions are not usually life threatening, they do have a negative effect on our quality of life. For example, many cannot venture far from home without mapping out restrooms. Some people are in pain from the simplest diet. Inflammatory bowel disease (IBD) can cause humiliation coupled with depression, isolation and nutritional malabsorption. Gastrointestinal disorders such as IBD, constipation, esophageal reflux and hemorrhoids have been successfully treated with homeopathy, nutritional supplements and dietary intervention. Many of these diseases are considered incurable in allopathic terms. Using traditional homeopathic wisdom and clinical findings, I hope to give the average person suffering with GI problems the tools to achieve health by using the simple, natural solutions outlined in this book.

CHAPTER ONE

UNDERSTANDING HOMEOPATHIC PHILOSOPHY AND PRESCRIBING

Homeopathy has been a healing art for over 200 years. It was founded by a German named Samuel Hahnemann. He was a maverick who challenged the medical system of his day. During these times, horrid practices such as blood letting and other cruel procedures were popular. Hahnemann had even recommended humane treatment of the insane and envisioned a place of solace for them, rather than the typical tortures and exorcisms they endured. He was considered both a hero and an outcast in his time. Upon his death he was recognized for being one of Saxony's greatest men.

Today, homeopathy is used worldwide by lay people and professional homeopaths. It is practiced in hospitals in many countries such as England, India and Germany. It is an inexpensive form of medicine that offers people a chance to heal deeply. Homeopathy has no side effects and is safe and gentle for any age or ailment. It can safely be used in conjunction with traditional medical treatment. Oftentimes a person will fare better when they use a complementary approach to their health care.

THE PRINCIPLES OF HOMEOPATHY

Like Cures Like

Homeopathy's foundation is built on a few basic principles. The first most popular principle is the theory that like cures like. If you give a dose of a crude substance to someone, it can produce certain symptoms. When you give the same thing to a sick person who suffers from these same symptoms, it can heal them. It works because a person cannot suffer from two similar diseases at the same time. For example, one cannot have cowpox and smallpox at the same time. This is why people were vaccinated with cow pox to successfully prevent small pox. A common remedy in homeopathic medicine, Allium Cepa, made from red onion, illustrates this principle. When we cut an onion, our nose and eyes water and burn. If you have a cold with these same symptoms, it will be cured with homeopathic doses of Allium Cepa. In healthy people the substance produces the same symptoms one wants to cure in the sick.

Many people are amazed that this principle is effective. However, many times in the news I have heard reports of so-called "medical breakthroughs." One was that low doses of Arsenic cure some cancers. We all know Arsenic is a poison in crude doses and actually causes symptoms like cancer. Diluted doses cure the symptoms it causes. Homeopaths have been preaching this for years!

The Minimum Dose

Another principle of homeopathic medicine is to use the smallest dose required to ellicit a cure. This is called the minimum dose. Homeopathic remedies are very diluted and carry an energetic quality to them, due to their preparation. Between each dilution remedies are succussed, which means shaken, 10 times. This gives the remedy potency yet it is still diluted. Despite being very dilute homeopathic medicine still remains effective.

The minimum dose affects the greatest cure. Less is more with homeopathic prescribing. When potencies are diluted, after a 12CH or 24X there are no molecules left of the original substance. This is called Avogadro's number, which is named after Amadeo Avogadro (1776-1856), a physicist who first recorded this principle in his own scientific studies unrelated to homeopathy.

The Symptoms, Not the Disease

Remedies must match the person's symptoms not the disease name. This differs greatly from traditional Western medicine. Homeopathy is more time consuming. However, if used correctly, it heals people at a very deep level. Such symptoms as a person's emotional state and physical symptoms are considered important in homeopathy. This stimulates one's unique healing mechanism. Symptoms that are important are often those that are considered strange, rare and peculiar. A person who has a sore foot, cannot walk on it and is exceedingly irritable may receive a dose of Bryonia Alba. Another person who claims they are well but are lame with an injured foot may receive Arnica Montana.

Our Vital Force Acts, Yet it is Intangible

Physical and emotional symptoms may be an expression of ill health through our vital force. Our vital force is an energy that maintains life, expression of health or disease. Everyone has a unique vital force that invisibly animates our existence.

Scientists have found that thoughts actually carry an energy that can be physically measured and documented by attaching electrodes on the head. We cannot see thoughts. It is said that what we put out, we attract. We seek things that confirm our way of being. Choosing certain friends, our clothes, our jobs and even our diseases match our "vibration". People look for certain events in their life, no matter how trivial to validate certain parts of their belief systems. Homeopathic medicine is congruently matched to one's symptoms, which deeply resonate on an energetic level to the person's healing core. After the correct homeopathic remedy, your body will be asking, "Where have you been all my life?"

I believe homeopathy works in the following manner: when we take a homeopathic substance that matches the totality of our symptoms or our vibration, it awakens our healing mechanism. Since we cannot accept two diseases of the same kind at the same time, our vital force is stimulated to rid itself of this foreign vibration that has been introduced. Along with the ridding of the foreign vibration comes healing, as the vital force's dormant healing powers have been awakened. The homeopathic medicine causes a medley of healing events.

From Within Outward and Top Down

Homeopathy cures from inside out and up to down. This means that the remedies act on the areas that are most crucial to survival first. For example, with a constitutional remedy, (meaning a remedy suided to one's emotional, mental and physical symptoms), the medicine will act on the inner organs before clearing up a skin disorder. This is because the body's natural healing mechanism will protect the heart or liver before the skin, because they are crucial for life. Symptoms heal from the mind or brain area first and then the lower extremities depending on the condition. This is the body's method of self preservation.

Order of Appearance

Remedies may act to cure symptoms in order of their appearance. This is called Hering's Law. This essentially means that if someone had asthma after they had eczema their asthma would be cured first and then their eczema. This is usually the case if someone has used suppressive treatments that did not cure. These treatments drive the symptoms deeper into the organism. With complicated cases, layers of disease like those of an onion present physically in reverse order of their appearance. One of my teachers used to say, "You do not outgrow your allergies, only your pants." Diseases that are suppressed can turn into other disorders. An example of suppression would be eczema which is a superficial ailment of the skin that when treated with steroids, often later manifests in asthma. The lungs are a deeper organ and are more pertinent for survival. The vital force is always looking for ways to express its disharmony. A non-suppressive treatment with a gentle constitutional remedy guides our unique vital force to heal deeply.

Types of Prescribing

Constitutional Prescribing

Homeopathic prescribing can be constitutional which means that the prescription is suited to all of a person's symptoms, physical and emotional. A prescriber would look at someone's history, heredity and susceptibility to disease as well as their current condition. Personality plays a role in homeopathic prescribing. Traits such as whether a person desires company or solitude, has irrational fears and how they express anger are accounted for. Diet, digestion, sleep, weather preferences, body temperature and sexual function are all considered important. This method empowers a healing mechanism (i.e. the vital force) and can prevent the expression of disease.

Even things that seem unrelated to a disease are important. Here is a good example to highlight this point. A woman with premenstrual syndrome had seen me for years. She would improve a bit and then relapse, but never experienced a complete cure. During her last appointment she told me she was separating from her husband. He had been living with another woman on weekends. This was a shock to me, because she had not let any emotional distress, heartbreak or anger come to the surface. I gave her the remedy, Natrum Muriaticum, for suppressed emotions. Her premenstrual discomfort swiftly went away. Homeopaths usually prescribe on the unusual symptoms if it is a chronic condition. If it had just happened and she was rightfully upset, an acute remedy like Ignatia for grief could be used.

Acute Prescribing

Acute prescribing is a type of homeopathic prescribing suited to ailments of rapid onset that last only a few days or weeks. The superficial symptoms of the acute ailment are considered. These complaints can be things such as viruses, parasites or bacterial infections. Acute injuries, shocks and traumas are successfully treated with homeopathic medicine. One of the most common acute injury remedies is Arnica Montana. It is an excellent remedy to keep on hand. Arnica speeds up the healing process and relieves pain. Keep a 6 or 30CH potency on hand and take four pellets every few hours as needed.

Combination Remedies

Combination remedies can be quite useful for healing. They are diluted and safe; however, they are not suited to a person's unique symptoms. These remedies are made by combining a few key homeopathic remedies in one bottle to target a particular ailment. For example, for liver trouble a combination of Lycopodium, Nux Vomica, Chelidonium and Taraxicum may help to effectively drain toxins from the liver. It will not however, offer deep healing so as to prevent the liver from soon becoming congested again.

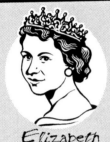

Elizabeth

Did you know...
Her Majesty Queen Elizabeth II and the Royal Family have a Homeopathic Doctor named Peter Fisher. They use homeopathy as their first line of defence from illness.
Ask yourself: If homeopathy is good enough for the Royal Family, could it be good enough for you too!
Source: *Homeopathic Revolution; Why Famous People and Cultural Heroes Choose Homeopathy,* by Dana Ullman MPH; www.homeopathicrevolution.com

Homeopathic Potency; what does "X", "D" and "CH" mean?

Homeopathic potency and frequency may vary. If you are a homeopathic novice, it is best to use the lower potencies, such as those ranging from a six CH to 30 CH. The CH refers to the Centesimal Hahnemann potency scale. This potency is diluted in the ratio of one part original substance to 99 parts carrier liquid. An X or D potency is the decimal potency, which is diluted one part original substance to nine parts carrier liquid. X potencies are used often and typically in a six or 30 X dilution.

CHAPTER TWO

HOMEOPATHIC SELF-PRESCRIBING; HOW TO CHOOSE THE CORRECT SINGLE REMEDY

Homeopathic self-prescribing can be a very rewarding thing. With any self-prescribing please keep in mind, that **you may need the help of a professional homeopath**. Some of the disorders named herein can be quite difficult to tame such as ulcerative colitis and Crohn's disease. These diseases and any other chronic condition are better treated by a professional. Since you are looking at this book and the remedies mentioned here, you must be made aware that there are **hundreds of homeopathic remedies that work well with digestive disorders.** I have not included all of the hundreds of them simply because that would require volumes, not a single book. Here are the most common for these types of disorders. You may suit one of the remedies listed here and have success.

WHAT YOU NEED TO KNOW ABOUT SELF-PRESCRIBING

Homeopathic case taking is an art and takes some skill to perfect with experience. Homeopathy requires a different manner of case assessment than traditional medicine. The more detailed information you acquire about the person's symptoms, the easier it is to prescribe accurately. One needs to write everything down. The following approach for prescribing for oneself is an adaption of the book "Homeopathic Self Care" by Robert Ullman and Judith Reichenberg-Ullman (see bibliography).

Observation
When taking a case, observe, listen and then ask questions. By observing you would note things such as their facial expression, skin tone (pale, flushed, sweaty), body posture, the throat, eyes, ears etc. You may notice that they have perspiration or discharges with a particular consistency, colour or odour. Make note of the person's facial expression, such as frowning, smiling or a pained look. Gestures such as scratching, repetitive movements, trembling and blinking are significant. Notice what environment is preferred such as a dark place, sauna, bathtub, under warm blankets, outdoors or in a mess.

Listening
Listen to the language the sick person uses to describe their symptoms. Asking open ended questions is better, such as "tell me more" to get information in the patient's words. If they say, "I feel like I am being threatened or attacked", write those symptoms down in their words. It is easier to research and review that information. It is hard to recall the subtleties of a case without good notes.

Ask Questions
Once your client has finished telling you about their problem in their own words, you can begin to ask questions. You can solicit more information by asking questions like:
- When did your symptoms start?

- How long have you had them?
- Do you know what caused your problem?
- When do your symptoms come on, time of day, season etc.?
- Is there anything that brings out the symptoms or makes you feel better or worse?
- Do you notice any difference in other environments?
- How is your mood with all that is going on?
- If you could rate the symptom on a scale of one out of ten, what would it be? 10 for very intense, 1 for barely there.
- How is your appetite or thirst? Do you have any cravings, aversion or aggravations from food and drink?
- Is there anything unusual about your symptoms?

Picking the Remedy

Write down your important symptoms and look up the remedies under the disorder that matches your condition. If the symptoms are strong, they must be covered in that remedy. If there are any mental or emotional symptoms present, they must also be included. It is easier to find a remedy when unusual symptoms are present as compared to only common ones. For example, there are at least a hundred remedies for the common cold. However, if there are a few strange, rare and peculiar symptoms, it can cut that list down considerably.

For example, people who have a cough who need the remedy Bryonia, tend to be very irritable and want to be left alone. They are thirsty and don't want to be moved. These symptoms are unusual for a cough and are found in only four remedies. That cuts the list down considerably. By reading the description of the remedies you can then differentiate between them.

Under each remedy heading, the symptoms that are strong or common to that remedy are marked in bold. If you match to a few of the bold symptoms, you may try that remedy. You will never match every single symptom of the remedy. Usually you would want at least three of your main symptoms to match a remedy. If none of the remedies match your symptoms, seek the help of a professional or do more research.

What Should I Expect from a Homeopathic Medicine?

Once you have taken the remedy, you must know what to expect for a response to know when to re-dose it or change your selection. There are a few scenarios that may appear:

- **No change:** After a few days of being on the remedy, you notice there is no change in the intensity of your symptoms. You likely do not have the right remedy. You can try a different remedy or you may need help from a professional homeopath.
- **There is some change for the better:** You have found some of your symptoms less intense or gone all together. The medicine has acted. You can stop the remedy and wait until you need another dose (when the symptoms return.)
- **There is complete relief:** The remedy has worked beautifully and all symptoms are gone. Only repeat this medicine if you have a relapse.
- **Symptoms are aggravated and there is no improvement:** If you find you have felt worse after taking the remedy and the symptoms are the same, you either have

the incorrect remedy or you have antidoted it, which results in no improvement after the aggravation. (Read on about antidotes to remedies) If you have antidoted it, meaning cancelled it, you can re-administer the remedy. If it is a chronic disease, you can wait a day or two to see if the symptoms abate. You can choose another remedy if there is no improvement or seek the help of a professional homeopath.

- **Symptoms are worse but improvement follows:** The medicine is correct and only repeat the dose as needed. Sometimes people have a slight aggravation from the remedies after they are prescribed. This is the body's way of fending off symptoms by recognizing them and then releasing them.

- **The original symptoms go away and then a new set appear:** The remedy picture has changed. Sometimes people have layers of symptoms like an onion. They may have released one layer and exposed a past layer that needs to be healed. It could also mean that a different remedy needs to be prescribed to cure the case.

What we gather from above is not to re-dose a remedy if it is acting. Only take the remedy again if you have a relapse or have antidoted it. You can take the remedy in a 6 to 30CH, four pellets under the tongue, two to three times a day. You can take them for a few days and then wait and see what happens. **If you have an improvement or aggravation, stop taking the remedy and wait.** Less is more with homeopathic prescribing.

Antidotes to Homeopathic Remedies

Some things such as camphor, mint, strong odours, coffee, drugs, X-rays, CAT scans, MRIs and electric blankets are known to antidote or counteract remedies. These strong flavours are said to antidote the remedies because the very gentle remedies can't compete with them. Coffee affects the nervous system but tea is said to be less injurious to the remedies.

Dosing the Remedy

Usually people would take their homeopathic remedy in a 30CH potency in a pellet or liquid form. Pellets are taken two or four at a time or drops are taken ten at a time, under the tongue. They have to be taken away from consuming meals or drinks by at least half an hour.

Lower potencies like those under a 6 CH dilution, have some molecules of the original mother tincture left. Therefore, a low potency is not suitable for remedies that are made from heavy metals or other potential poisons. Any dilution above a 6 CH has no potential side effects.

The higher the number of the potency, the more often it is used to treat the person's constitution, emotional or mental state. Lower potencies are more often used to treat the physical body. For example, if you sprain your ankle, you may use a Ledum 6 CH. Lower dilutions often have to be dosed more frequently than higher dilutions. However, it is best to start with a lower potency and increase it as needed. Start with a 12 or 30 CH initially. When taking a remedy over time, its effectiveness may wear off and a higher potency may be required.

Homeopathic remedies don't necessarily have to be prescribed daily; one dose may suffice. However, in an acute condition you may take the remedy every four hours as needed for a few days only. If there is an improvement or worsening, stop the remedy. When you are dealing with a chronic condition, you may take the remedy for a few weeks before you see a change. Be sure to read the previous section on what to expect when taking a homeopathic remedy to know when to stop or re-dose the remedy.

CHAPTER THREE

THE IMPORTANCE OF DIET
AND ITS ROLE IN DISEASE

Today's high paced lifestyle requires both parents to work to make ends meet. Cooking a meal from scratch isn't always a priority. Very few families eat together anymore, which is a sad reflection of our times. Most people of my era recall their mother as the archetypal housewife. She prepared the family meals from scratch and tended to her children. She may have bought a loaf of bread but would not hear of buying any baked good when she was capable of making it better at home. For most of us, that domestic matriarchal role is a memory. Luckily our family roles have expanded and fathers contribute to the home much more than ever before. We have little excuse for poor nutrition other than a lack of interest. Nutritional education of every family member is crucial.

Many people have a faulty idea of what a healthy diet is. Sometimes our best intentions fail because food labels are mysterious to the average person. The food industry's labeling distorts our perception of healthy foods. For example, packages state the contents are "low fat" yet they are high in refined carbohydrates, salt, sugar and chemicals. All the other ingredients may make us fat but the product itself contains less fat. We assume a low fat product is a healthy choice, but often it is not.

Did you know?
You are what you eat and do not excrete….
If you spread out the surface of the lining of your small intestine, it would fill the surface of a tennis court! The great surface of the small intestine aids in quick and efficient absorption of digestive products into the blood stream. This means that the intestines come in contact with the external world through what you consume! This is why one should be cautious with what one eats.

If someone has food sensitivities or allergies, labels can misguide them to consume products containing the offending food. This is because the food industry uses different names for common offenders or allergens to continue to sell product without changing the recipe. For example, monosodium glutamate (MSG) has several names such as hydrolyzed vegetable protein or anything with "protein" at the end may contain MSG. "Pea protein" on a label would mean it is a hydrolyzed protein rather than a plain pea. The label would just note "pea" if it was the vegetable. For most companies, food is a money making industry and our health is not their motivation. Usually, life threatening allergens such as nuts warrant conspicuous warnings on labels.

Do your own research on nutrition and beware of television claims. If you decide to enjoy a meal out, be aware that many restaurants don't disclose all the ingredients for their patrons. These ingredients may not be healthy for someone with gastrointestinal disorders. The cost of eating out may not be worth the pain. However, if you have to eat out, this book will arm you with the knowledge to make the right choices from the menu.

Many types of foods actually increase inflammation and dysbiosis in the body. These two states are the root cause of many diseases like inflammatory bowel disease, hypertension, headaches and even cancer. Dysbiosis is an excess or imbalance of bad bacteria in the gastrointestinal tract. Inflammation can cause a chain of cellular events that release inflammatory proteins into the body. Foods that cause this inflammation are high glycemic or high fat ones. High glycemic means the food quickly converts into a sugar in the bloodstream. Examples are white bread, white rice and sugar. Fats that cause inflammation are fried, trans or hydrogenated fats. Oils that are re-used for cooking become rancid which can cause oxidation. Oxidation causes damage to cells.

Although I don't believe in a completely low fat diet, I do believe one should be sensible about the quality, quantity and source of fats they use. We need fats for the health of our skin, hair, nails, brain and even our cells. Each cell in our body has a fatty membrane.

Imagine scenario number one: you eat fried eggs, bacon and white bread for breakfast. At lunch you eat some deep fried cut potatoes and chicken fingers with coleslaw. Then for dinner you eat a pork chop cooked in olive oil with potatoes and a beer.

Now, scenario number two: for breakfast you have toasted 100% rye bread with butter and almond paste. For lunch you eat a mixed greens salad with regular fat cottage cheese. At dinner you have wild salmon sautéed in coconut oil with wild rice and grilled peppers.

Now consider this. Both of these diets include saturated fats. Which one do you think is healthier? Of course number two is. One can still be healthy and eat certain fats in moderation. The studies that show that saturated fat in diets lead to cancer and heart disease may just be looking at the health of those in group one. As the old adage goes, "everything in moderation."

For year, the Mediterranean diet has toted benefits for cardiovascular health. It uses mainly olive oil and fish in this diet. Olive oil, like other plant-based fats have a heating point at which the oil tends to oxidize. Butter, lard and coconut oil are said to be saturated fats but they can be heated to a high temperature for cooking without turning into a trans-fat. However, many of us are averse to cooking with lard, butter or tallow. If you choose to cook with a vegetable-based oil, sauté food at a lower temperature to prevent oxidation. Do not re-use heated oils for other cooking projects.

Choose foods in their raw form, such as fruits and vegetables, whole grains, nuts and seeds. Choose low fat and low glycemic foods because they reduce inflammation and prevent many diseases. Healthy fats, such as fish oil, olive oil and flax are better sources of fat than deep fried oils. This way of eating is good for cardiovascular health, prevents cancer, promotes hormone balance and reduces inflammation and dysbiosis.

Organic foods are good choices when they are available. Organic foods tend to be more costly than regular foods, however, the increasing demand that is making organic mainstream is bringing down prices. Organic farming is not a big business like regular crop farming. If you have to choose only some organic foods, seek organic foods at your grocery store or health food store that have the skin that is thin or permeable, such as grapes or strawberries because they are more easily permeated by the pesticides. However, you cannot wash away all of the pesticides that is in a fruit that has been sprayed. Once it is contaminated, it stays that way. It is wise to try to consume only organic foods if you can. If you cannot buy fresh fruits and vegetables, you can use flash frozen vegetables. They have more nutrients and fewer additives than canned goods. It is a good idea to grow your own vegetables in the summer. It is an enjoyable pastime and stress reliever for many.

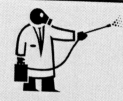

Did you know....
American children aged 6 to 11 years old had organophosphorus pesticide, chlorpyrifos at **four times the level** U.S. Environmental Protection Agency deems acceptable for long-term exposure. Chlorpyrifos is designed to kill insects by interfering with their nervous system. It also has been shown to be a nerve poison for rodents and humans alike. We have many other chemicals in our body both permitted and banned by our government for agricultural use. Agrochemical companies aggressively promote the use of many of the chemicals that our bodies are burdened with. **Ask yourself:** Would you want yourself or your kids to eat pesticides or carry neurotoxins for life?

Source: "Chemical Trespass: Pesticides in Our Bodies and Corporate Accountability" by Kristin Shafer   www.panna.org

It is wise to eat properly to ease the burden on the gastrointestinal tract. For portions, you can visually look at your plate and divide it into four equal parts. One part should be protein such as lean meats (chicken, turkey, fish) or legumes, one portion should be a whole grain (such as brown rice, whole wheat, rye, potatoes and whole grain pasta); and two portions should comprise fruits and vegetables.

The glycemic index is the rate at which food converts into a sugar in the bloodstream. High glycemic foods such as sugar, white bread and white rice quickly convert into a sugar. Low glycemic means the food flips into a sugar less quickly in the bloodstream. High glycemic foods support bacterial dysbiosis. See Table 1 for classification of low, medium and high glycemic and fat foods. In **column one**, you will see low glycemic and low or healthy fats, **column two** is medium glycemic and medium fat and **column three** is high glycemic and high or unhealthy fat. The best column to eat from for health in general is column one. Column two foods are fine to consume, but not more than one third of the daily food intake per day. Column three is best avoided or eaten only on special occasions.

Table 1: A Guide to Healthy Eating Via
Low Glycemic and Low Fat Foods

Key to understanding lists:
Food List 1: Eat freely from this column.
Food List 2: Eat from this column, about one third of daily food intake or less.
Food List 3: Avoid this column for optimum health.

See the following markers beside foods to achieve greater health, * + #

Foods marked with * beside it: Eat in moderation because these are high in glycemic load.

Foods marked with +: Eat in moderation because these increase your susceptibility to disease. They may contain food colouring, artificial preservatives or heavy metals for example. Please note some low fat foods, have been moved to third column, because they contain artificial sweeteners or trans fats.

Foods marked with #: Do not eat if you suffer from candida or dysbiosis

Food List One	Food List Two	Food List Three
BREAD PRODUCTS * Pita bread, whole wheat (1/2)*# Pumpernickel bread*# Sourdough bread*# Rye (100%) Bread*# Stone ground whole wheat (100%)*#	BREAD PRODUCTS:* Rye Crispbread* Breton wheat crackers*	BREAD PRODUCTS*# Bagels*# Baguettes*# Bread, white, french*# Buns, white (hot dog,hamburger etc)*# Cake*# Cookies*# Donuts*# Corn bread*# English Muffin*# Melba Toast* Tortilla* Muffins*# Pancakes*# Stuffing*# Waffles*# Pizza*#
CEREAL:* All Bran* Bran Buds* Fibre First* Oat Bran* Oatmeal (slow cooking)* Red River Cereal*	CEREAL* Grapenuts* Life* Oatmeal (quick cooking)* Cream of Wheat* Puffed Wheat* Special K* Raisin Bran*# Muesli*#	CEREAL* All cold cereals* Cheerios*# Corn Bran*# Corn Chex*# Cornflakes*# Rice Chex*# Granola*# Rice Krispies*# Total*# Shredded Wheat*# CRACKERS* Graham Crackers*# Melba toast* Stoned Wheat Thins* Ritz*# Rice cakes*
GRAINS:* Barley* Buckwheat* Bulgar* Quinoa* Rice (Basmati, Brown, Long and Wild)* Whole wheat pasta*	PASTA*# Fettuccine*# Macaroni*# Penne*# Linguine*# Spaghetti*# Vermicelli*#	PASTA* All canned pasta*# Gnocchi*# Macaroni and cheese*# Noodles, instant or canned*# Ravioli with meat sauce*# Tortellini with cheese or meat*# GRAINS* Rice (instant, white, long grain, jasmine)*# Rice noodles, white*#

Food List One

DAIRY PRODUCTS
Cottage cheese (light and fat free, 1%) #
Cream Cheese, fat free#
Feta cheese, light#
Goat cheese, light#
Parmesan, fat free#

Milk, skim, 1%
Sour cream, fat free#
Yogurt, fat free

FRUIT
Apple	Apricot, raw
Apricots, dried*	Blueberries
Cherries	Cranberries
Grapefruit	Grapes
Lemon	Mango*
Orange	Peaches
Pear	Plum
Raspberries	Strawberries

VEGETABLES
Asparagus	Artichokes
Broccoli	Brussel Sprouts
Cabbage	Carrots
Cauliflower	Celery
Corn*	Cucumber
Eggplant	Lettuce
Mushrooms#	Onion
Olives#	Pickles#
Peas	Pepper
Radishes	Spinach
Snow Peas	
Sweet Potato (Yam)*	
Squash	Tomato
Water Chestnut	Zucchini

Food List Two

DAIRY PRODUCTS
Butter (This is a saturated fat but withstands high temperature for cooking and does not turn into a trans fat. If used in moderation, it is a healthy choice as compared to margarine containing hydrogenated oil.)

Cheese, Cream# low fat#
Cottage Cheese Regular
Goat cheese, regular#
Ricotta Fat Free#,

Ice Cream, low fat with sugar#
Milk, 2%#
Sour Cream, light#
Yogurt, light
Yogurt, fat free with sugar#

FRUIT
Banana	Kiwi
Fruit cocktail, water cocktail	
Mangoes	Papaya
Pineapple (fresh and water packed)	

FRUIT JUICE (unsweetened)
Apple# Grapefruit# Pear#
Pineapple#

VEGETABLES
Artichokes	Beets
Potatoes, new boiled	
Pumpkin	

Food List Three

DAIRY PRODUCTS
Cheese, Brie#, Cheddar#,
Cream#, Feta#, Mozzarella#,
Mozzarella, shredded#
Parmesan, shredded#
Swiss#   Ricotta#

Cream, half and half#
Whipping cream, light and regular#
Sour Cream, regular#
Ice Cream, regular#
Ice Cream, fat free with sweetener+#
(please note this is low fat but contains artificial sweetener which is unhealthy)
Milk, homogenized#
Chocolate#
Margarine, regular
Yogurt, regular, plain and flavoured
Yogurt, fat free with sweetener+,
Yogurt, frozen, fat free with sweetener+
(please note this is low fat but contains artificial sweetener which is unhealthy)

FRUIT
Applesauce with sugar#
Cantaloupe
Fruits, canned in syrup#
Figs, dried*#
Honeydew melon
Lychee, canned in syrup#
Raisins# Watermelon

FRUIT JUICE
All sweetened juices#
Prune juice#

VEGETABLE
Broad Beans	French Fries#
Hash Browns#	
Instant Potatoes#	
Parsnips Potatoes, mashed#	
Rutabaga	Turnips

Food List One	**Food List Two**	**Food List Three**
LEGUMES AND NUTS	LEGUMES AND NUTS	LEGUMES AND NUTS
Beans: baked, in tomato sauce, black, butter, garbanzo (chickpeas)*, green, kidney, lima, mung, navy, pinto, soya, romano	Beans, kidney, canned	Beans, baked with pork#
	Lentils, canned	Broad beans
	Soya milk	Fava beans
Peas: black eyed, split	Split pea soup, canned	Peanut butter (regular, not
Lentils	Most nuts and seeds	peanuts only)
	Peanut butter# (peanuts only)	
PROTEINS	PROTEINS	PROTEINS
Eggs, whites and yolks	Bacon, turkey	Bacon#
Fish and shellfish+	Beef, liver, flank, top round,	Beef, broiled, porterhouse, short
(these may contain heavy metals	ground	ribs, ground, rib steak, sirloin,
and should be consumed one to	Chicken, leg with skin	T-bone, tenderloin
two times per week)	drumstick, thigh	Duck
Game meats (deer, caribou etc)	wing with skin	Fish, fish sticks, breaded fish
Roe	Cornish hen	Deep fried meats of any kind
Salmon (wild)+	Sardines, canned in olive oil	Ham#
Trout+(wild)	Luncheon Meats, roast beef,	Lamb, leg, rib
Tuna, blue and yellow fin+	Black Forest ham	Luncheon Meats#
canned in water+	Turkey	Organ Meats (kidney, heart,
Beef, extra lean	Rabbit	brain, giblets, liver)
Beef, eye of round	Tofu, regular	Pate de foie gras
Chicken, skinless, breast	Turkey, dark meat, with skin,	Pork, Hot-dogs# loin,
Pork, tenderloin Tofu, low fat	ground	sirloin, spare ribs
Turkey, breast, no skin		Sausages
Veal, leg		Veal, loin
FATS*	FATS*	FATS*
Fat Free Salad Dressings*#	Butter* Coconut Oil*	Canola Oil*
Flaxseed oil, do not heat*	(Butter and coconut oil are	Lard (lard is a saturated fat but it
Grapeseed oil	saturated fats but withstand high	withstands a high temperature for
Olive oil*	temperature for cooking and do	cooking without oxidizing)
	not turn into a trans fat. If used in	Margarine+*
	moderation, they are acceptable)	Mayonnaise#
	Corn Oil*	Peanut Butter*#
	Mayonnaise, light*#	Shortening* Palm Oil*
	Sunflower oil* Peanut Oil*	
	Salad Dressings, light*	
	Sesame Oil*	
SWEETENERS	SWEETENERS#	SWEETENERS#
Stevia	Honey#	Sugar, white, brown#
	Molasses, unprocessed,	Corn syrup#
	blackstrap#	Glucose#
	Maple syrup#	Maltose#
	Sucralose – Splenda+	Maltodextrin#
		Saccharine – Sweet N Low+
		Aspartame – Equal– Nutrasweet+

Food List One	Food List Two	Food List Three
	SNACKS	**SNACKS**
	Angel Food Cake#	Corn chips# Potato chips#
	Water Crackers#	Pretzels, thin# Rice cakes#
	Arrowroot Cookies#	Candy bars#
	Tortilla chips, baked, low fat#	Candy#
		Donuts#
		Popcorn, plain, microwave#
		Pizza#
		Desserts (pie, cakes, brownies, tarts)#
DRINKS	**DRINKS**	**DRINKS#**
Water	Wine, red and white#	Power drinks, Gatorade#
Mineral water	Beer, light, regular#	Soda pop#
Tea, green and herbal	Soda pop, diet+	Lemonade#
Herbal	Coffee, black#	Iced tea#
Greens drinks	Tea, black#	Fruit punch#
		Alcoholic beverages#

Food Combining for Optimum Digestion

Many people find food combining is very useful for digestive concerns. It is good for people who want to maximize their natural ability to digest and absorb nutrients from their foods. It is based on combining certain types of foods to utilize our digestive chemistry to the fullest. This is a particularly good idea for those who suffer with bloating, gas, constipation and diarrhea. Some people lose weight following the principles of food combining. In my practice, I use a very basic form of food combining. Eat fruit alone and at least half an hour or more away from other foods. Combine starches with vegetables and combine protein or fat with vegetables. Do not eat fruit with any other food and don't combine protein or fat with starches.

Fruits are a simple carbohydrate. They are digested very quickly if you eat them on an empty stomach. If you combine them with any other complex carbohydrate or fat you may find that you have a lot of gas, bloating and pain. This is because the fruit that is normally digested and absorbed very quickly ferments when it is mixed with other types of foods. It creates a gassy soup of bacteria which ferments and turns into alcohols, acetic acids and vinegars.

Starches are such things as potatoes, rice, bread, pasta and crackers. Proteins are fish, meats and legumes. Legumes also fall into the starch category. They are best combined with grains to get all the amino acids required. Usually these amino acids are found in meat and in combination with legumes and grains. Fats are things like nuts, seeds, oils and animal fats.

Conclusion

It is ideal to eat according to the columns one and two of Table One. The foods in column one are low glycemic and have less saturated or trans-fat which reduces inflammation and other inflammatory processes that lead to disease. This diet is helpful in preventing heart disease, hormone balance, blood sugar, dysbiosis and many other disorders. Eat a diet rich in fruits and vegetables, whole grains, legumes, lean meats and fish. Divide your plate in quarters, making one quarter protein, one quarter grains and half fruit or vegetables. If you suffer from bloating and distension, try the basic food combining.

CHAPTER FOUR

COULD HIDDEN FOOD ALLERGIES OR SENSITIVITIES BE MAKING YOU ILL?

Did you know that you may enjoy a food you are sensitive to? You can actually become addicted to foods that make you sick. This is not always the case with food sensitivities or allergies. Some people do not know what foods they are sensitive to and have a reaction to. Some hate the food they are sensitive to and some love it. It can be difficult to accurately diagnose food sensitivities and allergies. Food allergies are related to a number of factors such as heredity, dysbiosis, antibiotic use, susceptibility and others. They can be more pronounced at different times of the year and in certain situations. They can cause a number of diseases. The number of disorders that are commonly linked to foods is extensive and includes:

ADHD	Insomnia	Chronic Catarrh	Ear Infections
Celiac Disease	Depression	Glue Ear	Chronic Fatigue
Crohn's Disease	Allergies	Stomach Aches	Recurring Tonsillitis
Colitis	Eczema	Acne	Hives
Constipation	Asthma	Epilepsy	Bedwetting
Diarrhea	Obesity	Headaches	Migraines
Rheumatoid Arthritis	Lupus	Psoriasis	Psoriatic Arthritis
Heartburn	GERD	Flatulence	Belching

Food reactions can occur up to 72 hours after the food has been ingested. Some food intolerances make a person more susceptible to reactions to other foods. It can be quite a complicated venture to determine your own food sensitivities. Some people have a low susceptibility to a food and may have to eat pounds of it to get a reaction. Other people may get a reaction with very little of the food. The amount of food you require to have a reaction differs and depends on your susceptibility.

Some people have had food allergies or sensitivities since birth that may have manifested in diseases like chronic ear infections, eczema, colic, tonsillitis and hives. Recurrent antibiotic use causes secondary candida which in turn causes more intestinal troubles and allergies down the road. Some may develop food allergies later in life. Many are shocked to find that they can no longer tolerate a food they have eaten for years. (However, logically we know that we are not the same physiologically or emotionally at age 55 compared to age two; as we age, our bodies change.)

What is a Food Allergy versus a Food Sensitivity?

The most common food allergens are eggs, peanuts, cow's milk products, soy, tree nuts, shellfish, fish and wheat. A food allergy is a full blown immune reaction where one can detect an immune complex (a cluster of interconnected antigens and antibodies) in the blood. A food sensitivity can be more subtle and an immune complex may not be found in the blood. Detecting a food sensitivity or allergy can be difficult. IgE, the immunoglobulin that is related to food allergies or sensitivities, triggers mast cells (defined by Wikipedia as a resident cell of several types of tissues) to release histamine.

Typically IgE is found in the skin, the lining of the lungs and the intestinal tract. It is not always seen in abundance free floating in the blood and therefore some blood tests may show incorrect readings. The immunoglobulin IgG is present in some delayed food reactions. Delayed food reactions occur after 24 hours.

Histamine produces a range of allergic symptoms. Some symptoms are hoarseness and tingling lips, palate, tongue or throat. Nausea, vomiting with colicky pains and diarrhea may occur. Some people have skin symptoms such as hives, eczema, itching, redness and swelling. Respiratory symptoms are coughing, wheezing, tightness, pain and dyspnea. Mucous in the sinus and nasal cavity may be present. Sneezing, runny nose and eyes are common. Some people may lose consciousness and have a drop in blood pressure. Seek medical attention to rule out an allergy if you suffer from any of these symptoms. Many people are required to carry an EpiPen, which contains epinephrine. It is used when an allergy is life threatening.

A food intolerance is reproducible and causes undesirable negative reactions. It is not considered an allergy because immune complexes are not found in the blood. However, we do not yet fully understand the complex workings of the immune system. Research has shown that people with food sensitivities are helped by drugs that suppress IgE from releasing mast cells. Mast cells trigger histamine which, when released, causes a variety of allergic symptoms. If medication that decreases histamine works for food sensitivities, it would stand to reason that food sensitivities are somehow related to allergies.

WHAT CAUSES FOOD SENSITIVITIES?

1. Enzyme Deficiencies

Intolerances can be linked to a number of factors such as enzyme deficiencies, food as drugs and irritants. Enzyme deficiencies can cause food sensitivities. For example, people who are lacking in lactase, an enzyme that helps people to digest milk, will have negative reactions to dairy products. Some people are lactose intolerant. This can be acquired after an infection such as giardia or using antibiotics. Bifidobacteria, a beneficial bacterium found in the gut, is said to be helpful for those who have lactose intolerance.

2. Celiac Disease

Celiac disease is an intolerance to gluten found in wheat, oat, rye, spelt and barley. For some people, eating gluten causes an inflammatory reaction that actually destroys the villi in the lining of the small intestine. In this disorder, a biopsy of the small intestine will show blunting of villi, crypts, hyperplasia and lymphocyte infiltration. Symptoms of celiac disease are abdominal bloating, diarrhea, gas, ulcers and cramps. Some people can feel unwell emotionally and suffer from anxiety and depression. The only effective treatment for celiac disease is to avoid foods containing gluten.

3. Enzyme Deficiencies and Toxic Overload

People who suffer from migraines and hyperactivity are thought to be lacking certain enzymes that break down the chemical compounds in our environment. Some doctors of environmental medicine believe that we lack certain enzymes because the environment is burdened with toxins. This toxic load that we endure makes organs of elimination such as the liver work at full capacity. Picture our body's toxic load like a bucket of water with a few particles of dirt in it. Every particle is a toxin and an additional irritant. Once the bucket is full, we are overflowing with dirty water. Rather than contain all of this "dirt" in our bucket, it spills over the side and we manifest symptoms. We do not have the capacity to metabolize more toxins than we can tolerate. An example of a toxic burden is when children are exposed to secondhand smoke in the home and have an increased incidence of allergies.

4. Irritating Foods Equal an Irritated Reaction

Irritating foods, such as curry, hot peppers or Tabasco sauce, will naturally aggravate a person's GI tract. This usually clears up if these foods are not consumed in excess or are cut out altogether. Some foods act as drugs, such as caffeine and chocolate. Chocolate is said to have opiate-like properties. Caffeine in coffee and tea can cause dyspepsia, heartburn, diarrhea, irritability and the jitters.

5. Psychological State Influences Allergic Reactions and Vice Versa

Immune reactions have been linked to psychological states according to some psychoneuro-immunology studies. For example, asthma or eczema can be triggered by emotional traumas that cause a chain of events mediated by the immune system. Many people who come to my office were healthy until a great stress occurred: the breakup of a marriage or the death of a loved one, for example. Emotional factors are difficult to measure and study with regard to physical symptoms. However, you do not need a study to tell you that the start of your problems began with emotional stress.

Food sensitivities can also trigger strange psychological shifts such as sadness, irritability, mania and even schizophrenic symptoms. For example, someone who is sensitive to wheat products would become severely depressed whenever they ate wheat. They would feel down for days after eating ever so little of it.

6. Heredity

Heredity seems to play a role in the development of allergies. If you have two parents with allergies, you have a 40% to 60% chance of developing allergies. If you have one parent with allergies, you have a 20% to 40% chance of developing allergies. If you have a sibling with allergies you have a 25% to 35% chance. If none of your relatives have allergies, you still have a 5% to 15% chance of developing allergies. Thirty-five percent of kids who have asthma have at least one diagnosed food allergy.

7. The Hygiene Hypothesis

Another theory about the prevalence of food sensitivities or allergies is the "hygiene hypothesis." Studies have shown that kids who grew up in a sterile clean environment have more allergies than ones who lived with a dog or a mother who wasn't the best housekeeper. Research has also shown that kids who have been exposed to certain parasites actually show less allergy and asthma. We overuse antibiotics which kill all good and bad bacteria in the gut. In children, an early introduction of antibiotics prevents the development of a healthy immune system. It depletes both good and bad bacteria in the gastrointestinal tract. If our GI tract has an aseptic environment, without both good and bad bacteria, our immune system becomes deranged. It is thought that bad bacteria in balance with the good actually trains the immune system to function properly. If it doesn't function normally, it recognizes harmless things as potential allergens and organizes an inflammatory attack. We need a balance of both good and bad bacteria to be healthy.

8. Micro-organisms Affect Our Immunity

Food intolerance can also be caused by other factors such as dysbiosis, chronic infections such as candida, parasites and bacteria. For example, the bacterium that causes ulcers, Helicobacter Pylori, has been shown to also cause allergies. Certain microbes can encourage an overgrowth of bad gastrointestinal bacteria. Leaky gut syndrome may occur if these bad bacteria are out of proportion to the good bacteria. Also things such as stress and drugs (steroids, painkillers and antibiotics) can cause leaky gut. Leaky gut is characterized by the cell junctions in the GI tract separating. This allows partially digested food proteins to leak into the bloodstream. These particles of food start a medley of immune reactions. Immune cells start recognizing these particles as "non-self" and launch an attack. This process results in symptoms of inflammation, autoimmune disease, allergic and/or food reactions.

9. Over Consumption of the Same Foods

Foods that we consume most frequently are usually what we become sensitive to. Dogs fed the same kibble everyday have more incidences of food allergies. However, dogs in the wild rarely have such problems. The theory is that their food supply always varies. Foods that are consumed frequently become allergies. In Japan, rice allergies are common. In Scandinavia, fish allergies are prevalent. This is good advertising for food rotation diets.

Addiction and continual consumption of certain foods can cause an adaptation to it. For example, an offending food may give you an initial reaction but if you consume a small portion of it every day, you may become accustomed to it. After a while, you may feel sluggish if you do not have this food and when you have it, you feel picked up again. If this pattern persists over a period of time, you will need to eat more of the food to feel well. Once you get to a high dose of the offending food, you will start to suffer ill health. Some people are not willing to suffer withdrawal symptoms because it may feel worse than the symptoms of the allergy. However, these symptoms typically disappear after one week. Consider the following example.

Some people hate coffee when they first try it and they feel jittery and nervous. After a few days or weeks, they develop a resistance and have no symptoms. In time, they need coffee to be energized in the morning. After a while, they need to have 3 to 5 cups a day to keep their energy up. Over the course of a few years, they start to suffer with heartburn, osteoporosis, gastroesophageal reflux and stomach pain. If they stop consuming coffee, they will have withdrawal symptoms for about one or two weeks. Their stomach and energy improves. Some people without their coffee suffer from psychological symptoms such as depression and irritability. Have you ever given up a food for Lent or done a fast? Were you exceptionally cranky? These are physical and emotional withdrawal symptoms.

10. Oral Allergy Syndrome

Some people suffer from food intolerances or allergies that only occur at certain times of the year. This phenomenon is called oral allergy syndrome. Oral allergy is not usually caused by the typical allergy producing foods like shellfish, nuts, eggs, milk, soya and wheat. At certain times when pollen is at its peak, people may develop allergies to foods – particularly fruits, vegetables and nuts. If the food is cooked, it destroys some of the allergy provoking components. Some food and pollen combinations are responsible for oral allergy. For example, birch pollens may bring out allergies to almonds, anise, apples, apricots, beans, caraway, carrots, celery, cherries, coriander, cumin, dill, fennel, green peppers, hazelnuts, kiwi, lentils, nectarines, parsley, parsnips, peaches, peanuts, pears, plums, potatoes, sunflower seeds, tomatoes and walnuts. Grass pollens may bring out allergies to kiwi, melon, orange, tomatoes and watermelon. Ragweed pollens may bring out allergies to bananas, cantaloupe, cucumber, honeydew, watermelon and zucchini.

11. Exercise Induced Allergies

Another unusual phenomenon is food dependent exercise induced allergies. The rise in body temperature during exercise seems to trigger a release of histamine and other chemicals. Symptoms may include hives, itching, asthma and faintness. It is often associated with apples, cabbage, celery, chicken, parsnips, peaches, shellfish and wheat. An exercise-induced allergy typically happens three or four hours after ingesting the food. It can happen up to 24 hours later. You may try to exercise four hours or more after eating without suffering a reaction. This is an odd ailment for which we do not fully understand the triggering mechanism.

There are many factors to food allergies and sensitivities. The workings of the immune system are mysterious and scientists still do not have all of the answers. Some known causes of food allergies are an increasing toxic burden, dysbiosis, heredity, over consumption of certain foods and psychological stress. There are varying methods of detecting food allergies that will be discussed herein.

Ways of Detecting Food Intolerances and Allergies

Types of testing to detect food allergies or sensitivities are many and there is debate over which ones are most effective. Conventional allergists use skin prick tests and/or blood testing. Alternative health professionals may use blood tests, electrodermal screening (EDS) and applied kinesiology. Skin prick testing is considered by some to be less effective for foods than for environmental sensitivities such as pollens, dust and moulds. It seems to work better for those who have a strong history of food allergy. According to Dr. Julian Kenyon, the skin prick test is only 40% to 60% accurate. He claims the EDS testing is 70% accurate in the hands of a skilled practitioner.

RAST Testing

RAST testing is a type of test that measures IgE antibodies in the blood when a particular food is introduced. Some think that RAST tests are less accurate than skin prick tests because most IgE antibodies are attached to the mast cells in the surface of the skin, the lining of the nose and gastrointestinal tract. Usually IgE in the blood is attached to a basophil, a type of white blood cell. This type of blood test is very expensive. According to some researchers, these blood tests are about 20% accurate. The tests can show false positives or negatives. Results may depend on how much of a substance a person requires to produce an allergic reaction. Some people need to consume two pounds of chocolate to have a reaction and for others just a bite. Some blood tests detect Immunoglobulin G (IgG). IgG may be found in the blood when there is a delayed food reaction. One of these tests is called the ELISA test; this test is argued by some not to be reliable and produces unstable results.

Electrodermal Screening

EDS or electrodermal screening is a tool designed in the 1950s by a German physician named Reinhold Voll. EDS testing can detect food sensitivities by measuring a reflex on an acupuncture point. The machine has two attachments – a probe and a ground – which are attached to an Ohm metre for measurement. The practitioner places an electrode to a point on the subject that corresponds with an acupuncture point. The subject holds a ground and a complete circuit is made between the subject, the machine and the probe. The electrode measures a reflex on the skin called the galvanic skin response. (The galvanic skin response is also used in lie detector tests.) The resistance of the skin changes depending on the food substance put into the circuit of the machine. For example, a vial of corn may be put into the circuit and then challenged against the allergy acupuncture point. If you are sensitive you have a different reflex than if you are not sensitive. In the hands of a skilled practitioner EDS testing is very beneficial.

In 1998, a double blind study by Krop, Lewith, Gziut and Radulescu, entitled "Electrodermal Testing, Serial End Point Titration and Skin Prick Testing for Allergens," found that EAV testing was 89% accurate in detecting allergens versus non allergens. The traditional skin prick test was 25% accurate. They inferred that EAV testing was very time efficient, easy to perform, reliable, objective, cost effective and useful for sensitive patients. Arguably, any method can be less than 100% reliable in detecting food allergies and sensitivities.

Applied Kinesiology

Applied kinesiology is used by some alternative health practitioners. It is a method whereby food is placed on the client and muscles are tested for strength or weakness. The person's strength is measured by pressing down on his/her arm to determine whether the substance weakens or strengthens them. No scientific studies have been done to show its efficacy but many people attest to its validity and efficacy.

Food Challenge Testing

Food challenge tests require you to vigilantly stay away from a food for five days. You may feel ill for the first three days and by the fourth or fifth day, you begin to feel well. You may actually suffer from withdrawal reactions after the first few days. You must only avoid one food at a time and re-introduce only one food at a time. For example, when you avoid a food like milk, you must avoid all foods containing milk. This length of time is required to determine delayed food reactions and clear your digestive tract of it. It also gives some time for your body to heal from any ill effects of the food. To determine if your symptoms are caused by a food, you must fully eliminate it. You must prove which food, if any, is causing your symptoms. Start with one food at a time. If you do more than one, you will not be able to tell which one is the cause of your ill health. Do not use this method if you have severe or life threatening allergies. It is not worth the reaction when you re-introduce the food. **If you suffer from anaphylaxis, never attempt to challenge foods or you may die!**

If you do not have a life threatening allergy, but rather a mild problem or digestive disorder, select a food to eliminate. Start with common allergens like dairy products, wheat, corn, chocolate, soya, nuts, eggs and sugar. Most allergies are to these foods. When you avoid these products you must be a detective and read all labels. You must be vigilant not to consume even a little bit of the food you are sensitive to. You may be sensitive even to traces of the food. It may require some sacrifice but you can use alternative products. If you would like substitutes for these foods, see the list further on in this chapter.

Keep in mind that it is only for five days and a lifetime of suffering can be avoided if you find a food that bothers you. It is best to eat at home for these five days to ensure you do not have any of the foods you are trying to avoid.

You need to record your symptoms using the following checklist both before and after you have done an elimination diet. When you re-introduce the food, it will cause a greater reaction. When you eat a food you are sensitive to every day, you become accustomed to it. After avoiding it for a few days, you will notice a reaction up to 72 hours after ingesting it. You may feel well on the food elimination diet and not have an immediate aggravation of your symptoms, but they may show up again over a number of days. If your symptoms disappear during the five day elimination diet, continue to avoid the food.

After you have done the initial Allergy Sensitivity Survey which follows, you can begin an elimination diet. As mentioned earlier, if you have any severe allergies, do not do the food challenge test. Once you have completed the five days without the food, you can reintroduce it. If your symptoms vanish after the elimination of the food, continue to avoid it. You may find that you don't have food sensitivities at all.

Select which food you would like to start with. It is a good idea to choose the ones you most frequently consume or love because they are usually the culprit. Read all labels on packaged goods. See the complete list of ingredients or names of common foods. To do a milk challenge test, eliminate the following foods for five days: all milk products, dried, evaporated and skimmed milk, butter, calcium caseinate, casein, caseinates, cheese of any kind, cream, creamy sauces and soups, curds, dried milk solids, lactose, lactoalbumin, margarine (some may contain milk products), mayonnaise (some may contain milk products), puddings, whey and yogurt. Packaged foods such as muffin, pancake and cake mixes may contain dried milk.

To do a wheat challenge test, eliminate the following foods for five days: breads, cakes, cereal, couscous, pablum, modified corn starch, semolina, wheat germ, wheat bran, flour products, macaroni, spaghetti, vermicelli, ravioli, whole wheat flour, white flour, graham flour, pancakes, pies, bread crumbs, batter, cones, waffles, malted milk, certain soups, beer, ale, gravies and battered fish. Meat products such as sausage, hamburger, meat loaf and schnitzel may also contain wheat.

To do a corn challenge test, eliminate the following foods for five days: corn, corn nuts, corn flakes, corn meal, grits, popcorn, corn oil, corn syrup, corn sugar and kernel corn. Read labels for hidden sources of corn in packaged, canned and frozen goods. Medications and vitamins may contain traces of corn starch.

To do a soya challenge test, eliminate the following foods for five days: tamari, soy flour, soya beans, soy protein isolate, vegetable protein, soy flour, soya, vegetable broth, soy protein, hydrolyzed soy protein, soy oil, soya bean oil, lecithin and soya lecithin.

To do a nut challenge test, eliminate the following foods for five days: all nuts, almonds, brazil nuts, cashews, filberts, hazel nuts, macadamia nuts, pecans, peanuts and walnuts. Many foods are cross contaminated with nuts, so read the labels.

To do an egg challenge test, eliminate the following foods for five days: eggs, egg yolk, egg whites, albumin, ovomucoid, vitellin and ovovitellin. Read the labels on all packaged goods because many contain egg products.

To do a sugar challenge test, eliminate the following foods for five days: sugar, beet sugar, brown sugar, cane sugar, sucrose, succinate, turbinado, raw sugar and sugar cane.

To do a chocolate challenge test, eliminate the following foods for three weeks: chocolate candies, cookies and cakes, chocolate milk and hot chocolate, chocolate flavoring, chocolate liquors, coated nuts and raisins, cocoa products, cola drinks (check labels). Additionally, some dark rye breads contain cocoa (check labels).

ALLERGY SENSITIVITY SURVEY

Rate your symptoms before and after you have done the elimination diet. After the three week elimination period, assess your symptoms again before re-introducing the eliminated food.

Rating Scale from 0 to 4
0. Never have this symptom
1. Seldom have this symptom
2. Occasionally have this symptom
3. Frequently have this symptom
4. Always have this symptom

Beside each rating, put an "S" for a severe reaction and an "M" for a mild reaction. For example, if three times a week you get migraines that are so severe you cannot work, you would rate that a 3, S. Then, if after the elimination diet, you have only one mild headache, you would rate this a 1, M. Because many people forget how bad they felt, it is important to complete this survey *before* starting the elimination diet. It may be a good idea to make a few copies of the survey if you intend to eliminate more than one food.

DIGESTIVE SYMPTOMS   SKIN SYMPTOMS

___ ___ belching   ___ ___ acne

___ ___ blood in stools   ___ ___ body odour

___ ___ diarrhea   ___ ___ dandruff

___ ___ distension   ___ ___ dry skin

___ ___ flatulence   ___ ___ eczema

___ ___ heartburn

___ ___ haemorrhoids

___ ___ nausea

___ ___ rectal pain or itching

___ ___ smelly offensive stools

___ ___ stomach cramps

___ ___ vomiting

___ ___ other

___ ___ hair loss

___ ___ itching

___ ___ rashes or hives

___ ___ scaling

___ ___ sweating or perspiration

___ ___ swelling or edema

___ ___ other

EARS, NOSE, THROAT

___ ___ altered sense of taste or smell

___ ___ canker sores

___ ___ colds

___ ___ coughing

___ ___ dryness

___ ___ ear aches, infections

___ ___ fullness of ears, nose, throat

___ ___ hemming, throat clearing

___ ___ hoarse voice

___ ___ itching

___ ___ mucous build up, discharges

___ ___ post nasal drip

___ ___ redness

HEAD AND MOOD SYMPTOMS

___ ___ anxiety or fear

___ ___ depression

___ ___ faintness

___ ___ headaches

___ ___ fatigue or tiredness

___ ___ flushing or redness

___ ___ inattentive

___ ___ insomnia

___ ___ irritability

___ ___ lethargy

___ ___ memory loss

___ ___ migraines

___ ___ mood swings

___ ___ sneezing

___ ___ sinusitis

___ ___ sore throat

___ ___ swelling

___ ___ tinnitus

___ ___ other

___ ___ restlessness

___ ___ twitching or spasms

___ ___ vertigo or dizziness

___ ___ other

HORMONES OR METABOLIC

___ ___ binge eating

___ ___ dysmenorrhea or painful menses

___ ___ food cravings

___ ___ heavy menses or flow

___ ___ hot flushes

___ ___ low libido

___ ___ irregular menses

___ ___ premenstrual syndrome

___ ___ water retention

___ ___ yeast infections, discharges

RESPIRATORY OR HEART

___ ___ chest pains

___ ___ coughing

___ ___ difficulty getting a full breath

___ ___ difficult breathing during exercise

___ ___ mucous build up

___ ___ pounding heart

___ ___ quick heart rate

___ ___ shortness of breath

___ ___ wheezing

___ ___ other

JOINTS

___ ___ aching pains

___ ___ arthritis

___ ___ edema or water retention

___ ___ muscle cramps

OTHER SYMPTOMS OF IMPORTANCE TO YOU:

___ ___

___ ___

___ ___

___ ___

___ ___ numbness or tingling

___ ___ redness

___ ___ stiff joints

___ ___ weary limbs

___ ___ other

TIPS FOR EATING WITH FOOD ALLERGIES

Read labels on packaged foods. If there is less then 2% of a substance in a food, they are not always required by the FDA to list it. Some labels just say "flavouring or spices." This is when the toll free number on the package is handy. If you like a product and are unsure, give the company a call. They are quite happy to accommodate a consumer and would rather be safe than suffer a law suit from someone with an allergic reaction.

Become knowledgeable about alternative names for the food you are sensitive or allergic to. For example, monosodium glutamate can be called by other names such as hydrolyzed vegetable protein. Dairy products can be casein, caseinates, cheese, cream sauce, alfredo, etc. When in doubt, don't eat it!

When eating out, you may want to call ahead and speak to the manager. If you call ahead to book a reservation, be sure the staff is aware of your sensitivities. Be specific with your questions. Do not ask "Does this contain cow milk?" but "Does this contain milk, yogurt, cheese, casein or caseinates?" It is best to order plain food rather than those with sauces or stuffing. Plain food is easier and, if you like, you can add a garnish to it such as baked potato, rice or broiled meats.

Cross contamination happens when foods have come in contact with the sensitivity or allergen. Sometimes food can be cross contaminated in restaurants by cooking in the same pots. If the restaurant cannot guarantee no cross contamination, do not eat there. It is best to avoid buffets as well for this reason. If you are going to someone's house for a pot luck or picnic, bring a dish that you can safely enjoy. Avoid bulk foods as they can be easily cross contaminated, not to mention less than fresh. Deli meats may be sliced by the same cutter used for cheeses. Become a detective!

HIDDEN SOURCES OF FOOD ALLERGENS/SENSITIVITIES
AND THEIR ALTERNATIVES

<u>CORN</u>

<u>ALTERNATIVES</u>

Check labels for corn flakes, corn flakes, corn meal, corn sugar, corn oil, corn grits, kernel corn, corn starch, corn syrup, maize, popcorn, sorbitol

Some of these products may contain corn;

Barley, buckwheat, couscous, millet, quinoa, rice, rye, wheat.

Wheat flour can be used as a thickening agent.

aspirin, bacon, baking powder (most)
beer, ale, gin, whisky
biscuits, bread, brown sugar, cake, pancake
and pie mixes,
candied fruit, candy, canned fruits
(sweetened), canned or bottled juice drinks
capsules, carob, cereals (presweetened)
instant coffee, confectioner's sugar,
cookies, cranberry juice, custard, doughnut,
Fritos, frosting. frozen fruits (sweetened)
graham cracker, gravies, ham (cured),
hominy, hot dogs, ice cream, infant
formulas, hydrolyzed casein, gelatin mixes,
luncheon meat, monosodium glutamate
(MSG), ointments, orange juice (some
frozen or sweetened), peanut butter
(commercial sweetened), pie fillings,
pudding, sandwich spreads, sauces that
have been thickened but are transparent,
sausages, sherbet, tea (instant)
toothpastes/powders
vitamins and medicine, yogurt (thickened
or sweetened)

Read all labels.
MILK PRODUCTS

Check labels for binding agents, brown
sugar flavouring, butter fat, buttermilk,
butter oil, butter solids, calcium caseinate,
casein, cheese, cow milk products, cream,
cream sauces and soups, curds, custard,
dried milk solids, evaporated milk, frozen
yogurt, ghee, hydrolysates, hydrolyzed
casein, ice cream, lactate, lactulose, lactose,
lactoalbumin, margarine, milk, natural
butter flavour, potassium caseinate,
pudding, sour cream, whey, whey powder,
whey protein concentrate, whey protein
hydrolysate and yogurt.

Packaged foods such as muffin, pancake
and cake mixes may contain dried milk.

Read all labels.

ALTERNATIVES

Milk alternatives are: almond beverage,
amazake, cashew nut beverage, hazelnut
beverage, rice milk and soymilk.

Ice cream alternatives are: fresh fruit
sorbet, fruit smoothies, juice popsicles,
juice ice cubes, tofutti products, soy
delicious and rice dream

Mayonnaise alternatives are; avocado,
mustard, nut butter, soya yogurt, and tofu
sour cream.

Cheese alternatives are: ground nut butter,
tofu and soya cheese.

Butter alternatives are: non hydrogenated
margarine (check label for dairy free), flax

oil and olive oil.

EGGS

Check labels for albumin, dried egg, eggs, egg protein, egg solids, egg whites, egg white solids, egg yolk,

french toast, glazes, globulin, livetin, lyzozome, mayonnaise,

meringue, mousse, omelets, ovomucoid, ovovitellin, ovalbumin, ovotransferrin, ovovitella, powdered egg, silici albuminate,

Simplesse, vitellin, whole egg.

Read the labels on all packaged goods because many contain egg products.

ALTERNATIVES

When making your own recipes, use one of the following alternatives for an egg (they may be ineffective in recipes that require more than three eggs):

- 1 teaspoon baking powder, 1 tablespoon liquid, 1 tablespoon vinegar
- 1 teaspoon yeast dissolved in 1/4 cup warm water
- 1 1/2 tablespoons water, 1 1/2 tablespoons oil, 1 teaspoon baking powder
- 1 tablespoon pureed fruit such as apricots, apple sauce or bananas
- 1 packet gelatin, 2 tablespoons warm water (don't mix until ready to use)

WHEAT

Check labels for all purpose flour, bread crumbs, bulgur, couscous, durum wheat, farina, graham flour, gluten, plain and self raising flour, semolina, triticale (wheat and rye blend), whole wheat flour, white flour and wholemeal flour.

These foods may contain wheat products: baked goods, bagels, beer, biscuits, bread crumbs, bread, cakes, coffee substitute, cookies, crackers, dinner rolls, doughnuts, dumpling, gin, ice cream cones, gravy, hamburgers, hot dogs, luncheon meats, malt, muesli, muffins, pancakes, pasta, pies, pizza, soups, soya sauce, stock cubes, stuffing, vodka

Read all labels.

ALTERNATIVES

Substitutes for wheat flour are amaranth, arrowroot flour, bean flour (chickpea, lentil), buckwheat flour, corn flour, oat flour, rice flour, spelt flour, and tapioca.

Cereal substitutes – try cornflakes, kasha, Rice Crispies, millet, oatmeal, puffed rice, quinoa puffs.

Wheat bread substitutes: buckwheat bread, corn crispbread, kamut bread, tortilla, rice bread, rye bread and (100%), spelt bread.

Cracker substitutes: oat cakes, rice cakes and rice crackers.

Snacks such as corn chips, nachos and popcorn.

Pasta alternatives: buckwheat pasta, kamut pasta, quinoa pasta, rice pasta and soba noodles (buckwheat).

SUGAR

Check labels for sugar, brown sugar, sucrose, beet sugar, cane sugar, confectioners sugar, demerara sugar, dextrose, icing sugar, muscavado sugar, sucrose, sucanat, succinate, sugar, turbinado

Read all labels.
SOY

If you are sensitive to soy check labels for soybean, soy protein isolate, tamari, texturized vegetable protein, soy flour, soy grits, soya, tofu, bean curd, miso, vegetable broth, soy protein, hydrolyzed soy protein, soy oil, soy bean oil and lecithin

Read all labels as soy is often in packaged goods.

ALTERNATIVES

Substitutes for sugar: agave, dehydrated date pieces, honey, maple syrup (pure) and stevia.

Aspartame, saccharin, sorbitol, sucralose and xylitol may cause health problems because of their chemical nature.

TREATMENT FOR FOOD ALLERGIES/SENSITIVITIES

An ideal treatment for food allergies would be to correctly identify and avoid the offending food. It can be difficult to completely avoid certain foods that are hidden in many products. Foods like soya, wheat, eggs and milk tend to be hard to completely avoid. There are some effective medical treatments that temporarily reduce allergic reactions. Natural treatments may also help to reduce the inflammation that causes allergies.

Doctors sometimes use cortisone and anti-histamines to treat food allergies. Some side effects of cortisone are weight gain, hypertension, thinning of the skin and mood swings. They usually use cortisone for severe allergies and asthma. It is a good temporary fix, but has many damaging side effects. Anti-histamines may work temporarily to suppress an allergic reaction. This can be effective for environmental allergies but not always for foods. Other treatments may include "enzyme potentiated desensitization" where an injection is given of a food mixed with an enzyme beta glucuronide. This enzyme increases its effectiveness. This is said to desensitize the patient to the offending food.

Acute Allergic Reactions

For an acute allergic reaction, some doctors recommend taking baking soda in water. It is taken in the same manner as for heartburn. According to Arm & Hammer, the directions for heartburn are: add half a level teaspoon to half a glass (flour fl. oz.) of water every two hours, or as directed by a physician. Dissolve completely in water. Do not take more than 7.5 teaspoons at any age or 3.5 teaspoons if you are over 60 years old. Do not use the maximum dosage for more than two weeks. This is thought to work because allergic reactions are linked to acidity within the cells. This method is good for mild allergic reactions. If you suffer from anaphylactic shock to allergens, use a prescribed Epi-Pen and seek medical attention immediately. **Never eat a food that may cause anaphylaxis or you will be in trouble!**

Dysbiosis Diets

Some natural practitioners recommend dysbiosis diets to treat many diseases such as autoimmune disorders, migraines and leaky gut syndrome. Dysbiosis means an abnormal flora in the gastrointestinal system. There is always a balance of good and bad bacteria, but when the bad takes over, it is called dysbiosis. Treatment of dysbiosis or candida involves using natural anti-microbials and building up the beneficial flora. Follow a dysbiosis diet, and avoid foods that feed bad bacteria. In Chapter Three, you will see lists of foods. Eat from column one and two only and avoid any foods that have a # sign beside it. The foods with the # sign feed the bad bacteria. Use natural supplements that enhance your beneficial bacteria.

Some herbal supplements that work to kill bacteria, fungus, viruses and parasites are garlic and tea tree oil (which can be toxic). Remedies that kill candida are garlic, caprylic acid, berberine, black walnut, cinnamon bark oil, grapefruit seed extract, tea tree and oregano oil. According to studies by Nigel Plummer PhD, a microbiologist who works with Seroyal, only garlic and cinnamon have been shown to have no toxic effects in the body. Probiotics are also helpful in treating dysbiosis. They can be taken to improve one's own beneficial bacteria. It is best to use a standardized supplement that is kept in the fridge. (Acidophilus found in yogurt may not have any live culture left after delivery.) Some brands of acidophilus are made from cow strains and some are made from human strains. Cow strains of acidophilus do not mean they are made from dairy milk. They are made from the gut flora of a cow. Human strains have been cultured in a lab since the 1950s. Some claim human strains of acidophilus are superior and are indigenous to our natural flora and help our good bacteria to proliferate.

Probiotics must be nonpathogenic, (meaning that they do not grow bad bacteria uncontrollably), and capable of growing beneficial flora in the gut. They are useful in protection against infections, decreasing antibodies, nutritional absorption and aid in balancing the immune system. Lactobacillus acidophilus and Bifidobacteria are the most popular and most researched probiotics. According to a study by Ogionni et al in 1998, soil micro-organisms called bacillus subtilis may not be beneficial for autoimmune disease because they can grow out of control in a system with a depressed immune system.

Rotation Diets

According to a book entitled, *Healing the Planet, One Patient at a Time* by Dr. Josef Krop, a food rotary diet is the key to prevent food sensitivities and manage allergies. The basic principles of this diet are to rotate foods and their biological families on a four day cycle. This means that one person who ate eggs, chicken and chicken soup in one day would avoid chicken products for the next three days. The amount of food consumed is up to the individual. Then on day five, this person can eat them again. Therefore, this rotation diet is divided into four days. For further information and extensive lists of food families acquire Dr. Krop's above mentioned book (see Bibliography).

Change Your pH

Changing your alkaline and acid balance may keep allergic reactions at bay. If you have an allergic reaction, it is said to cause an increase in acidity of the cells during the inflammatory allergic response. Eating more alkaline foods, such as fruits and vegetables decreases the acid in the body which in turn inhibits the inflammatory process. Eating the food from column one and two in the diet outlined in Chapter Three is very helpful in decreasing inflammatory reactions which can lead to allergies. Eating healthy helps to decrease the toxic load that increases your susceptibility to allergies.

Decrease Your Toxic Load

To further decrease your toxic load, it is a good idea to use supplements that clear toxins from different organ systems. Eat a high fibre diet to cleanse the intestinal tract. High fibre foods are whole grains such as All Bran, psyllium buds, legumes and oat fibre. The fibre in these products cleans the waste from the lining of the intestinal tract. This helps you to better absorb nutrients and eliminate waste. Waste that sits in your intestinal tract creates bacteria and toxins. This leads to further health complications.

Drinking hot water with lemon upon rising is said to stimulate the liver. Some homeopathic remedies are gentle and cleansing for the liver. A very gentle and safe cleanser for the liver and kidneys is a mixture containing a 6 CH potency of the following remedies: Chelidonium, Carduus Marinarus, Taraxicum, Juniperus Communis, Solidago and Nux Vomica. It is a very effective and gentle detox. These remedies in a 6 CH potency are very mild and diluted. Take 10 drops twice daily for one month. Some practitioners recommend using homeopathic remedies made from the food allergen in a 3X or 6X potency. Some brand names such as Dr. Reckeweg or Bio Allers have the remedies already combined in a homeopathic potency. If you want to try the homeopathic desensitization, seek the help of a professional homeopath.

Reduce Inflammation

L-glutamine is an amino acid that helps to heal leaky gut syndrome. Leaky gut is a cause of many auto-immune diseases and allergies. The cells in the intestinal tract are open and leak proteins into the bloodstream which provokes an inflammatory reaction, be it histamine release or inflammation. If you use products that reduce inflammation such as L-glutamine, EPA and GLA, allergies often improve. EPA, eicosapentaeonic acid, is a compound found in fish oil. It has healing properties for the gut and is a powerful anti-inflammatory. A study done by Beluzzi et al in 1996, found that 59% of Crohn's patients had a remission by using 2.7 grams of fish oil per day. Only 26% of the control subjects, (those not taking fish oil), had a remission. Other supplements said to be useful for inflammation and allergies are digestive enzymes such as bromelain and protease. Bromelain is a useful anti-inflammatory. Protease helps to digest proteins such as antibodies that cause histamine reactions. Digestive enzymes are not good if you have an ulcer or gastritis. Quercitin and grapeseed extracts are also said to reduce the inflammatory reactions of allergies. You can take 500 mgs two to three times a day. Vitamin C with bioflavanoids is helpful to reduce an allergic response. Typical dosage of vitamin C is 1,000 mgs two to three times a day.

Homeopathic Solutions for Allergies

Some homeopathic remedies are useful for reducing the symptoms of an acute allergic reaction. A constitutional remedy is much better in preventing and reducing the occurrence of an allergy. These remedies suit all of your symptoms, both physical and emotional and should be prescribed by a homeopath who can spend time researching your case.

For an acute reaction, one can take four pellets of a 30 CH potency, every 15 minutes and every two hours for a general reaction. Of course, **seek the proper medical attention if your allergy is life threatening**.

Apis Mellifica is a remedy that suits reactions such as swelling of the tissues, painful burning and stinging pains. The throat, tongue and mouth may feel swollen, itchy, and show redness. There may be red and swollen hives or eruptions that look like a bee sting.
Histaminum is a homeopathic preparation of histamine. It can reduce your body's reaction to histamine. This remedy is usually given in a 9CH potency and taken only once a week.
Lycopodium is useful for reactions that occur in the digestive tract. The body's response to a food may be right sided abdominal pains, irritability, gas and bloating with constipation. Usually lycopodium types have a very full stomach which fills up quickly and to the throat. The lower abdomen may grumble and gurgle. They usually suffer from constipation or ineffectual urging with stool.
Nux Vomica types tend to be irritable with their digestive upset. They may overeat and tend to get hemorrhoids, constipation and indigestion. They may develop colicky pains in the stomach and intestinal tract. They may suffer from terrible digestive headaches. They may experience a stuffy nose and chronic nasal catarrh. They may have sour bitter belching and feel nauseated. They may wish to vomit but cannot.
Urtica Urens is another homeopathic remedy for food allergies. The typical symptoms alleviated by this remedy are hives, inflammation and edema. The gastrointestinal tract may be inflamed and cause nausea and vomiting with diarrhea. Usually, reactions to foods like strawberries and shellfish are treated with urtica urens. Lower potencies, from one to three X or CH work to clear out excess uric acid in the blood.
Seek professional help if you have a severe allergy. Homeopaths can prescribe a constitutional remedy and can oversee your natural treatments. There is a list of homeopathic doctors in Ontario online at www.ontariohomeopath.com. It is best to work with both your medical doctor and an alternative health professional. Patients who do this fare much better than those who just seek just one type of treatment.

CHAPTER FIVE

GASTROINTESTINAL DISORDERS A-Z

Acid Reflux/Heartburn

According to the National Institute of Health, 25 million U.S. citizens suffer from heartburn every day. That is big business for the makers of Tums and Zantac. Almost a third of heartburn sufferers feel they will never again be able to enjoy the foods they love. Another third of frequent heartburn sufferers say medication cost has an influence on their ability to effectively treat their heartburn. Why are we so dependent on drugs for answers? Diet is the most effective treatment of heartburn related symptoms.

WHAT IS ACID REFLUX OR HEARTBURN?

Acid Reflux is related to an incompetence of the lower esophageal sphincter. Food and acid may rise up into the esophagus (the tube that runs from the mouth into the stomach) from the stomach. Heartburn may cause a burning feeling behind the sternum, in the stomach, chest or throat. Accompanying symptoms are lack of appetite, gas, bloating, belching, sour risings, water brash, vomiting, shortness of breath and a bad taste in the mouth. It may be worse in pregnant women or those who take birth control pills. High estrogen or progesterone is linked to acidity.

WHAT ARE THE MAJOR CAUSES OF HEARTBURN?

Diet

Diet is often the key in treating heartburn. An overfilled stomach may be a factor in heartburn as the gastric contents push up into the esophagus. Too short an interval between meals can also cause heartburn. Foods that may aggravate heartburn are fried foods, fat, spices, salt, coffee, tea, sugar, vinegar, carbonated drinks, dried meats, alcoholic beverages, citrus fruits, tomatoes, chocolate and bread. It is fine to enjoy a luxury occasionally, but many continually try their digestion beyond its capacity. Drinking with meals is said to be inadvisable as it dilutes the stomach acid. Cold water is said to render enzymes less effective for adequate digestion.

Improper Chewing

Improper chewing of food may cause heartburn. This can be due to rushing whilst eating or not chewing due to pain in the teeth. Chewing your food not only breaks it down into smaller pieces but it also improves the digestion of starches. Saliva mixes with foods and produces an enzyme that helps to pre-digest starches before they enter the stomach.

Prescription and Narcotic Drugs

Certain drugs and stimulants increase the risk of heartburn, such as alcohol, tobacco, immuran, cortisone, iron, aspirin, antibiotics and pain killers.

Stress

Stress can cause heartburn. When we have chronic stress our blood supply travels to our extremities. This is because we have an evolutionary fight or flight response. This is to help us run when we are fearful of impending danger. We have no outlet for stress as we cannot ethically or socially attack or run. Thus, the blood supply travels away from the stomach and impacts our digestion. Any worry, stress, shock and anxiety can influence our digestion. Our nervous system is tightly connected to our digestion. For some people any stress manifests in digestive upset.

Digestive Insufficiencies

Digestive insufficiencies, such as a lack of hydrochloric acid (HCL), bile and enzymes, can cause acidity. Digestive enzymes are made by the pancreas and liver. Bile is made by the liver and stored in the gallbladder. Bile helps to emulsify fats. If you don't make enough bile, you don't digest fats as well. Many people who have their gallbladder removed do well taking digestive enzymes that include bile salts.

Hydrochloric acid is manufactured by the stomach and helps to break down proteins. Low stomach acid causes gas, bloating and heartburn. Sometimes low stomach acid has the same symptoms as high stomach acid. Excessive HCL can cause heartburn.

Quick Home Test for Acid

To establish if you lack hydrochloric acid (HCL) try this simple test. When you have heartburn, take a tablespoon of apple cider vinegar. If this alleviates your heartburn, then you need more HCL. If it aggravates it, you are too acidic and should avoid Betaine HCL and vinegar. Drink a large glass of water if this is the case. If you are low acid, take Betaine HCL or apple cider vinegar in water with your meals.

Structural Abnormalities

An incompetent esophageal sphincter may be the cause of heartburn. This sphincter is supposed to stay shut when we are not swallowing food. Some people with full stomach contents or on bending may have acid or water brash up into the throat. Their valve leaks out the stomach contents. Wearing clothes too tight around the waist actually pushes up the stomach contents. In the past, women were discouraged from wearing corsets, tight belts or pants for this reason.

Ulcers

Ulcers may add to the discomfort of heartburn. These ulcers can be caused by diet, stress or bacteria called Helicobacter pylori.

Heartburn as a Sign of Disease

Heartburn can be a sign of other diseases such as high estrogen or progesterone, gastric carcinoma, a stomach ulcer, gastritis and hiatal hernia. Other conditions that are associated with acid reflux are hypothyroidism, acne rosacea, malabsorption, aging and anemia. Complications of heartburn can lead to Barrett's Esophagitis and Dysphagia. A stricture can be caused from scar tissue that makes swallowing difficult.

DIETARY MEASURES

Heartburn sufferers should avoid sugar, tea, pop, spicy foods, coffee, fats, grease, pastries, tomatoes, citrus and alcohol. Lying down often aggravates heartburn. Some find elevating the head of the bed helpful.

Eat smaller meals every four hours and do not eat three hours before bed. Include fresh fruits, vegetables, lean meat, fish and whole grains in your diet. Some foods have healing properties. For example, papaya and pineapple have natural enzymes that aid in digestion. Raw potato and cabbage juice are said to heal the lining of the stomach and reduce acid.

Eat foods mostly from column one and two listed in Chapter Three. These foods are healthier fats and low to medium glycemic which help keep you healthy overall. Read over that chapter to ascertain how to eat healthy. Avoid foods that trigger your heartburn even if they are in these columns.

SUPPLEMENTS FOR HEARTBURN

For any of these treatments, stop the remedies if your heartburn gets worse. Seek professional help.

For Low HCL Use

Apple Cider Vinegar

Hippocrates touted vinegar as an antibiotic. It was used in the war to cure stomach disorders. There is a lot of promotion about the healing wonders of apple cider vinegar. It is an acidic substance, that when taken internally, aids in digestion. Typical dosage is one to two tablespoons in a glass of water, up to three times a day before a meal. This supplement is not suited to those with high acidity.

Betaine HCL

Betaine HCL is a supplement that is used as a digestive aid. Betaine HCL is made with beet sugar and attached to hydrochloric acid. This attachment makes it safe to swallow and doesn't damage the esophagus. The HCL makes a more acid environment in the stomach.

HCL helps with the digestion of proteins. It contributes to the protective barrier in the stomach. An acidic environment in the stomach protects against most microorganisms. It also prevents a bacterial overgrowth in the small intestine. An acidic environment in the stomach causes mucous production that acts as a barrier for it's lining. This barrier protects against microorganisms and acidity itself.

The typical dose for Betaine HCL is 500 - 650 mg right before a large meal. Dosage may vary depending on how little acid the stomach makes. You can test this by seeing how many capsules are required to cause a warm feeling in the stomach. If you take one right before a meal, the next day try two and so on. Then cut back depending on how many it took to feel the warmth. People typically require one to three tablets. It is wise to start with one capsule per day.

Digestive Enzymes that include HCL

Digestive enzymes are a means for the body to break down foods and absorb their nutrients. Our body naturally makes digestive enzymes through the liver, the pancreas and stomach. If you do not have good digestion, digestive enzymes act as insurance for proper absorption. Partially or improperly digested foods cause many health issues, such as heartburn, food allergies, constipation and the like.

Digestive enzymes usually include protease, which aids in protein digestion, lipase, which aids in fat digestion and amylases or cellulose which aids in carbohydrate digestion. Use a digestive enzyme that includes Betaine HCL. Take as directed on the package. This supplement is not suited to those with high acidity.

GENERAL SUPPLEMENTS FOR ACIDITY AND HEARTBURN

Aloe Vera Juice

Aloe Vera juice is very healing to the gastrointestinal tract. Aloe is said to be a tonic, laxative, to stimulate bile flow, eliminate parasites and heal the stomach. Typical dosage is one tablespoon to three ounces, one to three times daily. Start with the lowest dose until you find your comfort zone. If you take too much aloe vera, you may suffer with diarrhea. This supplement is not suited to those who suffer from diarrhea, heavy periods, pregnancy and/or kidney disease.

Calcium and Magnesium, 2:1 ratio

Take a 2:1 ratio of calcium to magnesium. It is an alkalinizing mineral that helps to absorb the stomach acid. Take in between meals. Typical daily dosage would be 800 to 1200 mgs of calcium and 400 to 600 mgs of magnesium. It is best to split this into two or three doses throughout the day. Calcium Carbonate is a better buffer for acid than Calcium Citrate or Calcium Hydroxyapatite.

Deglycyrrhizinated Licorice (DGL)

DGL is an excellent remedy for heartburn and healing the stomach and esophagus. It has been known since ancient Greek and Egyptian times. It is said to help heal ulcers of the gastrointestinal tract. It has anti-inflammatory, antiviral, antimicrobial, mucoprotective and expectorant properties. Typical dosage is 500 mgs a half hour before each meal, up to three times a day. Licorice decreases potassium which increases sodium in the body. This is why licorice is not suitable to those who have high blood pressure. Avoid licorice if you have low potassium, liver disease, kidney disease, heart failure or are pregnant. Avoid licorice if you are taking diuretics or prednisone-like drugs.

Garlic

Garlic is a great anti-microbial, which means it is effective in killing yeast, viruses and bacteria. It may be helpful in inhibiting the growth of bacteria that causes ulcers. Garlic is medicinal to the GI tract because it has antimicrobial, anti-dyspepsia and beneficial digestive properties.
Note: Avoid if you take blood thinners, have hypoglycemia or prior to surgery.

Papaya and Pineapple

You can consume these fruits. They contain beneficial enzymes that help with heartburn and digestion. Some people take a digestive supplement that contains Bromelain and Papain which is made from pineapple and papaya.

Probiotics

Probiotics such as acidophilus and bifidobacterium are beneficial bacteria. They help re-colonize the beneficial bacteria in the GI tract. You always have bad and good bacteria in your gut. If this bad and good flora become imbalanced, your stomach lining may become irritated. Bifidobacterium has also been shown to suppress Helicobacter pylori. The bacterium, Helicobacter pylori, causes peptic ulcers, anemia and gastric cancer. Products that are not refrigerated may be a dead culture, which does not help the beneficial flora to grow. Take as directed on the label.

HOMEOPATHIC REMEDIES FOR ACIDITY AND HEARTBURN

There are many homeopathic remedies for acidity and heartburn. Some of the more common remedies are listed with their symptoms here. For more information on how to self prescribe a homeopathic remedy, go to Chapter Two. If you cannot find a remedy suited to you, or find you are not improving or your symptoms get worse, seek the help of a professional homeopath or your medical doctor. As noted earlier, symptoms in bold are the most common.

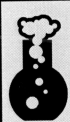

Did you know?
Your Digestive Juices are as Strong as Paint Stripper.
The lining of the stomach outputs gastric juices that contain strong hydrochloric acid. This is where the body digests proteins. This acid is corrosive enough to remove paint!

ABIES NIGRA
Common indications include:
- burning in stomach and abdomen, indigestion which may be accompanied by heart palpations or other **cardiac symptoms**
- acid belching
- **chronic indigestion of the elderly**
- sensation as if one had swallowed a hard boiled egg or rock and it lodged in the upper portion of the stomach
- constriction above the pit of the stomach
- aggravated by eating a hearty meal, tea or smoking

ANTIMONIUM CRUDUM
Common indications include:
- **white milky tongue, thick coating on tongue**
- burning in the pit of the stomach

- **empty belching**
- stomach always feels overloaded
- **overeating causes digestive distress**
- heartburn, nausea, vomiting, belching
- **rising of fluid tastes like food that was eaten**
- milk becomes curdled in the stomach
- vomits as soon as eats
- **mind symptoms include irritability and cannot bear to be touched or looked at**
- **cravings for pickles and acids, vinegar, wine**
- aggravated by fats, acids, sweets, vinegar, pork, alcohol

ARGENTUM NITRICUM
Common indications include:

- **much loud flatulence and belching**
- heartbeat may be affected by digestion
- **craving for sugar which aggravates the stomach**
- food lodges in the pharynx
- **expelling gas may or may not relieve symptoms**
- **pain after eating**
- tendency to stomach ulcers
- **mentally these types are nervous from anticipating an upcoming event, when alone or heights**
- **these types are hot blooded and worse from heat**
- relieved by warm drinks and alcohol
- **aggravated by eating sweets**, by pressure, any food, cold food and drinks
- worse one hour or immediately after eating

ARSENICUM ALBUM
Common indications include:

- **extreme burning sensations**
- **burning yet a desire to have small sips of hot liquids**
- **drinking milk helps stomach pains**
- may feel nauseated and low appetite
- heartburn feels like a fire, as if hot coals are against the affected parts
- cold water sits in the stomach like a stone
- **suited to chilly types**
- **mind symptoms includes restlessness, fear of disease and anxiety**
- **these types are aggravated after midnight**
- **improved by drinking small sips of hot liquids** despite suffering burning heat
- worsened by changing of weather, cold and damp, lying with the head low
- **aggravated by ice, cold drinks**, spoiled meat, alcohol, lobster, salad

BRYONIA
Common indications include:
- bitter taste in mouth from belching
- food and drink tastes bitter
- **dryness of all mucous membranes**
- water brash (a burp that is watery and goes into the throat)
- **thirsty for great quantities of cold drinks with a dry mouth**
- sensation of a stone in the pit of the stomach
- rheumatism may alternate with indigestion
- better after burping
- white coating on tongue
- heartburn from drinking cold water when the person is overheated
- stomach sensitive to touch
- lying still improves their symptoms
- **suited to irritable types who want to be left alone and quiet**
- craving for coffee and wine
- **aggravated by motion**, after eating and from vegetables, sauerkraut, cabbage, potatoes, acids, warm drinks

CALCAREA CARBONICA
Common indications include:
- **acid sour risings** and loud belching
- excessive stomach acid with burning
- rawness with a bitter taste in the throat
- stricture of the esophagus, food will not go down
- throat seems to contract on swallowing
- **craving for eggs**
- food tastes sour
- bloated abdomen requires loose clothing around the waist
- **may have sour perspiration and sweat profusely on the scalp**
- **mind symptoms includes stubbornness, fear of ill health, mice and insanity**
- **these types tend to be heavy and gain weight easily**
- aggravated by many foods, milk products, beans, sugar, pastries, oil and fats, cold drinks, vegetables, hard and dry foods
- worse while and after eating

CARBO VEGETABILIS
Common indications include:
- **belching offers temporary relief** (these types may even drink carbonated beverages to induce burping to feel some relief)
- **desires fanning, open air or windows**
- sour watery belching and risings
- violent burning stomach with external chilliness

- suited to sluggish people with weak and slow digestion
- sensation as if all food sits and putrefies before digesting
- sensation as if the stomach would burst
- desires whisky, brandy, coffee
- **these types tend to be indifferent, negative and depressed**
- aggravated by overeating, milk products, fat, tainted meats, fish, oysters, ice cream
- aggravated by lying down, warm sultry weather

LYCOPODIUM
Common indications include:
- sensation of fullness from the stomach up to throat
- **distended and full after least amount of food**
- burping or passing gas relieves distension
- **heavy sensation in the stomach**
- food may be regurgitated through the nose
- **water brash, sour, bitter or burning risings**
- **least pressure of clothes bothersome**
- **much flatulence,** distension and constipation
- may be suited to types **with low self esteem,** anger from contradiction, fear of public speaking
- **aggravated by fasting or missing a meal**
- **craving for sweets, olives,** alcohol, warm drinks and food
- **better in open air**
- **aggravated by cold drinks,** milk, cabbage, wheat, beans, onions, wine, rye, beer and **from 4:00 to 8:00 p.m.**

NATRUM PHOSPHORICUM
Common indications include:
- stomach pains, acid stomach and belching
- heartburn, **water brash with sour acid risings**
- trouble swallowing
- **yellow coated tongue**
- regurgitates fluid that is as sour as vinegar
- liquids are not tolerated as well as solid food
- **distension,** fullness after eating very little
- high uric acid in blood
- **cravings for eggs,** beer, fried fish and spices
- worse two hours after eating, sugar, milk, bitter and fatty foods

NUX VOMICA
Common indications include:
- **bitter, sour and watery belching**
- heartburn and sour taste in the morning before or after eating

- pain in the stomach like a weight or pressure, two or three hours after meals
- bloating and distension
- **sensation of a stone in the stomach after eating**
- putrid bitter taste in the mouth
- **sensitive to clothes around the waist**
- back of tongue is coated brown
- **digestive problems from overeating or overindulging** in alcohol, drugs or excessive spices
- **excessive appetite or aversion to food with hunger**
- reverse peristalsis, spasms from disordered peristalsis, pain when food passes down into the pyloric sphincter
- tightness of the abdomen after eating, must loosen pants
- altered sense of taste for milk, coffee, water and beer
- digestive complaints with accompanying headaches
- **may be suited to zealous, fiery temperaments who overindulge and overwork**
- cravings for fats and tolerates them well
- **cravings for tea, coffee, alcohol and spicy**
- worse after eating, drug use, tobacco poisoning, **overeating, overindulgence, alcohol, spices, stimulants, tea and coffee**

SULPHUR
Common indications include:
- **heartburn from overeating**
- **sour and watery risings**
- burning into the throat
- pressure in the throat like a lump, splinter or hair
- throat feels swollen like a ball that rises and closes the pharynx
- regurgitation of food tastes acid shortly after a meal
- water brash and saliva after eating
- **hearty appetite or vanishing at the sight of food**
- tendency to eat too quickly and not chew food well
- **hunger at 11 a.m.**
- taste in mouth like rotten eggs
- gastric complaints may alternate with skin conditions
- **may be suited to lazy, intellectual and/or slovenly types**
- **skin eruptions are common in this remedy**
- **cravings for sweets, fats, spices, raw food, alcohol, beer and ale**
- **aversion to meat and olives**
- worse in the morning, after eating, eggs, milk products, sweets, alcohol
- worse before the menstrual flow

Picture This….

You are a senior citizen and your digestion is not what it once was. You used to be able to eat anything. Now you are getting heart palpitations after eating. You eat and get great discomfort in your upper stomach with a racing heart at the same time. You have a history of arteriosclerosis and fear you may be in for more heart troubles. On the advice of your Homeopath, you take four pellets of Abies Nigra 6 CH a few times a day. After one month you feel much better but feel a pressure in your stomach after eating. The palpitations are gone. Adding in 500 mgs of Betaine HCL with each meal has helped you to digest your meals without discomfort! If you had known the natural route was so effective, you would have tried this sooner!

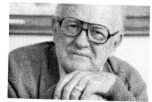

Bad Breath- see Halitosis

Barrett's Esophagus

Barrett's Esophagus is characterized by an abnormal cell lining of the esophagus. A normal esophagus or swallowing tube is lined with pinkish white cells called epithelium. In Barrett's Esophagus, this epithelium has changed into abnormal red cells. These cells have undergone changes and look like cells typical of the intestines. Lesion-like ulcers may be seen in the esophageal lining. This disorder is typically seen in people over the age of 60. Compared to the general population, the epithelium in Barrett's Esophagus has a 30 to 40 fold increase in becoming cancerous. However, only around five to 10% of people with this disorder ever develop esophageal cancer.

Diagnosis of Barrett's esophagus is done by doing an endoscopy and biopsy. An endoscopy is a long tube that is guided down the throat to better see the affected areas. A biopsy or tissue sample is taken to see if the cells are abnormal. This sample is sent to a lab for further investigation. Typical medical treatment for this condition includes antacids, surgery and a dilation procedure whereby they stretch any stricture in the throat.

It is considered a disorder that is related to acidity, heartburn and hiatal hernia. People who are overweight and smoke tend to suffer from Barrett's esophagus more often. Symptoms may include difficulty swallowing, which could be due to narrowing of the esophagus. Some suffer with burning, stabbing or sticking pains in the throat. They feel as if something is stuck there. Some may even vomit or expectorate blood that looks like coffee grounds. Unusual stools may be seen such as black, tarry or bloody stools. If you have any of these symptoms, see your doctor to rule out other diseases. Approximately half of all people who have this disorder suffer from no symptoms at all.

DIETARY MEASURES

People who suffer from Barrett's Esophagus should avoid the same foods that aggravate people with acidity/heartburn. Heartburn and Barrett's esophagus sufferers should avoid sugar, tea, pop, spicy foods, coffee, fats, grease, pastries, tomatoes, citrus and alcohol. Eat smaller meals every four hours and do not eat three hours before bed. Lying down after meals often aggravates heartburn. Some find elevating the head of the bed helpful. Include fresh fruits, vegetables, lean meat, fish and whole grains in your diet. Papaya and pineapple have natural enzymes that aid in digestion. Chewing your food well aids in digestion, is less work for the stomach and is easier on the esophagus. Reduce the use of unnecessary medications that may cause heartburn.

Eat foods mostly from column one and some from column two listed in the chart in Chapter Three. These foods are healthier fats and low glycemic which help keep you healthy overall. Avoid foods that trigger your heartburn even if they are in column one.

GENERAL TREATMENTS FOR BARRETT'S ESOPHAGUS

Aloe Vera Juice

Aloe Vera juice is very healing to the gastrointestinal tract. It helps to sooth the lining of the esophagus. Aloe is said to be a tonic, a laxative and stimulates bile flow, eliminates parasites and heals the stomach. Typical dosage is one tablespoon to three ounces, one to three times daily. Start with the lowest dose until you find your comfort zone. If you take too much aloe vera, you may suffer with diarrhea. This supplement is not suited to those who suffer from diarrhea, heavy periods, pregnancy and/or kidney disease.

Deglycyrrhizinated licorice (DGL)

DGL is an excellent remedy for heartburn and for healing the stomach and esophagus. It is very soothing to the lining of the esophagus. It is also useful for stomach ulcers. Typical dosage is 500 mgs half hour before each meal, up to three times a day. Take this in the form of a lozenge. Avoid licorice if you have low potassium, liver disease, kidney disease, heart failure or during pregnancy. Avoid licorice if you are taking diuretics or prednisone-like drugs.

Slippery Elm

Slippery elm is a herbal remedy that is used to soothe and heal the throat. The inside of the bark contains mucilage, which is a gel-like substance that expands with water. This gel is what coats and soothes the throat. Slippery Elm can be purchased in lozenge format which soothes the esophageal lining on the way to the stomach. This remedy has no known side effects.

Marshmallow Root

Marshmallow root contains mucilage, which coats and soothes esophageal lining. It may be harmful if taken by anyone with hypoglycemia, diabetes, pregnancy or nursing. As it may interfere with medication absorption, check with your doctor before taking marshmallow root. Typical dosage is 300 to 450 mgs taken one to three times daily with meals. Teas and tinctures are available. If you buy a tincture, get a non-alcohol based one because alcohol may further irritate the throat.

Cross reference treatments for acidity/heartburn, dysphagia, esophageal cancer and hiatal hernia.

HOMEOPATHIC REMEDIES FOR BARRETT'S ESOPHAGUS

There are many homeopathic remedies for Barrett's Esophagus. Some of the more common remedies are listed with their symptoms herein. For more information on how to self prescribe a homeopathic remedy, go to Chapter Two. If you cannot find a remedy suited to you, or find you are not improving or your symptoms get worse, seek the help of a professional homeopath or your medical doctor.

ARGENTUM NITRICUM
Common indications include:

- **sensation of a splinter lodged in the throat** when swallowing
- raw, sore, scraping in the throat, particularly in the trachea area
- choking feeling with constriction
- **belching very loud**
- **hoarseness and loss of voice**
- dark red areas in the esophageal lining
- **desires sugar but is aggravated by it**
- **these types are very hot**
- **emotionally these types are anxious, have anticipatory anxiety and fearful of heights**
- improved by cold drinks
- aggravated by sugar

ARSENICUM ALBUM
Common indications include:

- swallowing is very painful
- **burning sensation in the throat or stomach**
- sensation as if hot needles, wires or burning coals are in the esophagus
- throat is dry, sore, scraping and burning
- burning ulceration in the throat
- **tendency to be chilly and cannot be warm enough**
- **mentally these types are anxious, restless and worse after midnight**
- **improved by sipping hot drinks**
- aggravated by ice, cold drinks, vegetables and fruits, tobacco chewing and alcohol

CARBOLIC ACID
Common indications include:

- acid, burning in stomach and throat
- **throat is discoloured red**
- throat is ulcerated in patches with exudate (excretion of pus or serum)
- almost impossible to swallow because of burning dryness in the throat
- putrid foul smelling breath
- these types tend towards malignancy
- improvement is felt when smoking and after tea

CONIUM
Common indications include:

- pressure in the esophagus like a ball rising from the stomach
- spasmodic constriction of the esophagus
- sensation as if something was lodged in the throat

- constant tendency to swallow
- **irritated sensation of the throat**
- involuntary swallowing whilst walking in the wind
- frequent sour belching with distended abdomen
- **these types tend towards malignancy**
- bread does not go down and tastes bad
- **mental dullness and confusion called "brain fog"**
- **emotionally these people are flat or emotionally closed types**
- cravings for coffee, salt and acid
- aggravated by milk, bread, alcohol, while eating

KALI BICHROMICUM
Common indications include:
- burning in the esophagus that extends to the stomach
- ulcers with a red outline, which may have **yellowish exudate (discharge)**
- ulcers may be very deep, however slow in progressing
- **dryness of the throat**
- dark red shiny and swollen areas in the esophagus, may bleed
- left side of the throat tends to be more affected
- **these types tend to have a lot of thick yellowish discharges**
- dry mouth and lips temporarily relieved by drinking cold water
- **stomach symptoms alternate with rheumatism or asthma**
- sticking in the throat as if a fish bone is caught there
- **post nasal discharge**
- great thirst for cold drinks
- **cravings for sweets**
- food is swallowed and goes down slowly
- food sits like a heavy stone in the stomach after eating
- **mentally these types tend to be conformists and adhere to the "rules"**
- lessened by swallowing
- aggravated bymeat and after eating

LACHESIS MUTA
Common indications include:
- sensation of a plug in the throat with constant desire to swallow
- **these types hate to have their throat touched and are intolerant to tight collars, chokers or necklaces**
- ulcers of the throat
- **lesions tend to be purplish discolouration**
- **pain with empty swallowing or drinking liquids**
- **left sided symptoms**
- food seems to sit at the back of the throat and causes a pain
- sensation of a tight cord or constriction in the throat

- **emotionally these types tend to be passionate people with a high sex drive and a tendency towards jealousy or suspicion**
- improved by cold drinks, fruits and loose clothes
- aggravated by alcohol, hot drinks and the **slightest touch**

MERCURIUS SOLUBILUS
Common indications include:

- burning in the throat, like a hot vapor rising from the stomach
- pain as if a foreign body was swallowed
- **stitching pain on swallowing**
- pale ulcers with red edges
- sensation of a burning spot in the pharynx
- **copper coloured discolouration of the throat**
- throat feels too tight
- pains are raw, sore, burning, stings
- **glandular swellings**
- loss of voice
- very thirsty people
- constant desire to swallow with **excessive saliva in the mouth**
- bitter and sweet taste in the mouth
- **mentally these types may be introverted and intense**
- aggravated by empty swallowing and **worse from hot and cold**

NITRIC ACID
Common indications include:

- **ulcers with sharp splinter-like pains**
- burning and soreness in esophagus
- very sensitive to pain with pains here and there
- white spots in the esophagus
- ulcers bleed easily
- **foul breath**
- bitter taste after eating
- dry heat in the throat
- tongue very sensitive, mild foods may cause smarting
- **these types may be depressed, irritable and cross**
- **emotionally these types are unmoved by apology and hold grudges**
- **cravings for fat and salt**, herring, chalk
- improved by applying heat
- aggravated by milk, fat foods, eating

Picture This....
You have chronic heartburn and have recently been diagnosed with Barrett's Esophagus. After your doctor finds a strange lesion in your throat, you have a biopsy that confirms abnormal cells typical of this disorder. You have been a long-term smoker with

offensive breath and have an enlarged prostate. You have been taking Zantac for a number of years. You are anxious because your doctor recommends you just keep taking Zantac and recheck the lesion for further abnormality.

You go to your local Homeopath who recommends that you remove all caffeine, fried foods and tobacco from your diet. You are told to eat half of all of your foods in the form of fruits and vegetables and follow the diet outlined in Chapter Two.

You take Slippery Elm lozenges, three times a day and one tbsp of Aloe Vera juice daily. You are given a homeopathic remedy called Conium because it is thought to help the prostate in those who are widowers. Your Homeopath said that the lack of sexual outlet tends to affect Conium types' prostate and it is also useful for the throat symptoms.

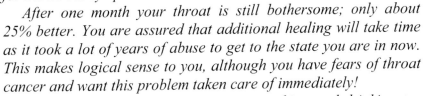

After one month your throat is still bothersome; only about 25% better. You are assured that additional healing will take time as it took a lot of years of abuse to get to the state you are in now. This makes logical sense to you, although you have fears of throat cancer and want this problem taken care of immediately!

Your Homeopath urged you to quit smoking and drinking tea but you told her that you feel really well with a cup of English breakfast tea and a smoke! She proceeded to tell you that you really needed to quit your bad habits. However, her eyes lit up when she found an unusual homeopathic remedy, called Carbolic Acid which suited your symptoms perfectly. You took that remedy along with the supplements and diet.

After one short month you had fewer cravings for tobacco and tea. Your breath problem and heartburn improved and rarely cause a problem now. Although you were sceptical in the beginning, you realize that have made more progress than you could have on your own.

Belching

In our society it is considered rude to belch in public. We all know a few ten-year-old boys who are very proud of their bodily functions. We typically shrug our shoulders in passive disapproval of their humour.

Studies have found that people typically expel gas between 10 to 20 times per day. We can only hold about one cup of gas in our gastrointestinal tract and the rest is expelled. If we are upright, we will expel the gas upwards or if we lay down it forces air into the intestinal tract. Expelling gas is not a negative occurrence but a normal gastrointestinal function.

Send My Regards to the Chef.....
In some cultures, such as the Middle Eastern Bedouin tribes, belching after a meal is considered a sign of politeness and an auditory way to salute your cook for doing a fine job!

Some people may simply be sensitive to the sensation of belching, although their symptoms are not out of the ordinary. It may cause psychological concern or physical discomfort. Usually belching is a transient symptom that may disappear on its own after a few days. However, if belching is uncomfortable and excessive, further investigation and treatment may be required.

The Causes of Belching

The typical causes of belching are as follows:

- air swallowing or aerophagia
- bacterial infection
- candida albicans overgrowth
- eating excessive gas forming foods such as artificial sweeteners, baking soda, beans, beer, carbonated drinks, cruciferous vegetables, fruits and milk
- eating quickly causes more air to be swallowed
- hyperventilation
- ill fitting dentures or sore teeth cause excessive saliva and swallowing of air
- obsessive compulsive disorder may cause excessive swallowing
- poor food choices causes gas, dyspepsia and heartburn
- post nasal drip may cause excess swallowing of air
- pregnancy causes pressure on the diaphragm which may stimulate belching to make room in the stomach
- stress causes excess swallowing and salivation
- sucking on candies causes swallowing of saliva and air
- swallowing, excessively

Belching Could be a Sign of Underlying Disease

Pains from distension should be dull, not sharp. If you have sharp pains, check with your doctor to rule out other disorders. Belching may be a sign of underlying disease or related to other disorders such as:

- Colitis
- Gallbladder disease
- Gastritis
- Gastroesophageal reflux disease
- Heart attack (belching is a rare symptom of a heart attack)
- Hiatal hernia
- Irritable bowel syndrome
- Lactose intolerance
- Obsessive compulsive disorder
- Pancreatitis
- Stomach cancer
- Ulcer

DIETARY MEASURES FOR BELCHING

Some gas-producing foods are healthy, like beans and cruciferous vegetables. It is normal to have a bit of gas after these foods. People who have excessive belching may benefit from avoiding foods that cause excessive gas such as artificial sweeteners, baking soda, beans, beer, carbonated drinks, cruciferous vegetables, fruits and milk.

Excessive gas may be related to a yeast overgrowth called candida albicans. It is wise to eat foods that are low glycemic to keep yeast to a minimum. High glycemic foods flip into a sugar quickly in the bloodstream and feed the bad bacteria. Examples of high glycemic foods are sugar, white bread and rice. If eaten in excess for a long period of time, these foods can cause other diseases like diabetes, hypoglycemia, hormone imbalance and heart disease. For a diet plan with listing of low, medium and high glycemic index foods, see Chapter Three. For more treatment options for Candida Albicans, refer to the Candidiasis section.

Food Combining

Food combining may be the key to controlling excessive gas. It is a good idea for people who want to maximize their natural ability to digest and absorb nutrients from their foods. It is based on the idea of combining certain types of foods to utilize digestive chemistry to the fullest. This is a particularly good idea for those who suffer with bloating, gas, constipation and diarrhea. In my practice, I recommend a basic form of food combining; the rules are as follows:

1) Eat fruit alone and at least half hour or more away from other foods.
2) Combine starches with vegetables. Starches are things like potatoes, rice, bread, pasta and crackers. Legumes fall into the starch category. They are best combined with grains to get all of the amino acids required. Usually these amino acids are found in meat and in combination with legumes and grains.
3) Combine protein or fat with vegetables. Proteins are fish, meats and legumes. (Legumes also fall into the starch category). Fats are things like nuts, seeds, oils and animal fats
4) Do not eat fruit with any other food. Fruits are a simple carbohydrate. They are digested very quickly if you eat them on an empty stomach. If you combine them with any other complex carbohydrate or fat you may find that you have a lot of gas, bloating and pain. This is because the fruit that is normally digested and absorbed very quickly ferments when it is mixed with other types of foods. It creates a gassy soup of bacteria which ferments and turns into alcohols, acetic acids and vinegars.
5) Do not combine protein or fat with starches.

Often simply improving the diet and avoiding high glycemic foods is enough to reduce the occurrence of belching. However, some natural supplements are useful for digestion and the tendency to burp.

GENERAL SUPPLEMENTS FOR BELCHING

Calcium and Magnesium, 2:1 ratio

Take a 2:1 ratio of calcium to magnesium. It is an alkalinizing mineral that helps to absorb the stomach acid which may cause excessive belching. Typical daily dosage would be 800 to 1200 mgs of calcium and 400 to 600 mgs of magnesium per day. It is best to split this into two or three doses throughout the day to get better digestion. Calcium Carbonate is a better buffer for acid than Calcium Citrate or a Calcium

Hydroxyapatite. However, Calcium Carbonate is harder to digest than the citrates or hydroxyapatite form. This is why it seems to buffer acid well, because it sits in the digestive tract longer and absorbs it. Citrates and hydroxyapatites are better for bone building.

Caraway Oil

Caraway has been used since Ancient Egyptian times for digestive distress. It is often used in combination with peppermint and fennel to relieve gas. It helps to improve bloating in stomach and spasms of the intestinal tract. Caraway should not be used on children under two years old or during pregnancy. Typical dosage of caraway oil is 0.05–0.2 ml of the essential oil taken three times daily.

Cinnamon

Cinnamon is useful to reduce gas from the gastrointestinal system. It aids in digestion, helps with ulcers, yeast infections and doesn't interfere with natural stomach acid. Typical dosage ranges from 150 mgs to 600 mgs, taken one to three times a day. Some people may experience a rash from cinnamon and it should not be taken during pregnancy.

Digestive enzymes

Digestive enzymes are a means for the body to break down foods and absorb their nutrients. Our body naturally makes digestive enzymes through the liver, the pancreas and stomach. If you do not have good digestion, digestive enzymes act as insurance for proper absorption. Partially or improperly digested foods cause many health issues, such as gas, heartburn, food allergies, constipation and the like.

Digestive enzymes usually include protease, which aids in protein digestion, lipase, which aids in fat digestion and amylases or cellulose which aids in carbohydrate digestion. Take as directed on the package. This supplement is not suited to those with high acidity.

Fennel Tea

Fennel tea relieves the feeling of fullness, gas and belching. It is used as an antispasmodic, antimicrobial and has mild estrogenic effects. Fennel relaxes the smooth muscle lining of the digestive tract, which aids in digestion. It helps with colic and the expulsion of gas. Typically fennel is taken in a tea form. It is not suitable for those who suffer with estrogen-related diseases such as breast cancer, uterine cancer, ovarian cysts or uterine fibroids or during pregnancy.

Ginger

Ginger improves digestion and helps with belching that is associated with nausea and upset stomach. Ginger is usually taken as tea. A fresh piece of ginger can be cut into a small piece and steeped in hot water. There are many commercial packages of ginger tea. It is not useful for those with a sensitive stomach, bleeding conditions, ulcers or inflammatory skin disease. If you are taking Coumadin or Warfarin do not use ginger. Don't take just prior to surgery.

Peppermint

Peppermint is a digestive aid that helps to relax the muscles of the digestive tract. It has been used since Roman times. It aids in expelling trapped gas, colic and dyspepsia. Peppermint is said to help sooth the gut and decrease inflammation. It is useful in reducing colic pains under the diaphragm. It is also useful for nausea and vomiting. Typically, peppermint is bought commercially as a tea. It is available in an oil, which tends to be much stronger than the tea. Typical dosage is two to three grams of fresh leaves, taken as an infusion. Large doses of peppermint may affect male libido by decreasing testosterone. Some people have allergic reactions to peppermint and it may worsen gastroesophageal reflux symptoms.

Probiotics

Probiotics such as Acidophilus and Bifidobacterium are beneficial bacteria. If these products are not refrigerated, they may be a dead culture, which does not help the beneficial flora to grow. Take as directed on the label. They help re-colonize the beneficial bacteria in the GI tract. You always have bad and good bacteria in your gut. If bad and good flora becomes imbalanced, your stomach may produce more gas than usual. Bifidobacterium has also been shown to suppress Helicobacter pylori. The bacterium, Helicobacter pylori, causes peptic ulcers, anemia and gastric cancer. Candida albicans, a naturally occurring yeast, is found in the gastrointestinal tract. If it is given the right conditions it can overgrow and cause many problems such as belching. This yeast is kept in check by using probiotics. See the Candidiasis section for more information on treatment protocols.

HOMEOPATHIC REMEDIES FOR BELCHING

There are many homeopathic remedies for belching. Some of the more common remedies are listed with their symptoms here. For more information on how to self prescribe a homeopathic remedy, go to Chapter Two. If you cannot find a remedy suited to you, or find you are not improving or your symptoms get worse, seek the help of a professional homeopath or your medical doctor.

ANTIMONIUM CRUDUM
Common indications include:
- belching that tastes like the food ingested
- constant burping
- stomach feels distended but may not be visibly bloated
- **cravings for acids and pickles, which aggravates their symptoms**
- **digestive powers are weak and easily disturbed**
- **tongue tends to be coated white**
- sensation as if something is lodged in the throat
- constant desire to swallow
- **these types are hot blooded and feel worse in the heat**
- **suited to types who put on weight easily**
- **mentally these types can feel irritable and cannot bear to be looked at or touched**

- aggravated by overloading the stomach, in the afternoon and at night, from bread, candy, vinegar, pastry, sour wine, acids and pork

ARGENTUM NITRICUM
Common indications include:
- **loud and copious belching**
- air is expelled with great violence
- shortness of breath is experienced with gas pressure
- burps may be tasteless or food may be belched into the mouth
- belching occurs after every meal
- stomach is very distended, as if it would burst with gas
- esophagus may feel closed and air is trapped
- **these types have great cravings for sugar and candy but this aggravates their symptoms**
- **suited to nervous types who have anxiety for upcoming events, health or when passing over a bridge or high places**
- **aggravated by sugar**, cold foods and ice cream
- lessened by empty burping, passing gas and dilute alcoholic drinks
- lessened by bending double or putting hard pressure on the abdomen

ASAFOETIDA
Common indications include:
- burps that smell odd, like garlic or feces
- **bursting feeling in the stomach that presses upwards or as if a lump in the stomach is rising into the throat**
- an amazing amount of air is produced
- **stomach is filled with air but nothing much passes despite belching**
- expulsion of wind with the sound of a pop gun going off
- **empty and ineffectual burping**
- pulsation in the pit of the stomach
- hysterical spasm of the trachea and esophagus

BRYONIA ALBA
Common indications include:
- frequent bitter or empty eructation (or belching) after eating
- **there is a great dryness of all mucous membranes in this remedy**
- regurgitation of food with belching
- **great thirst for large quantities of liquids**
- sour, watery belching
- pressure in the stomach after eating, which is sensitive to touch or force
- stomach is distended and feels as if food is pushed to the left side
- **these types tend to dislike being moved and are irritable**
- **these types fear financial stress and tend to be preoccupied with business**
- aggravated by bread, cabbage, potatoes, sour food

- lessened by **pressure, cold drinks** and food

CALCAREA CARBONICA
Common indications include:
- belching can be empty or sour, acidic and watery
- eructation may be burning, bitter and taste of the food eaten
- loud belching with heartburn
- pressure in the pit of the stomach with sensation of a lump
- **these types tend to be sweaty or clammy** and have a good appetite
- **these types may tend to gain weight easily and be heavy set**
- **mentally these types are stubborn, hard working and responsible**
- **cravings for eggs, sweets** and indigestible things like chalk
- worse after meals and from milk and meat

CARBO VEGETABILIS
Common indications include:
- **frequent belching that offers relief**
- sour, rancid burping
- **shortness of breath from gas or overeating**
- chronic dyspepsia of the aged or those with weak digestive powers
- food seems to sit and putrefy
- **distension is better from burping**
- fullness after a few bites
- sensation as if the abdomen is full to bursting
- stomach pains with burning
- **these types like open air, a fan or open window**
- **may faint easily from indigestion or gas**
- dislikes anything tight around the waistline
- **emotionally these types can be apathetic, negative and depressed**
- aggravated by fats, alcohol, rich food, poultry, pork, milk, decayed food and high living
- lessened by loosening the clothes, belching and cool air.

CHINA
Common indications include:
- **belching with persistent bitter taste** of food eaten
- enormous distension of the abdomen
- **fullness is not relieved by belching**
- food seems to sit in the stomach
- **frequent rumbling, belching and flatus**
- eructation may be air only
- **these types may become ill after losing a lot of fluids, such as after diarrhea, vomiting, sweating or bleeding**
- **craving for sweets** and acids

- **mentally these types may be sensitive or touchy and be fearful of animals, even house pets**
- aggravated by milk, fruits, excessive tea drinking
- lessened by hard pressure or bending double

LYCOPODIUM
Common indications include:
- excessive accumulation of gas
- **sour belching with heartburn**
- **loud noises from the abdomen**
- **these types eat very little and become full**
- violent hiccoughs
- pressure from gas causes shortness of breath
- **distension and gas is relieved by belching or flatulence**
- bitter taste in the mouth at night
- these types tend to have poor digestion and flatulence
- intolerance to tight clothing around the abdomen
- **cravings for sugar and sweets**
- **mentally these types may have low confidence or excessive ego and suffer from stage fright**
- worse after eating, **from 4:00 to 8:00p.m.**, cold food, cabbage, onions or oysters
- lessened by belching, warm food and drinks, loosening garments

NUX VOMICA
Common indications include:
- bitter, sour and watery eructations
- rising of water and bitter fluid from the stomach
- stomach is distended two to three hours after eating
- violent hiccoughs with rancid heartburn
- overeating is a regular occurrence which causes shortness of breath
- **cravings for alcohol, spices, fat and coffee**
- loosening of the clothes after meals
- **colic and sharp spasmodic pains in the stomach**
- **tendency towards painful constipation**
- **these types tend to be zealous types, angry or anxious**
- **they have a competitive, impatient, workaholic side to them**
- these types are oversensitive to noise and are chilly
- **worse after meals, from overeating, alcoholic drinks, coffee**, fat and sour foods

SULPHUR
Common indications include:
- sour and acidic belching that ameliorates gastric distress
- burps taste like rotten eggs
- belching when the stomach has any pressure on it

- **thirsty for ice cold drinks**
- sour eructations all day
- pain from incarcerated flatus
- fullness after meals with abdominal tenderness
- **these types have a hearty appetite**
- **cravings for sweets, chocolate, spices, alcohol and fats**
- **hunger usually strikes them at 11 a.m.**
- **these types may tend to suffer from skin conditions such as eczema, sweating, acne, body odor etc.**
- suited to types who drink too much alcohol and suffer from dyspepsia
- may suffer from diarrhea or constipation
- **mentally these types are messy, lazy, intellectual types who are extroverted**
- aggravated by acids, farinaceous foods, fat, meat, milk and sweets
- lessened by belching

Picture This....

You are a 35 year-old-man who has been suffering with incessant belching for at least six months. A year ago you had heartburn which changed into this annoying burping. Your diaphragm hurts from burping so much. You have this "stopped- up" sensation in your throat, like your stomach contents are pushing up on it.

You are feeling fed up with it. You see your uncle's Homeopath because he had said

he had some good luck with that type of treatment. At this point you are willing to try anything.

The Homeopath spends almost two hours on your case and even asks questions about the odour and type of burping you have. They seem to have a garlic odour even when you do not eat garlic. You are prescribed Asafoetida 30 CH to take as needed.

After the first month you check in with the Homeopath and report that the belching is gone and the pain is much better. You reveal that you eat a lot of spices and still have the odd bout of heartburn. You are asked to cut back on the spicy and fried foods. The Homeopath recommends a Calcium Magnesium supplement 2:1 ratio, 800:400 mgs per day. This really does the trick. You haven't had another belching bout in the past year.

Bile, lacking

In the mid sixteenth century, people who had too much bile were called cholerics or bilious and were typically considered ill humoured or irritable. The humours in medieval science and medicine refer to any of the four main fluids of the human body: blood, yellow bile, black bile and lymph. These determined a person's mood and temperament However, people who are deficient in bile are not cheerful. They may be irritable as well due to the number of problems it causes, such as constipation, greasy and pale coloured stools (due to indigestion of fats), distension, itching, pains and fatty deposits.

WHAT IS BILE?

Bile is a yellow green coloured substance that is made of bile acids, water, electrolytes, bilirubin, cholesterol and phospholipids. The liver usually manufactures about a quart of bile per day. The gallbladder also stores and excretes it into the duodenum. Bile has a few key functions. It aids in the absorption of fat soluble nutrients like vitamin A, D, E and K. It binds and removes toxic substances (such as drugs, hormones and toxins) from the intestinal tract. Bile absorbs water into the bowels to promote bowel movements. It helps to excrete destroyed red blood cells (bilirubin) in the stool. Bile helps to make stomach acid more alkaline and has bacteria killing properties.

CONDITIONS THAT HINDER BILE FLOW

Certain conditions may predispose one to a bile deficiency which will be discussed herein. Bile duct obstruction or scarring is often a symptom of gallbladder disease, gallstones, tumours or cirrhosis of the liver. These disorders are characterized by a lack of bile because the duct is blocked or damaged and hinders or halts bile flow altogether.

Cirrhosis is a disease that causes scarring and hardening of the liver cells. The liver is unable to maintain its duties because of cellular destruction. This may be caused by alcoholism, hepatitis C or malnutrition. A lack of bile is a byproduct of cirrhosis, simply because the liver is too damaged to produce or excrete it. Gallstones and tumours may physically block the bile duct and prevent it from descending into the duodenum. Removal of this obstruction should result in improved bile flow. Occasionally, the gallbladder may develop an infection which can cause spasmodic pains, fever and a deficiency of bile excretion. Antibiotics may be prescribed for the infection but surgery may be necessary in far gone cases. Surgical removal of the gallbladder causes a lack of bile excretion. Although the liver still manufactures it, it is not as effective as when the two organs work together. Many people require digestive support after their gallbladder is removed.

Usually people who are fair, female, forty and flabby tend to get gallstones. This is called the Four F's in the medical community. Maintaining a healthy body weight seems to help with proper digestion and bile flow. People who are overweight tend to eat foods that are high in fat or high glycemic.

DIETARY MEASURES FOR BILE PRODUCTION

Diet is crucial for health and proper digestion. Drink eight to 10 glasses of water per day. Coffee and tea do not count, as they have a dehydrating affect on the tissues. Water is perfect and has no calories. Consume low to medium glycemic and healthy fats, found in column one or two of the chart outlined in Chapter Three. Column One is low glycemic and lower fat, which is the best column to eat from. These foods are higher in fibre and decrease the prevalence of many other diseases such as heart disease, diabetes, cancer and hormone imbalances.

When you are filling your plate, visualize it like a pie. Grains should represent only a quarter of your plate. Another quarter should be lean protein or legumes. The other half should be fruits and vegetables. Eat a wide variety of colours of fruits and vegetables to ensure that you are getting optimum nutrition from your food. For example, orange vegetables are high in beta carotene and dark leafy vegetables contain folic acid. Try to consume mostly raw fruits and vegetables because they have more nutrients than cooked.

Bitter vegetables such as globe artichokes, dandelion and beet greens help with bile production. Higher fibre foods help to cleanse the gastrointestinal tract and clear the toxins which ease the burden on the liver. They also help to remove cholesterol via the intestinal tract. As mentioned previously, cholesterol deposits in the gallbladder cause gallstones. Examples of high fibre foods are listed in the constipation chapter. Eat a high fibre, low glycemic and low fat diet with lots of fresh fruits and vegetables. It is crucial to be your own health advocate. You are what you eat!

Foods to limit and/or avoid

A high fat and high animal protein diet requires more bile to aid in digestion. This may tax the liver and gallbladder's supply. If you overeat these foods, it stands to reason that you may simply not have enough bile. Eating this way makes your system more acidic and causes inflammation. Inflammatory conditions are arthritis, gout, heart disease, irritable bowel and muscle pains. Another downside of eating high fat and high protein diets is that over time gallstones may develop. This happens when the gallbladder excretes a lot of bile and it becomes stagnant and crystallizes. These crystals made of cholesterol or calcium turn into gallstones. Surgical removal of the gallbladder may be necessary, but this further reduces the excretion of bile. Make wise food choices and your body will reward you!

GENERAL SUPPLEMENTS FOR BILE PRODUCTION

Bile Salts

Ox bile is often used as a digestive aid. This supplement is useful for those who lack bile, have had their gallbladder removed or other liver disorders. Typical dosage is 250 to 500 mgs with meals.

Bile salts may be included in digestive enzymes. Enzyme supplements usually include protease, which aids in protein digestion, lipase, which aids in fat digestion and amylase or cellulose which aids in carbohydrate digestion. Some digestive enzymes contain Betaine HCL, which helps with protein digestion. Take it as directed on the package. This supplement is not suited to those with high acidity, intestinal or stomach ulcers.

Dandelion

Dandelion is a bitter herb that supports the digestion and function of the liver and gallbladder. It stimulates bile flow and aids in fat digestion. It also acts as a tonic for the intestines which helps alleviate the symptoms of constipation.

Some people eat dandelion greens as a salad which is very beneficial. Dosage varies depending on which form you purchase. Dandelion comes fresh or as a tea, capsules or tincture. This herb is best taken right before a meal to aid in digestion.

Goldenseal

Goldenseal is a gentle, bitter herb. It improves digestion, increases bile flow and tones the gallbladder. Goldenseal is also a useful anti-microbial that kills candida and other bacteria that cause stomach and gastrointestinal disorders. Typical dosage of Goldenseal is 300 to 450 mgs taken three times a day.

Goldenseal has mild anti-bacterial properties, it may deplete your body of the beneficial bacteria in the gut. Take probiotics when you take Goldenseal to maintain healthy gut flora. Do not take Goldenseal for longer than two weeks at a time. Goldenseal is contraindicated during pregnancy, if you take blood thinners or have a peptic ulcer.

Lecithin

Lecithin is a supplement that is useful to aid in liver support and cognitive function. It helps to support the liver with liver damage caused by alcohol, toxins, viruses and disease. It binds to cholesterol and reduces it in the blood stream. Studies have shown that lecithin is protective of liver diseases like fibrosis and cirrhosis in groups of rats that were fed a lot of alcohol. Typical dosage is 1 to 3 grams per day. There is no reported toxicity with Lecithin use.

Milk Thistle

Milk thistle is a fabulous herb that is known to protect, cleanse and stimulate the liver to release toxins and manufacture bile. This herb has a detoxifying affect and is often used for jaundice, cirrhosis or hepatitis. It is better used in the early stages of cirrhosis than the late stages of liver failure. Typical dosage is 200 to 250 mgs per day with each meal. Drink lots of water whilst using milk thistle to flush your system of toxins.

Swedish Bitters

Bitters preparations are made by an infusion and/or distillation process using aromatic herbs, bark, roots, and/or fruit. Bitters may contain herbs like aloe, myrrh, saffron, orange peel, gentian, quinine, angostura bark, cassia, senna leaves, camphor, angelica roots, manna, rhubarb roots, goldenseal, artichoke leaf, blessed thistle, wormwood and yarrow flowers.

Historically, Bitters were taken as a dinnertime aperitif to stimulate the digestive juices. Swedish Bitters are useful to aid in digestion, to settle a stomach before eating and to ward off the ill effects of alcohol. They were used as a tonic and taken in a shot glass. The liquor variety of bitters has a high percentage of alcohol. Purchase your bitters from a health food store, not the liquor store. Typical dosage is one tablespoon before meals. Follow the directions on the individual package.

Vitamin C

Vitamin C is required to convert cholesterol into bile. Typical dosage of vitamin C is 500 mgs to 3,000 mgs per day with meals.

HOMEOPATHIC REMEDIES FOR BILE PRODUCTION

There are many homeopathic remedies for bile production. Some of the more common remedies are listed with their symptoms here. For more information on how to self prescribe a homeopathic remedy, go to Chapter Two. If you cannot find a remedy suited to you, or find you are not improving or your symptoms get worse, seek the help of a professional homeopath or your medical doctor.

BERBERIS VULGARIS
Common indications include:
- biliary and gallbladder colic
- these types are sleepy after eating
- pains in the lumbar region, gallbladder and liver
- **pains are sharp, stitching and radiate outward or downward**
- stools are hard, round, tough and may be watery
- gouty and rheumatic complaints
- these types are easily mentally and physically fatigued
- suited to fleshy people

CALCAREA CARBONICA
Common indications include:
- **chronic painless constipation without urging**
- stools are hard, white or pale colour, chalky or grey
- painful and large stools
- undigested food in the stools
- sour, acid stools and belching
- distension of the abdomen
- itching in the rectum which is worse at nighttime
- **cravings for eggs and sweets**
- gurgling in the right side of the abdomen
- **these types tend to be heavy set and good eaters**
- **mentally these types are stubborn, hard working and reliable types**
- **perspiration of the head** during sleep with a **sensitivity to damp, cold weather**
- aversion to and aggravated by fatty food

CHELIDONIUM
Common indications include:
- the need to decrease inflammation in the common bile duct
- **a good remedy for jaundice**, gallbladder pains from stones or infection
- yellow eyes, face, urine and stool with liver disturbance such as jaundice
- needs to lie down after eating
- constipation with hard, small and round stools
- flatulence with cutting colicky pains
- diarrhea that is slimy, light grey, yellow, white or pasty
- burning and itching in the rectum
- tongue may be coated yellow
- **right sided symptoms such as: pains in the right side of the abdomen which are better lying on the left side, pain inside the right shoulder blade, right sided headaches or pains under the right rib cage**
- **these types may be domineering**, forgetful, anxious and depressed
- suited to people who are weary and feel lazy

- ameliorations from pains with warmth, hot drinks, pressure and bending backwards, walking
- **worse on the right side, 4:00 a.m**. or p.m., change of weather

CHINA
Common indications include:
- **colic from gallstones and bile duct obstruction**
- weight felt after eating a small amount of food
- pain comes on alternating days
- painful liver sensitive to light touch but better by hard pressure
- eating at night causes food to not digest at all
- **frequent gurgling, belching and flatulence**
- diarrhea can be watery and contain undigested food
- involuntary stool with fruits
- loosens the belt after eating
- **lessened by hard pressure on the abdomen**, bending double
- **aggravated by loss of fluids,** eating late, light touch
- aggravated by eating fruits, diarrhea, milk, night, fish, tea

LYCOPODIUM
Common indications include:
- **liver affections, right sided pains**
- sensitive to touch in the region of the liver
- gallbladder attacks and gallstones
- always hungry and headaches if not appeased
- inactivity of the gastrointestinal tract
- sleepy after eating
- **heartburn with sour belching**
- bitter taste in the mouth on waking
- sensitive to tight pants or belts
- constipation with stools that are difficult to pass
- **cravings for sweets**
- distention with much gas and fermentation in the bowels
- **mentally these types suffer from low self esteem or excessive bravado and have stage fright**
- these types are tired, annoyed easily, weak physically, sensitive
- lessened by warm foods and drinks, loosening pants
- **aggravated by cold drinks, right side, from 4:00 to 8:00 p.m.**, heavy meals

NUX VOMICA
Common indications include:
- **ailments from over indulgence (food, alcohol, coffee, tea, drugs)**
- digestion easily disturbed
- **these types are easily angered, irritable and impatient**

- painful constipation with colicky pains
- enlarged liver, alcoholic cirrhosis
- nauseated in the morning on waking
- **colicky pains that are worse from anger and tight clothes**
- fatty foods seem to be tolerated well
- nervous dyspepsia with mental work
- **these types may wake up at 3:00 a.m. with thoughts of work**
- **these types may be competitive, impatient and workaholic types**
- **lessened by hot drinks and warm applications**
- aggravated by bread, sour foods, alcohol, drugs, tobacco
- aggravated by high living, morning, sedentary habits

PHOSPHORUS
Common indications include:

- fatty liver, hepatitis, jaundice
- jaundice with congestion of the liver
- stools are thin, hard and difficult to expel
- pain in the left shoulder and hypogastria
- **great hunger and thirst for cold things**
- gas pain felt in the short ribs of the abdomen
- suited to tall, slender types
- **mentally these types are open, anxious and sympathetic types**
- **these types may fear thunderstorms or that something bad will happen**
- **amelioration cold drinks and food, eating**
- **aggravated by fasting**, left side, fruit, **warm drinks and food**, coffee, garlic, boiled milk, potatoes and tea

PULSATILLA
Common indications include:

- **changeable symptoms are typical of this remedy**, (for example no two stools are alike, the mood changes from happy to sad)
- skin rash after eating rich, fatty, greasy foods
- pain in the stomach after eating
- dragging pain in the liver that extends to the back and between the shoulder blades
- **thirstless people despite having a dry mouth**
- mouth has a bitter, sour and fatty taste in it
- bread especially tastes sour or bitter
- jaundice with a white coated tongue
- **desires peanut butter and ice cream**
- **feels better in cool air or with an open window**
- suited to women who tend to be fleshy, fair and freckled
- **mentally these types are timid, weep easily and desire consolation**
- **lessened by open air**, lemonade

- **aggravated by fat, rich, greasy foods, pork**, meat, pastry

SULPHUR
Common indications include:

- feels hungry but is opposed to eating as soon as they reach the table
- **ailments from suppressed discharges** such as skin eruptions, constipation, diarrhea stopped by medications, suppressed sweat
- abdomen is full and distended with incarcerated flatus
- **these types have a hearty appetite**
- wakes early morning to rush to a bowel movement
- constipation alternating with diarrhea
- **hunger felt at 11:00 a.m.**
- **these types may suffer from skin conditions such as eczema, hives, acne, perspiration or body odor**
- tendency to redness of the mucous membranes
- burning felt in the stomach and rectum
- **cravings for sweets. beer, fat, spices and whiskey**
- **desires ice cold drinks**
- ailments of drunkards
- **mentally these types can be lazy, messy, intellectual and extroverted**
- aggravated by milk, sweets, alcohol and spices
- lessened by free discharges, bowel movements, belching, open air

Picture This....

You have young kids at home and have been on the run with all of their activities. You 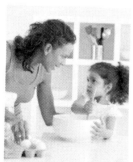 *have no time to relax and your digestion is really getting to be a problem. You have been suffering from hard and pale-coloured stools. You rarely have any desire to go to the bathroom. When you do go, the stools seem to be too large and painful to pass.*

Your regular love of sweets and eating in general is starting to bite you back! Your digestion is on the fritz and now the simplest of meals is giving you heartburn. You have gained about 10 lbs and every night your head perspires so much that you soak your pillow. You are wondering if you have some kind of virus. Time to take action!

You had brought your kids to a Homeopath for their earaches with great success so you go to hear what she has to say about your case. After a few hours of assessment you are prescribed Calcarea Carbonica 200CH. You are to take it once a night for a week and to stop if you see positive or negative action. In other words, if you start to have normal bowel movements or sweating or your condition gets worse, you should stop the remedy and wait for things to settle. Your Homeopath also recommends that you smarten up with your diet and eat higher fibre foods, such as whole grains, veggies and fruits and steer clear of white bread and sugar.

The day after your first dose of Calcarea Carbonica you had a normal bowel movement – in fact, many! This was great! After one month your digestion has never been better. The annoying perspiration stopped in the first week. You have a normal consistency and frequency of bowel movements. From time to time, you take a dose of Calcarea Carbonica but only on an as needed basis.

Biliousness

Biliousness refers to a liver or bile duct dysfunction that causes excess secretion of bile. This excess secretion fills the digestive tract with bile and can cause a number of problems. There are many symptoms that excess bile causes such as:

- bitter taste in the mouth
- burning in the stomach and intestines
- coated tongue
- diarrhea (may be green or yellow bile colour)
- furry tongue
- headaches with nausea
- irritability
- loss of appetite
- nausea and vomiting
- colicky, sharp pains in the stomach or bowels
- vomiting yellow or green bile

Conditions that cause excess bile are an improper diet, medication, stress, disorders of the bile ducts, liver and/or gallbladder. Overeating, eating late and the wrong types of food trigger this condition. Foods that are no-no's for those who suffer with sensitive digestion are as follows: alcohol, fat, unripe fruits, sweets and pastries, coffee and tea. Leading a sedentary life triggers digestive difficulties. This could be related to the fact that most people who do not exercise do not burn the food they eat. This taxes the digestive tract. Weak digestion inherently contributes to biliousness. If the liver, gallbladder and bile ducts malfunction, oversecretion causes problems.

In medieval times, a bilious or choleric temperament was said to be bitter and exceedingly irritated. Stress may cause an excess of acid in the digestive tract. It also causes blood to travel away from the stomach and go to the extremities for the person to run. This is an evolutionary mechanism termed the "fight or flight" response. It was an innate survival mechanism for us to run from a predator. When less blood is in our abdominal region, digestion is impeded.

A few interesting recommendations from some turn of the century homeopathic texts were to apply heat and friction to the abdomen. Warmth could be applied using wet towels. Friction would be applied using a "flesh" brush. This flesh brush is likely the same type of brush we use today for skin brushing. One antique medical book had a funny recommendation for biliousness: crab's eyes. Imagine how many it would take to make medicine! (Don't try this at home.)

DIETARY MEASURES FOR BILIOUSNESS

Common sense dietary measures for biliousness are a bland, basic diet with lukewarm drinks, fresh fruits and vegetables. Eat during the day, not at night because digestion is better in the morning and declines as the day progresses. Avoid nicotine and dietary triggers mentioned in the previous paragraphs.

Exercising burns calories, stimulates bowel movements and improves lymphatic drainage. Eating more than you need burdens the digestive tract. The stomach labours to break down this mass of food for excretion. Eat smaller meals to relieve digestive strain.

People who overindulge in the pleasures of the table are prone to digestive upset. Bile is made to break down fats. Greasy foods will stimulate bile secretion. Follow a healthy diet that is low in fat, sugars and refined carbohydrates. Dietary recommendations, found in Chapter Three, contain a list of low, medium and high glycemic and fat foods. The low glycemic and low fat foods in Column One are best for health.

Food combining is another great tool for optimum digestive function. It maximizes one's digestive powers to absorb nutrients from foods. It is based on combining types of foods to utilize our digestive chemistry to the fullest. The principles are as follows: eat fruit alone and at least half hour or more away from other foods. Combine starches with vegetables and protein or fat with vegetables. Do not eat fruit with any other food and don't combine protein or fat with starches.

Fruits are a simple carbohydrate. They are digested very quickly if you eat them on an empty stomach. If you combine them with any other complex carbohydrate or fat you may find that you have a lot of gas, bloating and pains. This is because the fruit that is normally digested and absorbed very quickly ferments when it is mixed with other types of foods. It creates a gassy soup of bacteria which ferments and turns into alcohols, acetic acids and vinegars.

Starches are items like potatoes, rice, bread, pasta and crackers. Proteins are fish, meats and legumes. Legumes also fall into the starch category. They are best combined with grains to get all of the amino acids required. Usually these amino acids are found in meat and in combination with legumes and grains. Fats are things like nuts, seeds, oils and animal fats.

GENERAL SUPPLEMENTS FOR BILIOUSNESS

Calcium and Magnesium, 2:1 ratio

Take a 2:1 ratio of calcium to magnesium. It is an alkalinizing mineral that helps to absorb acid. Take in between meals. Typical daily dosage would be 800 to 1200 mgs of calcium and 400 to 600 mgs of magnesium. It is best to split this into two or three doses throughout the day. Calcium Carbonate is a better buffer for acid than Calcium Citrate or Calcium Hydroxyapatite.

Deglycyrrhizinated Licorice (DGL)

DGL is an excellent remedy for heartburn and healing the stomach and esophagus. It has been known since ancient Greek and Egyptian times. It is said to help heal ulcers of the gastrointestinal tract. It has anti-inflammatory, antiviral, antimicrobial, mucoprotective and expectorant properties. Typical dosage is 500 mgs half hour before each meal, up to three times a day. Licorice decreases potassium which increases sodium in the body. This is why licorice is not suitable to those who have high blood pressure. Avoid licorice if you have low potassium, liver disease, kidney disease, heart failure or are pregnant. Avoid licorice if you are taking diuretics or prednisone-like drugs.

Fibre

Foods that are high in fibre help with constipation but also clear bile, cholesterol and toxic debris from the gastrointestinal tract. Certain types of fibre are particularly beneficial for cleaning up the system. Fibre that contains gums, mucilages, lignans and pectin is useful to absorb and excrete excess acid, bile and cholesterol. It also prevents gallstones. Examples of high fibre foods are apples, brussel sprouts, kale, cabbage, cooked legumes, ground flaxseed and whole grains. Whole grains that are high in fibre are brown rice, bulgar, millet, oat bran, slow cooked oatmeal, quinoa, whole wheat and wheat bran.

Papaya and Pineapple

You can consume these fruits. They contain beneficial enzymes that help with heartburn and digestion. Some people take a digestive supplement that contains Bromelain and Papain which is made from pineapple and papaya.

HOMEOPATHIC REMEDIES FOR BILIOUSNESS

There are many homeopathic remedies for biliousness. Some of the more common remedies are listed with their symptoms here. For more information on how to self prescribe a homeopathic remedy, go to Chapter Two. If you cannot find a remedy suited to you, or find you are not improving or your symptoms get worse, seek the help of a professional homeopath or your medical doctor.

Did you know….
According to the notes of Charles Darwin, the father of science, he may not have been healthy enough to write "The Origin of the Species" without the water and powders from his homeopath, Dr. James Manby Gully.

Note to self: Darwin was not a slave to conformist thinking or a dummy with regards to scientific matters!

Source: *Homeopathic Revolution: Why Famous People and Cultural Heroes Choose Homeopathy,* by Dana Ullman   www.homeopathicrevolution.org

ANTIMONIUM CRUDUM

Common indications include:
- **thick white coated tongue**
- burning in the pit of the stomach
- **overeating causes digestive distress**
- **weak digestion**
- emotions are felt in the stomach
- belching, heartburn, nausea and vomiting
- rising of fluid tastes like food that was eaten
- stool composed of undigested foods, hard lumps with water
- sensation of something lodged in throat which makes him swallow

- **hot blooded people who are worse from heat**
- milk becomes curdled in the stomach
- **these types tend to be heavy set**
- vomits as soon as eats
- **irritable types who cannot bear to be touched or looked at**
- **cravings for pickles, acids, cucumbers, vinegar** and wine
- aggravated by fats, acids, sweets, vinegar, pork, alcohol and overeating

BRYONIA
Common indications include:

- splitting, bursting and nauseous headaches that are relieved by closing the eyes
- headaches start in the morning and increase as the day goes on
- **constipation and dryness**
- **dryness of all mucous membranes**
- nausea and vomiting of bile
- water brash with bitter taste
- sharp pains after eating that may extend to the shoulders
- heartburn from drinking cold water when the person is overheated
- stomach sensitive to touch
- white or brown coated tongue
- **intense thirst for large quantities of water with dry lips and mouth**
- food tastes bitter
- craving for coffee and wine
- **these types may have rheumatic complaints that are worse from movement**
- **mental symptoms include irritability, wants to be left alone in a quiet environment, preoccupied with thoughts of finances and business**
- worse after eating and from vegetables, sauerkraut, cabbage, potatoes, acids, warm drinks, bread
- **aggravated by motion** and hot weather
- **lessened by pressure**, resting and being left alone

CHAMOMILLA
Common indications include:

- spells of painful colic
- bitter bilious vomiting
- **spasmodic colicky cramps in the bowels and stomach**
- stomach is tender and distended
- **stool like cut grass or spinach**
- **stools or belching smells like rotten eggs**
- undigested food in the stools
- **ill humour from pains (these types are abnormally sensitive to pains)**
- one cheek red and the other pale

- **very irritable, cannot be civil**
- **children want to be carried but cannot be consoled**
- addicted to strong coffee, which increases bile flow
- aggravated by strong emotions, coffee

COLOCYNTHIS
Common indications include:
- bitter taste in the mouth
- vomiting yellow or green bile
- spasmodic pains in the stomach that extend to the throat
- waves of pain that feel like the intestines are squeezed between stones
- stools are frothy, watery and yellow
- **pain compels them to bend double which improves their condition**
- great restlessness and sadness **during pains**
- **emotionally these types are impatient and easily angered**
- **aggravated by anger and/or indignation**, upset by eating the least amount food and drink
- **lessened by hard pressure**, lying face down, **bending double**, heat and belching

IRIS
Common indications include:
- bilious headaches
- **burning of the whole alimentary canal, from mouth to anus**
- acidic, bilious, bitter, sour, watery belching and vomit
- nausea with or without vomiting
- stomach contents feel like vinegar
- low appetite
- stools are fatty
- severe pain in the head with diarrhea
- **one sided headache, typically the right side above the temple or eye**
- **sick headache begins with blurred vision**
- **vomiting with the headaches**
- temporary improvement from drinking cold water
- worse in the spring and summer
- aggravated by milk but with the sensation it curdles in the stomach

LYCOPODIUM
Common indications include:
- sensation of fullness from the stomach up to the throat
- food tastes sour
- **water brash and sour belching**
- **distended and full after least amount of food**
- flatulence and constipation

- **may be suited to types with low self-esteem, anger from contradiction, fear of public speaking**
- least pressure of clothes bothersome
- **right sided complaints or right to left**
- **craving for sweet**s, alcohol, warm drinks and food
- **aggravated from cold drinks**, milk, cabbage, wheat, beans, onions, wine, rye, beer, morning and fasting
- better with open air, belching

NATRUM PHOSPHORICUM
Common indications include:
- stomach pains
- heartburn, water brash
- trouble swallowing
- acid stomach and belching
- **yellow coated tongue**
- regurgitates fluid that is as sour as vinegar
- vomiting sour, acid fluids
- liquids are not tolerated as well as solid food
- fullness after eating very little
- high uric acid in blood
- **cravings for fried eggs**, beer, fried fish and spices
- worse two hours after eating and from sugar, milk, bitter and fatty foods

NUX VOMICA
Common indications include:
- helps bile be reabsorbed
- primary remedy for **aggravations from overindulgence**
- sour taste in the morning after eating
- cramps in the stomach, bowels and even cramping headaches
- pain in the stomach like a weight or pressure, two or three hours after meals
- bloating and distension
- vomits sour mucous
- putrid bitter taste in the mouth
- **back of tongue is coated brown**
- squeezing stomachaches, tender stomach
- aversion to food with nausea
- **these types tend to be chilly**
- tightness of the abdomen after eating, must loosen pants
- diarrhea and constipation with painful urging
- **suited to zealous, fiery temperaments who overindulge and overwork**
- cravings for fats and tolerates them well
- **cravings for tea, coffee, alcohol and spicy food**

- **aggravated by tight clothes**, after eating, drug use, tobacco poisoning, overeating, overindulgence, alcohol, spices, stimulants, tea and coffee
- **lessened by warmth, warm drinks**

PULSATILLA
Common indications include:

- water brash and heartburn
- sour, bitter, putrid belching
- thick, white, coated tongue, flat taste in mouth
- nothing tastes good, aversion to food
- sensation of a lump in mid sternum, food seems stuck there
- **stools change consistency**
- green or yellow watery stools
- indigestion with a disordered stomach
- **thirstless with a dry mouth**
- **these types are said to be easily moved to tears or laughter**
- **craving for butter, cream, cheese, ice cream and/or peanut butter**
- worse one hour after eating
- **aggravated by rich fat foods, pork**, ice cream and pastry
- lessened by cold and open air

SULPHUR
Common indications include:

- sick headache every week or two
- **hungry feeling around 11:00 a.m.**
- tendency to constipation and hemorrhoids
- burning, sour, watery belching after eating
- regurgitation of food tastes acid shortly after a meal
- tendency to eat too quickly and not chew food well
- **hearty appetite**
- taste in mouth like rotten eggs
- **warm blooded types who are worse from heat**
- diarrhea drives them out of bed in the morning
- flatus and stools have a foul odor
- gastric complaints may alternate with skin conditions
- **may be suited to lazy, intellectual and/or slovenly types**
- **skin eruptions are common in this remedy**
- **cravings for sweets, fats, alcohol, beer and ale**
- aggravated in the morning, after eating, eggs, milk products, sweets, alcohol
- aggravated before the menstrual flow

Bloating
See Flatulence and Dyspepsia

Candidiasis/Thrush

Candida Albicans is a single cell microbe that is an opportunistic fungus. It overgrows if it is given the right conditions. It affects the gastrointestinal and genitourinary tract, endocrine, nervous and immune system. The skin, mouth, ears, nose, toe and finger nails are also affected. This fungus weakens the immune system, causes hyper-reactivity to allergens and may be worse in damp moldy environments. It also causes chemical sensitivities such as to petroleum, oil, rubbers, exhaust fumes and perfumes.

Causes of Candida Overgrowth

- **Medications:** antibiotics, birth control pills, chemotherapy, steroids
- **Diet:** sugars, refined carbohydrates, mouldy foods, foods containing yeast
- **Poor digestion:** deficiency in hydrochloric acid or digestive enzymes do not kill excessive yeast in the gut
- **Diseases:** diabetes, immune deficiencies like AIDS and HIV
- **Hormones:** pregnancy

Symptoms that may be caused by Candida Overgrowth

- **Gastrointestinal:** abdominal pains, burning tongue, canker sores, colitis, diarrhea, halitosis, heartburn, rectal itching, white spots on the tongue, thrush
- **Genitourinary:** bladder infections, impotency, prostatitis, night sweats, premenstrual syndrome, vaginitis
- **Mind/Nervous symptoms:** adrenal insufficiency, alcohol abuse, depression, drunken feeling, erratic behavior, foggy thinking, hyperactivity, lethargy, memory loss, numbness, mood swings, underachievement
- **Immune system symptoms:** congestion, ear infections, recurrent infections, sore throats, sinusitis
- **Skin symptoms:** acne, eczema, hives, itching, psoriasis, toe and fingernail infections
- **Musculoskeletal symptoms:** arthritis, joint pains, muscular aches

Recommendations for Candida Overgrowth

- Replace your toothbrush once per month
- Wear cotton clothes to help the skin breath and prevents rashes
- Follow a candida diet
- Avoid medications such as antibiotics, birth control pills, chemotherapy and steroids
- Be checked for food allergies, sometimes food allergies are masked as candida symptoms
- Follow a candida diet (See below)
- Replenish the good bacteria lactobacillus and Bifidobacteria

DIETARY MEASURES FOR CANDIDIASIS

The diet outlined in Chapter Three lists groups of foods according to low, medium and high glycemic and fat. Avoid high glycemic and fat foods. Also if you want to do the candida diet, any food listed with a "#" sign beside it should be avoided. The foods that have "#" beside it feed the bad bacteria. It is a strict diet, but it works. Examples of foods to avoid are sugars, yeast containing foods, mouldy foods (cheese, wine, beer), dried fruits, melons, peanuts, vinegar, smoked meats, pickles, mushrooms, soya sauce, citrus fruits (lemon, orange, lime, grapefruits, tomatoes), milk and all milk products, honey, maple syrup and sugar. This bad bacterium, Candida Albicans, feeds off of sugars and moldy foods. Anything that is high glycemic, mouldy or has sugar added is not acceptable. If it is given the right environment, candida flourishes. Many people find this diet very strict, but the vast majority feel better after they get over negative food withdrawal symptoms.

GENERAL SUPPLEMENTS FOR CANDIDIASIS

Biotin

Biotin is a member of the B vitamin family. It helps with many processes in the body. People with biotin deficiencies are prone to candida infections and elevated bad cholesterol. This could be because biotin is involved in fatty-acid assimilation and production of antibodies and enzymes. It also helps with hair loss, alopecia, skin and nail growth. Our bodies need 30 mcgs per day of biotin, however, supplement dosage may vary. There is no known toxicity with this supplement.

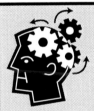 According to Dr. Joseph Mercola's website, high glycemic foods and/or being diabetic leads to a greater incidence of Alzheimer's, memory loss and dementia!
Being diabetic ups your risk of alzheimers by 65 percent!
Ask yourself: Is eating refined carbohydrates and sugar worth losing your mind over?
Source: www.mercola.com

Caprylic Acid

This supplement is an anti-fungal that destroys candida and is said to be beneficial for streptococcus and staphylococcus aureus infections. Caprylic acid has also the common name Octanoic Acid and is an eight-carbon straight chain fatty acid. This acid can easily permeate fatty cell membranes of microbes, thus it is very effective against bacteria because it can break into its hard cell membrane. It is naturally found in coconuts and breast milk. Typical dosage for caprylic acid is 500 to 1200 mgs per day. Avoid if you are pregnant or nursing. It may cause some gastrointestinal upset because it alters the body's natural flora. Be sure to use probiotics while you use this product.

Fibre

Foods that are high fibre help with constipation but also clear bile, cholesterol and toxic debris from the gastrointestinal tract. Fibre is particularly beneficial for sweeping out yeast from the gut. Many candida cleansing kits contain psyllium, a type of soluble fibre. This is an inexpensive supplement that works well. Drink a large amount of water whilst you use it, to prevent an intestinal blockage. It is healthy to include more fibre in your diet. Examples of high fibre foods are apples, brussel sprouts, kale, cabbage, cooked legumes, ground flaxseed and whole grains. Whole grains that are high in fibre are brown rice, bulgar, millet, oat bran, slow cooked oatmeal, quinoa, whole wheat and wheat bran.

Garlic

Garlic helps to improve the immune system by stimulating bad bacteria eating cells. It has antibacterial, antifungal and antiviral properties and has a good long term effect on those with chronic yeast infections. It is not as strong as antibiotics and has only a modest effect on bacteria. Garlic has been shown effective for cancer, heart disease, immunity, candida, ulcers and parasites.

Typical dosage of garlic is 500 mgs to 1000 mgs per day. Avoid garlic if you take blood thinners or are undergoing surgery.

Goldenseal

Goldenseal is a gentle, bitter herb. It improves the digestion, increases bile flow and tones the gallbladder. Goldenseal is also a useful anti-microbial that kills candida and other bacteria that cause stomach and gastrointestinal disorders. Typical dosage of Goldenseal is 300 to 450 mgs taken three times a day.

Since Goldenseal has mild anti-bacterial properties, it may deplete your body of the beneficial bacteria in the gut. Take probiotics when you take Goldenseal to maintain healthy gut flora. Do not take Goldenseal for longer then two weeks at a time. Goldenseal is contraindicated during pregnancy, if you take blood thinners or have a peptic ulcer.

Oil of Oregano

Oregano oil has a strong anti-microbial effect and acts as an anti-inflammatory, antiseptic and diaphoretic (causes sweating). It comes in oil or capsule form and potency varies, so follow the directions on the individual labels. Side effects may include mild stomach upset and interference with iron absorption. Do not take oregano if you are pregnant or breast feeding, as studies have not confirmed its effect.

Pau D'Arco

Pau D'Arco is a rainforest herb, also known as Lapacho or Taheebo, made from the inner bark of a tree. It is an immune enhancer that is anti-microbial and useful in killing candida albicans. Like garlic it stimulates macrophages, bacteria-eating cells. This herb also helps with diabetes, ulcers, parasites, ringworm and boils. Avoid this herb if you are pregnant or nursing. Typical dosage of Pau D'Arco in capsule form is 1,000 mgs per day. It also comes in a liquid or tea form. Follow the directions on the individual labels.

Probiotics

Probiotics such as Acidophilus and Bifidobacterium are beneficial bacteria which are found in kefir and yogurt. If you like these products, use an unsweetened variety. These bacteria help to re-colonize the beneficial bacteria in the gut and keep bad bacteria in check. They also help the intestine to metabolize and eliminate toxins.

If these products are not refrigerated, they may be a dead culture which does not help the beneficial flora to grow. They can be purchased in a standardized capsule to ensure the number of live bacteria per capsule. Follow the directions on the package.

Note: Any of these supplements that kill candida should be taken with probiotics to replenish the good bacteria. They may kill some of the good bacteria, like an antibiotic.

HOMEOPATHIC REMEDIES FOR CANDIDIASIS

There are many homeopathic remedies for candidiasis. Some of the more common remedies are listed with their symptoms here. For more information on how to self-prescribe a homeopathic remedy, go to Chapter Two. If you cannot find a remedy suited to you, or find you are not improving or your symptoms get worse, seek the help of a professional homeopath or your medical doctor.

BORAX
Common indications include:
- **hot ulcers or canker sores** in the mouth and inner surface of the cheek, that bleed easily
- heat and dryness in the mouth
- salivation
- sore mouth when chewing or in nursing babies
- redness of the margins of the eyelids
- much clear mucous vaginal discharges
- extreme pain before urinating
- cramping and diarrhea from fruits
- brown, green, mucous or watery stools
- **headache at 10:00 a.m.**
- colicky pains before diarrhea
- **mentally these types are easily startled and sensitive to noise**
- **aggravated by fear in descending or a downward motion**

HYDRASTIS
Common indications include:
- mouth is sore (in nursing)
- tongue burned as if raw
- tongue feels too large or flabby, shows the imprint of the teeth
- **thick, stringy yellow discharge from mucous membranes**
- stools mixed with mucous
- offensive sweat
- low appetite with aversion to food
- chronic ear infections
- constipation
- fissures and ulcers may form on lining of mouth, throat, stomach, vagina
- pus-like discharge from the ears
- worse after bowel elimination
- aggravated by use of wine and drugs
- lessened by pressure

KREOSOTUM
Common indications include:
- severe itching in the margins of the eyelids, worse by rubbing
- small wounds bleed profusely
- **excoriation and inflammation of the mucous membranes**
- itching so intense that it drives people mad
- **burning and foul vaginal discharge** that stains the clothes yellow
- **discharges causes swelling and burning of the vulva**
- burning as if red hot coals in the vaginal tract
- **hemorrhages and abnormal bleeding**
- colicky pains
- **gums are painful, spongy, ulcerated, bleeding**, dark red or blue
- incontinence of urine
- urine burns on passing it
- foul breath
- stool is very painful from excoriation
- aggravated by washing in cold water, cold food and drink, lying, eating and pregnancy
- lessened by warmth, hot food and motion

SILICEA
Common indications include:
- **crippled nails, ingrown toenails, poor bone and hair growth**
- frequent infections, urinary tract, sinus, ears
- chronic low grade infections
- **chronic sinus infections** and meneire's disease (inner ear disease)
- **abscesses, boils, acne that leaves pitting scars**
- **enlarged glands**
- **constipation with straining, stools seem to recede after coming out**
- weakness and collapse
- **sour perspiration, sweats on the head**
- **these types tend to be delicate, timid, anxious and stubborn**
- **aggravated by cold weather, drafts and uncovering**

SULPHUR
Common indications include:
- **all skin symptoms**
- heartburn, diarrhea
- **itching and redness of mucous membranes** or around margins of eyes, nose, mouth, rectum
- burning in all symptoms
- headaches
- **foot sweat is offensive with burning, they must put their feet out the covers**
- itching worse from heat and bathing

- craving for sweets, alcohol, chocolate, overeating

THUJA OCCIDENTALIS
Common indications include:
- eczema, psoriasis, tinea, ringworm
- **sweet, oily or offensive perspiration**
- nails are distorted from fungus
- nose is running during stools
- rectal fissures
- **may have tendency for warts or tumours**
- greenish discharges from the urethra or vagina
- **craving, intolerance or aversion to onions**
- foot sweat is offensive
- **mentally these types feel unattractive and have low self esteem**

Celiac Disease

Celiac Disease, otherwise known as celiac, endemic or non-tropical sprue and gluten intolerance, is considered a metabolic malfunction whereby the body is not able to break down peptides containing gluten. It is a hereditary disorder without any cure except avoiding gluten products. People can be affected at any stage of life, from infancy to adulthood. According to the National Institute for Health, www.nih.org, if you have celiac disease, five to 15% of your first-degree relatives will also have it. About three to 8% of people with Type 1 diabetes will have biopsy-confirmed Celiac Disease, and five to 10% of people with Downs Syndrome will also be diagnosed with it.

The mechanism that causes damage in Celiac Disease is the immune system, which reacts with bowel tissue causing inflammation. This, in turn, causes a flattening of the lining of the small intestine, which impedes nutrient absorption. The flattened lining, called the villi, can heal and absorb nutrients if a proper diet is followed.

Celiac Disease is related to other conditions such as thyroid disease, systemic lupus erythematosus, Type 1 diabetes, liver disease, collagen vascular disease, rheumatoid arthritis and Sjögren's Syndrome. Long term consequences of unchecked celiac disease are cancer such as lymphoma or adenocarcinoma and osteoporosis. Osteoporosis is a condition where the bones weaken, become brittle and are prone to breaking. Miscarriage and birth defects, such as neural tube defects may be a result of untreated celiac disease. This could be due to poor nutrient absorption and depletion. Long term cases may also suffer from bone pain, malnutrition, edema and unexplained skin sensations, such as burning, tingling or pricking, strictures of the intestines and ulcer formation in the lower bowel.

Some hypothesize that low spleen function causes immune complexes to go unchecked and bind in the intestines. The body reacts by mounting an attack on these complexes and damages the intestinal wall. The spleen's reticuloendothelial system produces cells that are said to remove these immune complexes from the blood. People who have their spleen surgically removed go on to develop autoimmune diseases more often then the general public. Some people with autoimmune diseases improve when given spleen extract or supplements that support the spleen function.

Following a gluten-free diet, children can heal the small intestine in three to six months and adults sometimes up to two years. Healing of the villi means that the small intestine can properly absorb nutrients. However, improvement begins as soon as the diet is adhered to. Although one must avoid gluten to stay healthy, certain remedies can help the intestinal tract to heal much faster if they are given in conjunction with a gluten free diet.

SYMPTOMS OF CELIAC DISEASE

- vomiting and diarrhea
- anemia, B6, B12, iron, zinc and folic acid deficiency
- distension/bloating in the abdomen
- muscle wasting and fatigue
- a lack of weight gain and stunted growth in children
- infertility, puberty delay
- canker sores and dermatitis herpetiformis (itchy skin lesions)
- stools may be pale, foul smelling and float due to the high fat content
- often a secondary lactose intolerance may occur due to the irritated intestinal tract

HOW IS CELIAC DISEASE DIAGNOSED?

Some of the symptoms of Celiac Disease are similar to other diseases. Diseases usually confused with Celiac are irritable bowel syndrome, anemia, Crohn's disease, diverticulitis and chronic fatigue syndrome. It can be difficult to diagnose accurately. However, celiac sufferers have a higher then normal level of auto-antibodies in their blood. Auto-antibodies are protein molecules that react against the body's own tissues or cells. For a diagnosis of celiac, your medical doctor can test the blood for levels of Immunoglobulin A (IgA), anti-tissue transglutaminase (tTGA) and IgA anti-endomysium antibodies (AEA). These are all immune system cells that may indicate celiac disease. If all of these tests point to Celiac Disease you may be sent for a biopsy of the small bowel. This biopsy is done using an endoscope that takes a very small piece of tissue from the small intestine and checks it for damage to the villi. The villi line the small bowel and aid in nutrient absorption. Damaged and flattened villi will confirm Celiac Disease.

FOODS TO AVOID THAT CONTAIN GLUTEN

According to the Canadian Celiac Association, www.celiac.ca, the following foods contain gluten and should be avoided:
- barley
- bulgar
- cereal binding
- couscous
- durum (type of wheat)
- einkorn (type of wheat)
- emmer (type of wheat)

- faro (type of wheat)
- farina (type of wheat)
- graham flour
- kamut (type of wheat)
- malt (contains barley)
- oats (oats are thought to be cross contaminated with wheat products. According to the Canadian Celiac Association, adults can consume ½ to ¾ cup of uncontaminated dry rolled oats and children can have ¼ cup. If you are unsure of contamination, do not eat them.)
- rye
- semolina
- spelt or dinkel (type of wheat)
- triticale (is a cross between wheat and rye)
- wheat

CARBOHYDRATES AND GRAINS THAT ARE SUITABLE FOR CELIAC DISEASE

- amaranth
- arrowroot
- buckwheat
- cassava
- corn
- flax
- Indian rice grass
- legumes
- millet
- nuts
- potatoes
- quinoa
- rice
- sago
- seeds
- soy
- sorghum
- tapioca
- wild Rice
- yucca

Please note: any of these foods may be cross contaminated and if any of them cause you symptoms, avoid them.

PROCESSED FOODS THAT MAY CONTAIN WHEAT

This is not an extensive list. These foods may or may not contain wheat. Please read all labels and consult your doctor for a complete list of foods that may contain gluten in the form of wheat, barley or oat. These foods may contain gluten thickeners, extracts, syrups, starches or sauces. Read all labels.

- baked beans
- baking powder
- bouillon cubes
- brown rice syrup
- buckwheat flour (pure buckwheat is fine; be sure it is not mixed with wheat flour)
- cheese spread
- chips, potato or corn
- candy
- chocolate milk
- cold cuts, hot dogs, salami, sausage
- communion wafer
- corn cereals
- dried fruits (may be dusted with wheat to prevent sticking)
- French fries
- gravy
- hydrolyzed vegetable or plant protein
- icing sugar
- imitation fish/crab
- matzo
- nuts, dry roasted
- pie fillings
- puddings
- rice cakes
- rice drinks
- rice mixes (cereals may contain barley malt)
- salad dressing
- sauces
- seasoning mixes
- self-basting turkey
- soups, canned, dried and bouillon
- sour cream (may contain modified food starch)
- soy sauce, beverages and nuts
- vegetables in sauce
- yogurt, flavoured or frozen (may contain wheat thickeners)

IDEAS TO AVOID CROSS CONTAMINATION

Often gluten-free products come in contact with gluten and cause an aggravation. This is called "cross contamination." Some simple things can save you from suffering. Use your own butter dish, cutting board and toaster. The Canadian Celiac association recommends using a toaster oven with a removable rack that can be washed between uses. Use your own packaged goods, like peanut butter, jam, butter, mustard, relish, etc.

Your company may use the same cutlery twice from a jar that has come in contact with gluten. Clean any dishes well after baking. Clean the BBQ rack before cooking on it, as it may have cooked some breaded goods prior. Make your gluten free goods first in the kitchen and wrap them before others begin using the kitchen. Wrapping up your gluten free products keeps them away from possible sources of gluten. Do not use foods from a bulk bin. They can be cross contaminated by others using the same scoop or bin. Avoid buffets, deli counters and restaurants. They are not as careful as you are. It is easier to control your home environment and cook for yourself.

GENERAL SUPPLEMENTS FOR CELIAC DISEASE

Aloe Vera Juice

Aloe Vera juice is very healing to the lining of the gastrointestinal tract. It is said to be a tonic, laxative, stimulate bile flow, eliminate parasites and heal the stomach. Start with a low dose of one to three tablespoons per day. Start with the lowest dose and increase it until you find your comfort zone. If you take too much Aloe Vera, you may suffer from cramps and diarrhea. Take Aloe Vera three or more hours away from medication because it may reduce the absorption of some prescription drugs. This supplement is not suited to those who suffer from diarrhea, heavy periods, kidney disease and/or are pregnant.

Vitamin A

Vitamin A is an excellent supplement to aid in the healing of the epithelial cells of the intestinal tract lining. It helps to heal ulcers, skin lesions and aids in vision. It is known as an antioxidant which hinders cellular damage that leads to the aging process. The typical dosage for Vitamin A is 10,000 IU per day. Vitamin A in high doses, such as over 100,000 international units can be toxic. Beta carotene is a precursor to vitamin A and has no toxic effects if taken in larger doses. The skin may turn an orange tinge, however it is not harmful.

B Complex and Folic Acid

B vitamins are necessary for intestinal health. Each B vitamin has a special function in the body. There are many more properties of these vitamins (too many to list here.) A few relevant properties include:

1. B1 or thiamine is required for proper muscle tone in the intestinal tract and aids in the production of hydrochloric acid (HCL) or digestive juices in the stomach.
2. B2 or riboflavin is used for red blood cell formation and helps the body to metabolize carbohydrates, protein and fats. Along with vitamin A it helps to heal and nourish the lining of the digestive tract.
3. B3 or niacin is also a good aid for forming enzymes to break down protein, carbohydrates and fats. It also helps with hydrochloric acid synthesis.
4. B5 or pantothenic acid is used for the conversion of fats, carbohydrates and proteins into energy.
5. B6 or pyridoxine is necessary for the absorption of fats and proteins. It also is great for hydrochloric acid production. It aids in absorption of B12 and plays a role in immunity.

6. B12 or cyanocobalamin is required to prevent anemia and helps with the metabolism of carbohydrates and fats. It helps with nervous system disorders, such as depression, lethargy and irritability. It prevents anemia and is typically deficient in celiacs.
7. Folic acid is needed for the formation of red blood cells. It is involved in the metabolism of proteins. It is necessary in the treatment of anemia.

Calcium and Magnesium with Vitamin D

Calcium, magnesium and vitamin D are excellent supplements for everyone to take. Celiac disease often causes a deficiency in these minerals, due to their poor digestion and absorption. A consequence of this disease is osteoporosis and poor bone health. Typical daily dosage for calcium is 1,200 mgs, magnesium 600 mgs and 1000 International Units of vitamin D per day.

DGL

DGL or deglycyrrhizinated licorice has a potent anti-inflammatory and healing effect. It aids in healing of ulcers and lesions in the digestive tract. It protects the mucous membranes or the lining of the intestines. It acts as an antioxidant, which slows cellular aging. Licorice should not be used long term, in pregnancy or with diuretics. Over time, it can increase blood pressure and affect estrogen receptors. DGL is said to not increase the blood pressure as the unadulterated herb, licorice does. It should not be taken with steroid drugs, such as Prednisone because it may increase its affects on the body.

Vitamin E

Vitamin E is a fat soluble vitamin that may be low in those with celiac disease. Vitamin E acts as an anti-oxidant. It improves circulation and is necessary for tissue repair. It can reduce scarring from lesions and aids in healing the intestinal mucosa. Typical dosage of vitamin E ranges from 200 to 400 international units per day.

L-Glutamine

L-glutamine is an amino acid that is useful for fuel for the intestinal and brain cells. It helps prevent muscle wasting in metabolic disease. It aids in the healing of the intestinal tract and reduces inflammation. Typical dosage of L-glutamine is 1,000 to 3,000 mgs per day. People who have Reye's syndrome, liver or kidney disease or any condition resulting in ammonia accumulation should avoid glutamine supplementation. Glutamine interferes with ammonia and nitrogen in these cases which could prove harmful.

Probiotics

Every person has billions of bacteria in their intestinal tract. Most bacteria are beneficial and maintain health. There is a fine balance of good and bad bacteria in everyone's digestive tract. Celiac disease tends to cause an overgrowth of bad bacteria in the bowel. This bad bacteria inhibits proper digestion and causes foul smelling stools and gas.

Good flora helps to maintain the immune system and displace the bad bacteria in the gut. They also help to sustain normal arrangement and function of the intestine's cells.

The most popular beneficial bacteria are lactobacillus acidophilus and bifidobacteria. The lactobacilli can be found in fermented foods such as yogurt, miso, tempeh and kefir. However, the number of bacteria is not standardized. The bacteria may not be an active culture if they are not stored properly. Also many people who suffer from celiac disease become lactose intolerant which is an intolerance to dairy products such as milk, cheese and yogurt.

It is best to use a standardized capsule of probiotics. It should be stored in the refrigerator which helps ensure that it is a live culture. Follow the directions on the package. Typical dosage for a probiotic supplement is one to 10 billion cells per capsule. One to three capsules can be taken daily. There are no known side effects from probiotics.

Zinc

Often celiac disease causes a zinc deficiency due to poor absorption. Zinc aids in immunity and is required for healing of wounds. It aids in the absorption of vitamin A and E. Zinc is not a water soluble vitamin, which means it is not excreted in the urine if too much is taken. Typical dosage of zinc ranges from 15 to 50 mgs per day.

HOMEOPATHIC REMEDIES FOR CELIAC DISEASE

There are many homeopathic remedies that suit the symptoms of celiac disease. Some of the more common remedies are listed with their indications here. For more information on how to self prescribe a homeopathic remedy, go to Chapter Two. If you cannot find a remedy suited to you, or find you are not improving or your symptoms get worse, seek the help of a professional homeopath or your medical doctor.

ARSENICUM ALBUM
Common indications include:
- **great restlessness, anxiety and despair**
- **burning in any area of the body**
- ulceration of the duodenum, which may involve the pancreatic ducts
- **diarrhea with burning, smelly and watery stools**
- **diarrhea worse from anxiety, fruit, cold drinks and ice cream**
- stools undigested, containing fat
- **refuses to eat**
- stools cause a weak feeling afterward
- **burning pain in the abdomen**
- **desire for sips of hot drinks**
- burning hives and swelling
- **these types tend to be chilly and worse for cold**
- **these types have many fears about health, death, disease, cancer and robbers**
- **relieved by warmth, sipping hot drinks,** passing stool and motion
- **worse after midnight,** cold drinks

CHINA
Common indications include:

- **suited to people who become exhausted or have ailments from excessive diarrhea**
- people may feel apathetic with no desire to live
- faces may be pale, sickly and sunken
- excessive gas and gurgling
- abdomen packed full with no relief passing gas
- diarrhea is watery, undigested food which is worse at night
- **passing gas provides no relief**
- colic pain occurs every hour or at a certain time every day
- dermatitis
- **anemia**
- **aggravated by slightest touch**, at night, after eating
- **relieved by hard pressure**

LYCOPODIUM
Common indications include:

- persons who are flatulent
- **fullness is felt after only a few bites of food**
- painful bloating of the lower abdomen
- loud grumbling and motions in the abdomen
- sleepy after eating
- bitter taste in the mouth at night
- **abdomen bloated and intolerant to clothing**
- **heartburn, sour vomiting,** water brash
- **canine hunger, the more one eats, the more one craves**
- constipation alternates with diarrhea
- eruptions about the anus, bleeding, moist and tender
- skin itches violently, becomes fissured or ulcerated
- **cravings for sweets**
- **suited to personalities with low self esteem, fear of public speaking or bullying behavior**
- **worse from 4:00 to 8:00 p.m.**

MAGNESIA CARBONICA
Common indications include:

- irritability and nervous types
- green frothy diarrhea
- **sour smelling stools**
- pain in the rectum
- much gas and diarrhea
- colic pains that are better by bending double
- pain in the left side under the ribs
- itching over the whole body
- itching vesicles on the hands

- hair and nails are unhealthy
- **craving for vegetables, bread and butter**
- relieved with motion, walking around, warmth
- aggravated by milk, starches, warm food

PHOSPHORUS

Common indications include:
- stools contain undigested particles of fat
- stools are watery with yellow or white lumps
- profuse diarrhea that pours out like a hydrant
- sensation as if the anus remains open, involuntary diarrhea
- great weakness after stool
- **vomiting of drinks as soon as they warm up in the stomach**
- **thirst for cold drinks and food**
- pale, yellow face, thin types
- anemia and great emaciation
- **tendency to have bleeding with discharges**
- **mentally these types are easily fearful with great anxiety**
- friendly and sympathetic types
- **craving for ice cream, cold food, spices and alcohol**
- **relieved by cold food and drink, being rubbed and cared for**
- aggravated by warm drinks and food

Constipation

Constipation is a North American epidemic. Laxative sales are booming. According to some U.S. statistics, 3.1 million people suffer with constipation. One million are on prescription drugs for it. Our bowels are a holding tank for our body's waste. Our waste is not only what we eat and drink but our manufactured toxins such as hormones, acids, alcohols and cholesterol. There are environmental toxins that we absorb such as pesticides, heavy metals and pollution. A popular revision of the old proverb is "You are what you eat and don't excrete." We are exposed to many toxins every day and we must ensure our organs work effectively to eliminate these poisons.

Constipation is a serious health concern and can lead to many other health disorders. These disorders are appendicitis, arthritis, bad breath, bloating, body odour, cancer, candida, colitis, depression, diverticulitis, fatigue, gas, headaches, hemorrhoids, hernia insomnia and indigestion. If constipation becomes chronic, stool builds up and stretches the bowel. Over time, the muscles and tissue of the intestine lose elasticity and become stretched. An irreversible pouch called a "diverticula" is formed. This can be a trap for stool and bad bacteria. An infection in this pouch is called diverticulosis. With this long list of diseases caused by constipation it is a wonder why more people do not seek an immediate and natural cure.

Constipation is basically defined as difficult and/or infrequent bowel movements, hard stools and a feeling of incomplete elimination. Some health authorities recommend a bowel movement after every meal. There is room for individual variation, however, it is unhealthy to have less then three bowel movements per week.

THE CAUSES OF CONSTIPATION

There are many causes of constipation, the primary two are a lack of fibre in the diet and not enough water intake. The following list is not complete, but includes the main causes of constipation:

- inadequate water intake
- candida
- nervous system disorders
- laxative and enema abuse
- a low fibre diet
- poor liver and gallbladder function
- hypothyroidism
- vitamin deficiencies
- stress
- diverticulitis
- tumours
- parasites
- medications
- physical inactivity
- endometriosis

Low Fibre Diet

A low fibre diet contributes to many diseases such as constipation, hemorrhoids, high cholesterol, colon, breast and prostate cancer. Fibre binds up toxins, negative hormones and cholesterol and excretes them via the intestinal tract. Constipation allows a build up of toxins that can cause headaches, bloating and flatulence.

Dehydration

We require water to have a normal soft consistency to the stools. If we are dehydrated, our stools become hard and difficult to pass. Water is the best liquid to hydrate your body. Drinking eight to 10 glasses of pure water a day is often enough to stimulate a normal bowel movement. Water also helps to flush toxins out through the kidneys.

Laxative, Enema and Colonic Abuse

Chronic use of enemas, colonic irrigation and laxatives can cause a lazy bowel. A colonic irrigation flushes gallons of water into the intestinal tract. Many people report they feel well after a treatment. A few authorities recommend caution in the elderly as the water can stretch the bowel and perforations may result from the equipment. This treatment depletes the intestines of bile salts and good flora. Some colon hydrotherapists use distilled water mixed with probiotics for the flush. Home enemas using a colema board are very popular. It is a helpful temporary solution for constipation. Laxatives irritate the lining of the intestine, which stimulate muscle contractions. This chronic irritation can damage the bowel and cause a laxative dependency. If your bowel is chronically sluggish, you should find the cause and eradicate it.

Sedentary Lifestyle

A lack of exercise contributes to constipation. Exercise has been shown to help with constipation in a number of ways. Motion helps to move food along which stimulates muscle contractions. Hormones that are released during exercise help to relax the nervous system. This relaxation of the nervous system helps the intestinal tract. Stress can be a trigger for constipation. Exercise also helps with elimination of toxins through lymphatic drainage and increased circulation.

Liver and Gallbladder Insufficiency

Constipation may be caused by a sluggish liver or gallbladder. The liver and gallbladder make bile that helps to lubricate the stools. These bile salts actually bind fats for excretion and aid in their digestion.

Medication and Vitamin Side Effects

Vitamins and medications may cause sluggish bowels and/or hard stools. Typically these are pills like iron, calcium, painkillers, antidepressants, blood pressure drugs and cough syrup. Talk to your doctor about reducing or eliminating unnecessary medications.

Did you know...
Constipation with straining not only aggravates hemorrhoids; it is dangerous for those with aneurysms and heart disease?
 We may even know of loved ones who actually had a stroke or heart attack whilst straining to pass stool.
Catherine the Great died of a stroke in 1796 that was rumoured to be whilst on the toilet. **George II** of Great Britain died on the loo on October 25, 1760 from a ruptured aneurysm.

Note to self: Keep your health and dignity intact. Prevent constipation and eat properly!
Source: www.wikipedia.org

Candida and Parasites

Parasites and candida can cause constipation. Parasites block the intestinal tract and bile ducts. Bile acts as a lubricant for stools and binds up cholesterol. Parasites alter our bowel flora and rob our nutrients. Candida is part of our natural bowel flora. When it overgrows it displaces the good bacteria. Our good and bad bacteria should be in perfect balance to be healthy and have normal bowel movements. An imbalanced intestinal flora can weaken the immune system. According to some authorities 60 to 80% of the body's immune system is found in the gastrointestinal tract.

Vitamin or Mineral Deficiencies

A deficiency in vitamin C and magnesium causes constipation. Vitamin C is found in many fruits and vegetables, such as asparagus, berries, broccoli, citrus fruits, melons, peppers and tomatoes. Typical dosage for a vitamin C supplement is 500 to 1,500 mgs per day. Magnesium food sources are brussel sprouts, green leafy vegetables, legumes, nuts, soy, spinach and whole grains. Typical dosage of magnesium is 400 to 600 mgs per day. People with kidney problems or heart disease should check with their doctor before taking magnesium.

Hypothyroid

Hypothyroidism is a hormonal condition characterized by the thyroid not absorbing and utilizing hormones such as TSH, T3 and T4 properly. Symptoms of this disorder are sluggish bowels, fatigue, dry skin, obesity, depression, water retention and premenstrual syndrome. Major causes of an underactive thyroid are an overactive adrenal gland, nutritional deficiencies and poor liver function. The thyroid requires certain minerals to properly function, such as copper, iodine, selenium and zinc. Sea vegetables, such as kelp, dulse, wakame, laver, konbu and irish moss, are excellent sources of minerals that support the thyroid. During stressful times your adrenal glands produce adrenalin and cortisol. These hormones can worsen hypothyroid symptoms and depress thyroid function. Nutritional and emotional support for stress is particularly beneficial in these cases. Examples of common adrenal gland supplements are licorice, pantothenic acid and vitamin C.

There are many causes of constipation. It is best to identify the cause and treat it naturally to prevent toxic build up in the body. Many people have suffered with constipation for years. In some cases, very hard stools form a blockage or tough layer along the intestinal tract. This layer prevents nutrients and water from being properly absorbed. Stools may block the intestinal tract. An emergency intervention may be required. Many doctors recommend a healthy diet and colon cleansing as keys to health and longevity.

DIETARY MEASURES FOR CONSTIPATION

Diet is crucial for health and proper digestion. Drink eight to 10 glasses of water per day. Coffee and tea do not count, as they have a dehydrating affect on the tissues. Water is perfect and has no calories. Consult Chapter Three for recommendations on a healthy diet. Those listed mostly in column one are higher in fibre and decrease the prevalence of many other diseases such as heart disease, diabetes, cancer and hormone imbalances.

When you are filling your plate, visualize it like a pie. Grains should represent only a quarter of your plate. Another quarter should be a lean protein or legumes. The other half should be fruits and vegetables. Eat a wide variety of colours of fruits and vegetables to ensure that you are getting optimum nutrition from your food. For example, orange vegetables are high in beta carotene and dark leafy vegetables contain folic acid. Try to consume mostly raw fruits and vegetables because they have more nutrients than cooked.

Foods to limit and/or avoid

Sugar, alcohol and refined carbohydrates feed bad bacteria in the gut that cause constipation and candida. These foods do not contain fibre. Animal protein and fat can make your system more acidic. An acidic condition can lead to inflammatory conditions such as arthritis, gout, heart disease, irritable bowel and muscle pains.

Foods that are beneficial for constipation

Foods that are high fibre help with constipation. Increase your fibre slowly every day. Some people experience cramps or diarrhea if they have a steep increase in fibre at once. Examples of high fibre foods are

- Vegetables: beets, brussel sprouts, cabbage, carrots, cauliflower, celery, green beans, kale, okra, potato skins
- Fruits: apples, apricots, blackberry, citrus fruits, cranberry, figs, peaches and prunes, pears
- Beans: cooked legumes such as adzuki beans, garbanzo beans, kidney beans, lentils, lima beans, navy beans, split pea
- Whole grains that are high in fibre are brown rice, bulgur, millet, oat bran, slow cooked oatmeal, quinoa, whole wheat and wheat bran

Categories of Fibre Types

There are different types of fibre such as soluble and insoluble, cellulose, hemicellulose, lignans, mucilage and pectin. Often more than one type of fibre is found in a food.

Two Main Types of Fibre: Soluble and Insoluble

Insoluble fibre does not break down in the process of digestion. It is found in foods like whole grains, fruits and vegetables. Insoluble fibre shortens the duration of time that food spends in the bowel. It scrubs the edges of the intestinal tract to clear toxic debris from it. This irritates the lining of the intestinal tract and stimulates bowel movements. Insoluble fibre is found in foods like whole wheat, brown rice, flaxseed, carrots, celery, potato skins and green beans.

Soluble fibre swells in the digestive tract by absorbing water. This swelling increases pressure on the sides of the digestive tract which stimulate a bowel movement. This type of fibre makes the stools softer and easier to pass. It also makes us feel full and aids in weight loss. Soluble fibre forms a gel in the intestines that help slow the absorption of glucose, which aids in blood sugar stability. It is found in pectin and gums. Food sources of soluble fibre are adzuki beans, apples, apricots, barley, beets, blackberry, cabbage, carrots, citrus fruits, cranberry, dried beans, figs, okra, peaches and prunes.

Subcategories of Fibre

According to the excellent book called *Prescription for Dietary Wellness* by Balch and Balch, (see bibliography), there are different fibre subcategories that have many healing benefits and they all aid in eliminating constipation.

1. Cellulose

Cellulose is a type of fibre that is found in apples, beets, brazil nuts, brussel sprouts, cabbage, carrots, cauliflower, green beans, kale, lima beans and pears. This type of fibre is said to have cancer protective qualities. It removes carcinogens from the lining of the intestinal tract. It helps with constipation and aids in weight loss.

2. Gums and Mucilages

Gums and mucilages help to regulate blood glucose levels. They aid in lowering cholesterol and remove toxins. They can be found in legumes, oat bran, oatmeal and sesame seeds.

3. Hemicellulose

Hemicellulose is found in apples, bananas, beets, broccoli, brussel sprouts, cabbage, cauliflower, corn, mustard greens, pears, peppers and whole grains. It helps with weight loss, colon cancer and constipation.

4. Lignans

Lignans are found in the cabbage family, carrots, flax seeds, green beans, peaches, peas, potatoes, strawberries, tomatoes and whole grains. The lignans in ground flax seed are said to help with constipation and prevention of colon, prostate and breast cancer. They also aid in reducing blood cholesterol and preventing gallstones.

5. Pectin

Pectin is a source of fibre found in foods such as apples, bananas, beets, brussel sprouts, cabbage, carrots, grapefruits, kale, lemons, okra, oranges and dried peas. Pectin is good for removing toxins, reducing cholesterol, helping with gallstones and stabilizing blood sugar. Some authorities claim it lowers the risk for cardiovascular disease.

It has been said that most of our disease comes from our own table. There are many underlying causes and disorders that cause constipation. It is important to figure out your cause and eradicate it.

GENERAL SUPPLEMENTS FOR CONSTIPATION

Aloe Vera Juice

Aloe vera juice is very healing to the lining of the gastrointestinal tract. It is said to be a tonic, laxative, stimulate bile flow, eliminate parasites and heal the stomach. Aloe works as a cathartic laxative which stimulates intestinal contractions that cause bowel movements.

Typical dosage is one tablespoon to three ounces, one to three times daily. Start with the lowest dose and increase it until you find your comfort zone. If you take too much aloe vera, you may suffer from cramps and diarrhea. Take aloe vera three or more hours away from medication because it may reduce the absorption of some prescription drugs. This supplement is not suited to those who suffer from diarrhea, heavy periods, kidney disease and/or are pregnant.

Cascara Sagrada

This herb is a laxative made from the bark of cascara sagrada. Native Americans called it cascara or "sacred bark" because of its effectiveness in treating intestinal problems like constipation, hemorrhoids and gallbladder disorders.

Cascara stimulates regular intestinal contractions and stops absorption of water from the bowel. This improves the size and softness of the stool. Cascara sagrada comes in tea form, tincture or capsules. Typical dosage ranges from 100 to 300 mg a day. Do not take for more than seven days without medical supervision. It can create a dependency. Follow the instructions on the individual package.

If you suffer from intestinal obstruction, diarrhea, dehydration, inflammatory bowel disease or are pregnant, do not take cascara sagrada.

Dandelion Extract

Dandelion roots and leaves are bitter. They help to support digestion and the function of the liver and gallbladder. Dandelion stimulates bile flow and removal of excess fluids in the body. Bile helps to break down fats and lubricates the intestinal tract.

Some people eat dandelion greens as a salad which is very beneficial. Dosage varies depending on which form you purchase. Dandelion comes fresh or as a tea, capsules or tincture. This herb is best taken right before a meal to aid in digestion.

Digestive Enzymes

Digestive enzymes are a means for the body to break down foods and absorb their nutrients. Our body naturally makes digestive enzymes through the liver, the pancreas and stomach. If you do not have good digestion, digestive enzymes act as insurance for proper absorption. Partially or improperly digested foods cause many health issues, such as heartburn, food allergies and constipation.

Digestive enzymes usually include protease, which aids in protein digestion, lipase, which aids in fat digestion and amylase or cellulose which aids in carbohydrate digestion. Some digestive enzymes contain Betaine HCL, which helps with protein digestion. Take digestive enzymes as directed on the package. This supplement is not suited to those with high acidity, intestinal or stomach ulcers.

Magnesium

Magnesium is a mineral that can be used as a laxative. A common constipation drug is called "Milk of Magnesia." A magnesium deficiency manifests itself with symptoms of constipation, cramps, heart palpitations and allergies. Typical dosage of magnesium ranges from 400 to 600 mgs per day with meals. Do not take magnesium if you have kidney disease.

Milk Thistle

Milk thistle helps to improve liver function and stimulate bile flow. This herb has a detoxifying effect on the liver and gallbladder. It is often used in conjunction with dandelion. Drink plenty of water to flush the system of toxins. Typical dosage is 200 to 250 mgs per day with each meal.

Probiotics

Every person has billions of bacteria in their intestinal tract. Most bacteria are beneficial and maintain health. A small percentage of bacteria in our intestines are harmful if they spread. If these bad bacteria overgrow it may have negative health consequences such as immune dysfunction, infections, constipation and/or diarrhea.

Good flora helps to maintain the immune system and displace the bad bacteria in the gut. They also help to sustain normal arrangement and function of the intestine's cells. The most popular beneficial bacteria are lactobacillus acidophilus and bifidobacteria. The lactobacilli can be found in fermented foods such as yogurt, miso, tempeh and kefir. However, the number of bacteria is not standardized. The bacteria may not be an active culture if they are not stored properly.

It is best to use a standardized capsule of probiotics. It should be stored in the refrigerator which helps ensure that it is a live culture. Follow the directions on the package. Typical dosage for a probiotic supplement is one to 10 billion cells per capsule. One to three capsules can be taken daily. There are no known side effects from probiotics.

Psyllium

Psyllium is an inexpensive source of soluble fibre and a mild bulking agent. When mixed with water, psyllium expands and forms a gel in the intestinal tract. This expansion stimulates bowel movements. This bulk gently scrubs along the intestines and makes stools softer. Psyllium absorbs water so drink at least eight to 10 glasses of water per day. If you do not, expect to become more constipated.

In addition to its benefits for the bowels, psyllium is useful for diabetes. It helps to lower cholesterol and reduces high blood pressure and elevated blood sugar. Take psyllium away from meals with a large glass of water. If you have a spastic bowel, impacted feces or a narrowed intestinal tract avoid psyllium. Psyllium comes in powder or capsule form. Typical dosage is one teaspoon or five grams of psyllium husks, in 10 ounces of water, twice a day or as instructed on the label.

Senna Tea

Like Cascara sagrada, senna increases the intestinal contractions that stimulate bowel movements. It increases the water in the stool to soften the bowel movements. It should only be used for a period of a week. It is a habit-forming laxative. It comes in the form of a tea or capsules. It is found in popular drugs like Senokot and Exlax.

Vitamin C

Vitamin C has a colon flushing ability. Take 1,000 mgs of powdered Ester or buffered vitamin C in a glass of water. Take this dose every half an hour. Record how many milligrams it takes to produce loose stools. Then reduce the dose by one spoonful every day, until a dose is found where the stools are a comfortable consistency. Alternatively some people start with 500 mgs of Vitamin C per day and work up to 5,000 mgs a day. Do not take vitamin C if you have inflammatory bowel disease, kidney stones, ulcers or are undergoing surgery.

HOMEOPATHIC REMEDIES FOR CONSTIPATION

There are many homeopathic remedies for constipation. Some of the more common remedies are listed with their symptoms herein. For more information on how to self prescribe a homeopathic remedy, go to Chapter Two. If you cannot find a remedy suited to you, or find you are not improving or your symptoms get worse, seek the help of a professional homeopath or your medical doctor.

ALUMINA

Common indications include:
- stools may be hard, dry, pale coloured, knotted like sheep's dung
- stools may be soft and clay like, adhere to parts
- straining even with soft and small stools
- **constipation is so stubborn that they may use their fingers to assist with the expulsion of stool**
- sensation of an inactive rectum
- **extreme dryness of the intestinal tract and rectum**
- before stool has frequent urgings to pass stool
- bleeding from passing hard stools
- **no desire for stools** until there is a large accumulation of it
- rectum feels dry and constricted during stool
- pressure and sharp pains in the anus with bloody discharge
- pain and itching in the anus
- after stools there is a long lasting pain in the rectum
- constipation of pregnant women
- urine only can be passed during stools
- suited to sedentary and elderly people

- mentally these types may be dull, slow to answer and have an abnormal fear of knives
- **aggravated by an aversion to potatoes** and artificial foods like formula

BRYONIA
Common indications include:
- **stools are dry, hard**, dark brown as if burnt
- stools are too large
- pain during stools which are passed after much straining
- constipation associated with rheumatism
- constant chilliness
- **tongue is coated brown**
- **dryness of the rectum**
- may suffer from headaches and irritability
- **dry lips and unquenchable thirst**
- constipation from a sedentary lifestyle
- **these types tend to have left-sided headaches**
- **emotionally, bryonia types can be irritable and want to be alone alone and quiet**
- **preoccupation with business and money matters**
- aggravated by summer heat or becoming overheated
- **relieved by pressure** and drawing up the knees

CALCAREA CARBONICA
Common indications include:
- stools are large and hard
- stool is first hard then mushy or liquid
- stool may be clay like or chalky
- diarrhea alternates with constipation
- before elimination, has an ineffectual desire with pain
- **constipation without any desire for elimination**
- heavy sensation in the lower rectum
- after stools intense burning pain in the rectum
- feels faint after stools
- feels well when constipated
- for obstinate constipation of infants
- sour heartburn
- these types tend to have a hearty appetite and may **crave eggs and sweets**
- may be suited to those who perspire easily and are clammy
- **these types are heavy set and gain weight easily**
- aggravated by from milk

LYCOPODIUM
Common indications include:

- stool is hard, difficult and small
- stool seems broken and may be mixed with or followed by liquid
- strong desire to pass stool; ineffectual urging
- flatulent colicky pains before stool and after
- constipation with much flatulence
- pain in the anus
- has a tight feeling in the anus which keeps stools behind, sensation of incomplete bowel movements
- these types have much rumbling and distension
- **full after eating a few bites** because of bloating
- tends to have heartburn and water brash
- pit of stomach is swollen and sensitive to belts and tight clothes
- constipation may be present since puberty, traveling or since giving birth
- **cravings for sweets**
- indigestion after eating too many farinaceous foods or a heavy diet
- **these types have right sided symptoms**
- fatigue after dinner and **aggravated from 4:00 until 8:00 p.m.**
- **mentally these people have low self esteem, fear of public speaking or can be arrogant**
- **worse in the morning on waking** and from wheat foods
- **relieved by open air**, hot food and drinks, loosening the clothes

MAGNESIA MURIATICUM
Common indications include:
- stools are hard, crumbling at the verge of the anus
- stools are large, lumpy and covered with mucous or blood
- before stools have painful urgings
- during stools a sense of pressure with very little stool passing or just wind
- after stools burning in the anus is felt with trembling
- swollen abdomen with sharp and pinching pains
- pains felt in the liver when walking or touching it
- constipation with a yellow tongue and bad taste in the mouth
- constipation of infants during teething
- suited to children who cannot tolerate milk products
- aggravated by milk and salty foods
- relieved by motion, exercise and hard pressure

NATRUM MURIATICUM
Common indications include:
- stools are large, hard and crumbling
- **passive types and aversion to quarrels**
- stools may be irregular or alternate with diarrhea
- before stool the person has frequent desire with no affect
- sensation that the rectum is lazy

- rectum is constricted with sharp and burning pains
- painful urging for stools with rectal bleeding
- anal fissures and hemorrhoids that bleed and sting
- these types tend to have a very dry mouth and intestinal tract
- these types can tend to be depressed and gloomy
- stools are dry and crumbling
- gurgling of wind through the bowels
- **these types may feel unrefreshed on waking and need an hour to wake up**
- these types crave salt
- **craving for vegetables and fruits**
- **anxiety at night when lying down or on closing eyes**
- **aggravated by milk**
- inactive intestines with no urging for days or weeks

NUX VOMICA
Common indications include:
- stools are black and hard, blood streaked
- constant desire for stool with urging
- irregularity of the peristaltic action of the intestines
- pressing in the rectum with low back pain, relieved after stools
- sensation as if the rectum is shut or narrow and some stool remains behind
- relief is felt after stools
- **cutting pains** in the lower bowels
- flatulence and belching relieves pain a little
- painful bleeding hemorrhoids
- **chilly and worse for cold air**
- **ailments from anger**
- excessive use of alcoholic beverages, coffee, stimulants, drugs
- spasmodic pains of the intestinal tract
- **suited to hard working irritable types who are hypersensitive**
- **these types are competitive and impatient**
- **cravings for spices, fats, alcohol and coffee**
- **relieved by warmth**
- **aggravated by anger, tight clothes**, sedentary lifestyle, alcoholic drinks, drugs and overwork

SEPIA
Common indications include:
- stools are hard, knotty, small and covered with mucous
- often urging to stools with only mucous or wind passing
- pain in the rectum extending upwards to the vagina or perineum
- pain in the rectum felt long after a stool
- **stomach has an empty feeling that is not helped by eating**
- these types may have a prolapsed rectum, bladder or vagina

- blood passes with stools
- **itching rectum**
- **sensation of a ball remaining in the rectum, not helped by passing stool**
- these types may tend to hormonal troubles and low libido
- suited to women with headaches or rheumatism
- hemorrhoids
- **this remedy is suited to women who are worn out, have a low libido and tend to be irritable or weepy**
- **worse during pregnancy, menopause, before or during the menstrual flow**
- aggravated by drinking milk, standing and doing housework

Picture This....

You are a pre-menopausal woman. You suffer from weight issues, fatigue and constipation. You love carbs like cookies, white bread and salty chips. You always feel parched even though you drink a ton of water. You had a lot of grief at one point in your life and did tend towards depression. You can get feeling pretty gloomy and ruminate on the past. You are a very chilly person and always tend to painless constipation. Going once a week is the norm for you, although you have read that one should go after every meal.

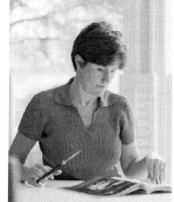

After reading an article on high fibre foods, you decide to try it. You start to go once every four days which is an improvement. However, you had read a magazine article about a homeopathic remedy that suited you. It is called Natrum Muriaticum. It is suited to salt cravings, brooding, cold body temperature, thirst and constipation. It seems you were meant to read that article. You had taken the remedy as directed on the package and lo and behold, your bowels are moving every day. Some days you may miss the odd one but your bowels are on track!

Crohn's Disease

Autoimmune conditions are becoming more and more prevalent today. They are illnesses characterized by the body's immune system marking a particular organ as the enemy and attacking it. Many alternative health practitioners believe that autoimmune diseases are related to an event(s) that happened before age 7, even in utero. Many types of autoimmune diseases exist, such as lupus, rheumatoid arthritis, Hashimoto's thyroiditis, Crohn's disease, and multiple sclerosis. Despite the different symptoms, there is often a common thread in all of these disorders. The immune system becomes abnormally reactive to a particular organ in the body. Autoimmune sufferers have had a series of toxic insults to their system, whether they are subtle or obvious. Some of these include physical injuries, psychological stress, food sensitivities, parasites, viruses, fungi, vaccinations and heavy metal toxicity.

What is Crohn's Disease?

Crohn's disease is an autoimmune inflammatory bowel disease. Like most autoimmune diseases it has active periods followed by remission. It is characterized by inflammation that can affect any part of the digestive tract from the mouth to the anus, not just the small intestine. However, it usually affects the ileum and the colon. This disease causes ulcer-like lesions of the gastrointestinal tract's mucous membrane lining. These lesions can be superficial or extend deep into the underlying layers. The lesion can also cause a thickening of the intestinal wall with scarring. The immune and lymphatic system are involved causing lymph nodes to swell and cause water retention in the affected area. In chronic cases, bowel obstruction may result from thickening and scarring in the intestinal tract. Surrounding areas may show signs of inflammation such as the bladder, uterus and skin. Fatty stools may be present and are a sign of malabsorption. This is usually because the ileum portion of the intestine is affected by Crohn's. This is where the body absorbs bile salts and helps to break down fats.

Diagnosis and Medical Treatment

Most cases occur before age 30 with a rise in incidence between the ages of 14 to 24. It is more common in families where one person has already been diagnosed. If a sibling has Crohn's disease the risk increases to 30% of also being diagnosed with it.

Medical diagnosis is done using several blood tests to determine an elevated white blood cell count, elevated sedimentation rate and C-reactive protein. A barium X-ray, colonoscopy, biopsy and upper GI series are useful to detect lesions associated with Crohn's disease. Often a Medical Doctor will then differentiate Crohn's disease from Ulcerative Colitis, enterocolitis and cancer.

Typical medical treatment includes the use of corticosteroid drugs, immunosuppressive drugs, salfasalazine and broad spectrum antibiotics. Surgery may be necessary in some cases of obstruction or a stricture but is not a viable option for a cure. Immunosupressive drugs may be necessary but they leave a person open to more infections. Sulfasalazine decreases folic acid and iron stores. Steroids such as Prednisone expend more vitamin C, calcium and magnesium. Antibiotics kill the beneficial bacteria in the gut. Supplementation may be necessary to counteract the affects of the medication and to aid in vitamin deficiencies.

What are the Symptoms of Crohn's Disease?
- rectal bleeding
- malnutrition
- inflammation anywhere from the mouth to the anus
- ulcers and scar tissue in the intestinal tract
- anemia
- gas and bloating
- fever and high white blood cell count
- weight loss and loss of appetite
- diarrhea and stools that have fat or blood in them
- lower abdominal pain
- fatigue
- arthritis
- fistulas and abscesses
- mouth ulcers or canker sores
- erythema nodosum (red, elevated, hard patches on the skin)

- intestinal strictures
- kidney and gall stones
- stunted growth in young children
- increased incidence of intestinal cancer

Seek Professional Help for Autoimmune Diseases

Autoimmune conditions are difficult to treat and there is no overnight cure. For an autoimmune condition to be healed it can take an upwards of six months to halt the condition and another six to heal. For this reason you have to have confidence in your practitioner and their method of healing. Steer clear of any overnight success claims. Seek the help of a professional when taking any remedies. There can be interactions between prescription medications and natural supplements. Medications can cause other health problems. Immune suppressants, anti-inflammatories, steroids and Prednisone all have side effects. For example, immune suppressants can leave the body open to serious infections and cancer. Steroids can weaken bone strength, skin integrity and eyesight. They can also sap the energy from the adrenal glands.

What Causes Crohn's Disease?

There is no known single cause of Crohn's disease. There are many factors that may contribute to the development of a faulty immune system that turns on itself. Some of the main factors that contribute to autoimmune conditions are imbalanced intestinal flora, dysbiosis, leaky gut syndrome, improper diet, hygiene hypothesis and external toxic insults.

1) Imbalanced Intestinal Flora

The intestinal flora is comprised of delicately balanced healthy and non-healthy bacteria. It is said that 60% of our immune system comes from our intestinal tract. This is our gut associated lymphoid tissue (GALT). If our natural flora is compromised, our GALT may not be as effective at maintaining proper health.

There are immune system cells throughout the gut that influence the body's capability to fight off invaders. It is important to note that the gastrointestinal tract is in contact with the outside world. It is an open passage for food, toxins and the like to enter our system. Without a healthy gut flora, we can fall prey to outside offenders such as parasites, viruses, fungi and environmental toxins (such as pesticides, heavy metals and pollution).

In utero, children acquire their intestinal flora from their mother. Neonates also acquire part of their healthy gastrointestinal flora from breastfeeding. Often newborns or breast-feeding mothers are required to take antibiotics that strip the healthy flora of the gastrointestinal system. This creates an imbalance of the good and bad bacteria in the gut if not properly replenished with probiotics. A person's natural flora is usually set in the first few years of life. Thus, if a child is exposed to a variety of toxic insults or the mother's flora was imbalanced, the child may have more of a chance of developing other disorders later in life. These disorders can be allergies, immune dysfunction, ADHD, intestinal problems and the like.

2) Dysbiosis and Leaky Gut Syndrome

A couple of hypotheses for the cause of autoimmune disorders are leaky gut syndrome and dysbiosis. Leaky gut syndrome is characterized by the gut lining of the intestinal tract having small perforations or opening in the tight junctions of the cells that allow waste and food particles into the blood stream. Due to the nature of the body's immune system, it mounts an inflammatory attack on these particles. Particles circulated in the blood may also be deposited into unsuspecting organs such as the liver, kidneys or joints. This inflammatory reaction causes the body to unknowingly mount an attack on itself.

Dysbiosis is characterized by an imbalance of the gut flora as discussed. Dysbiosis can lead to leaky gut syndrome. It also creates dysfunction by not properly protecting the gastrointestinal lining that provides a safe barrier between the environment and your internal organs. This is a very basic explanation of the complexities of autoimmune disorders. Nevertheless, it provides basic information for those to understand and heal autoimmune problems.

3) The Hygiene Hypothesis

Another theory about the prevalence of food sensitivities, allergies and autoimmune disease, is the "hygiene hypothesis". Studies have shown that kids who grew up in a sterile clean environment have more immune reactions and allergies than ones who live with a dog or a mother who wasn't the best housekeeper. Research has also shown that kids who have been exposed to certain parasites actually show less allergy and asthma. We overuse antibiotics which kill all good and bad bacteria in the gut. In children, an early introduction of antibiotics prevents the development of a healthy immune system. It depletes both good and bad bacteria in the gastrointestinal (GI) tract. If our GI tract has an aseptic environment, without both good and bad bacteria, our immune system becomes deranged. It is thought that bad bacteria in balance with the good actually trains the immune system to properly function. If it doesn't function normally, it recognizes harmless things as potential allergens and organizes an inflammatory attack. We need a balance of both good and bad bacteria to be healthy.

4) Improper Diet

Many types of foods actually increase inflammation and dysbiosis in the body. These two factors are the root cause of many diseases like inflammatory bowel disease, hypertension, arthritis and even cancer. Inflammation causes a chain of cellular events that release inflammatory proteins in the body. These proteins cause immune system reactions which include the destruction of healthy cells called oxidation. Both high fat and high glycemic foods increase inflammatory reactions and feed the bad bacteria which cause dysbiosis.

The term "high glycemic" means the food such as refined carbohydrates like white bread, white rice and sugar quickly converts into a sugar in the bloodstream. For a list of low, medium and high glycemic and fat foods see the chart in Chapter Three. Fats that cause inflammation are saturated, hydrogenated fats or those high in arachadonic acid (A.A.). A.A. is said to be one of the major players in inflammatory responses and is found in animal products such as organ meats, red meats, pork, animal fat and skin. Oils that are re-used for cooking become rancid and cause oxidation which also damages the cells. Stimulants such as caffeine, nicotine and alcohol affect the nervous system. The nervous system and the gut are tightly connected. When it is stimulated it can cause a chain reaction of gastrointestinal upset, gas, bloating, constipation and diarrhea.

Food sensitivities may play a role in autoimmune conditions. If you have a reaction to certain foods, you may inadvertently be causing an inflammatory reaction in your body. Take care to avoid certain foods that are triggers for your condition.

5) External Insults

External insults from our environment such as stress, vaccines and heavy metal toxicity can weaken our immune system. The nervous system and the gastrointestinal tract are tightly connected. Stress hormones can cause bowel disruptions such as constipation and diarrhea. Heavy metal toxins such as lead, mercury, aluminum, arsenic and barium can cause intestinal and immune system abnormalities. Detection of heavy metals can be done using a hair mineral analysis. Some medical doctors use a chelating drug to bind heavy metals and then test the urine for their excretion. Vaccinations are thought to prime our immune system to recognize a virus so that we will not succumb to it. This is a good theory and has prevented many merciless diseases. However, some vaccines still contain toxic ingredients such as mercury and formaldehyde. What happens with those toxins when we are injected with them? How can we excrete something injected right into our blood without it being deposited into some of our tissues? Obviously we cannot.

DIETARY MEASURES FOR CROHN'S DISEASE

Crohn's Disease is a condition that has a great deal of individuality. Some may have a severe case and others may have a very mild one. Food restrictions are very individual as well. In the Caruso Homeopathic Clinic, everyone is usually prescribed a diet, outlined in Chapter Three, because it reduces inflammation, dysbiosis and prevents many other diseases. Any food on this list that has a "#" sign beside it should be avoided. These foods contribute to intestinal dysbiosis, which is an inappropriate balance of bad and good bacteria in the intestinal tract.

Food sensitivities are a factor in most Crohn's cases. Try the food challenge test as outlined in Chapter Three or be tested by a professional for food sensitivities. With either method, you will have more knowledge to control your symptoms. Typical offenders are wheat, dairy, citrus, gluten, peanuts, corn, soya or sugar. In practice, wheat and dairy are the top two culprits because people tend to overeat them which creates sensitivity. For more information about food sensitivities see Chapter Three.

A book that contains beneficial dietary information for inflammatory bowel disease (IBD) is called, *Breaking the Vicious Cycle* by Elaine Gottschall (*see bibliography*). It is for inflammatory bowel conditions such as Crohn's, colitis, irritable bowel syndrome and celiac disease. Although the diet outlined in this book is very restrictive, it helps most people with IBD. Some of the foods to avoid that are mentioned in this book are all canned foods, processed meats, sugar and grains like barley, corn, rye, oats, rice, buckwheat, millet, triticale, bulgur and spelt. Potatoes, yams, parsnips, okra, chickpeas, bean sprouts, turnips, soy, mung, fava and garbanzo beans are not acceptable. No milk products, yogurt, soya milk or coffee substitutes can be used. The list of foods to avoid is longer than mentioned here. However, it is a good option for those who do not have such resources as those found in the bibliography to see a Homeopath or do the home food challenge test.

GENERAL SUPPLEMENTS FOR TREATING CROHN'S DISEASE

With serious illness, often a liquid or powdered variety is more readily absorbed than a tablet form. If a pill is taken, a capsule is preferred to a tablet.

Aloe Vera

Aloe Vera juice is very healing to the gastrointestinal tract. It helps to sooth and repair the intestines. Aloe is said to be a tonic, laxative and to stimulate bile flow, eliminate parasites and heal the stomach. Typical dosage is three tablespoons to three ounces, one to three times daily. Start with the lowest dose until you find your comfort zone. If you take too much aloe vera, you may suffer with diarrhea. This supplement is not suited to those who suffer from acute diarrhea, heavy periods, pregnancy and/or kidney disease.

Antioxidants

Antioxidants are useful for Crohn's disease sufferers because they do not assimilate nutrients well and they have an increased risk for cancer. They prevent oxidative damage which helps slow the cycle of cellular destruction. They also help to heal the gastrointestinal lining.

   i.   **Vitamin A**

Vitamin A helps to heal the lining of the gastrointestinal tract, aids in immunity and helps the lining of the mucous membranes. It is necessary for the maintenance and repair of the mucous membrane lining, thus it heals ulcers. It is needed for new cell growth and is said to slow the aging process. Beta Carotene is converted into vitamin A in the liver. If the liver is not working well, it is best to take vitamin A. In high doses, beta carotene does not have any side effects, other than turning one's skin orange. Typical dosage of vitamin A is 10,000 IU per day. Taking more than 100,000 IU has been known to cause liver damage.

   ii.   **Vitamin C**

Vitamin C is a powerful antioxidant that helps with tissue growth and repair. It attacks free radicals that can cause cell destruction. This wonder vitamin protects the blood vessels, decreases cholesterol, decreases inflammation and enhances immunity. It also helps one to absorb iron, L-glutamine and B vitamins. Use an "Esterified" vitamin C because it is easier on the stomach, not as acidic and is more readily absorbed than a regular vitamin C. Typical dosage for vitamin C is 500 to 3000 mgs per day.

   iii.   **Vitamin E**

Vitamin E helps to heal the mucous membrane lining of the gastrointestinal tract and is good for the cardiovascular system and the skin. It helps selenium be absorbed more readily. Typical dosage for vitamin E is 200 to 400 IU per day.

   iv.   **Selenium**

Selenium is helpful for inflammatory conditions, maintaining proper immune function, protecting the liver, preventing heart disease and cancer. Typical dosage is 200 to 400 micrograms (mcgs). Do not take selenium in doses higher then 40 mcgs if you are pregnant.

B Vitamins

B complex is useful for people who suffer from autoimmune disease. It aids in toning the muscles of the gastrointestinal tract, nerves and acts to combat the effects of emotional stress. Certain medications such as steroids deplete vitamin B. One can safely take 100 mgs of B Complex daily with meals.

B12 and Folic Acid are useful to better absorb iron and reduce high homocysteine levels. High levels of the amino acid, homocysteine, in the colon and blood may predispose people to both ulcerative colitis and Crohn's disease. It is said to influence other diseases as well, such as Alzheimer's, dementia, depression, ischemic heart disease and stroke, osteoporosis and cancer. Vitamin B6, B12 and folic acid work to decrease homocysteine levels.

Calcium and Magnesium

Calcium and magnesium are useful for people using steroids because steroids decrease bone mass. Calcium is also one of the more difficult minerals to absorb; however calcium citrate tends to be better absorbed than carbonate. Calcium carbonate was studied and is thought to prevent colon cancer. This is likely because it is not absorbed well and binds intestinal toxins and excretes them. One can take up to 1,200 mgs of calcium with 600 mgs of magnesium daily. Check with your doctor for interactions between calcium and your medications.

Essential Fatty Acids (EFAs)

Essential fatty acids, mainly flax and fish oil, are good for pain, inflammation, dry skin, gas, bloating, gastrointestinal function and secretion, and immune system deficiency. They can also help with allergic symptoms, depression, concentration problems, joint pains, inflammation, skin eruptions and cardiovascular disease. Be sure to keep your EFAs in the fridge to prevent rancidity. Do not use your EFA liquid for cooking. Once it is heated, it releases free radicals.

Eicosapentaenoic acid (EPA) found in fish oil is most beneficial for inflammatory bowel disease. Some studies have shown that it may reduce the need for corticosteroids and ensure longer remission. EPA can be found in cold water fish such as herring, trout, salmon and mackerel. It increases a type of prostaglandin that actually decreases inflammatory proteins. EPA improves blood flow and reduces inflammation. Cod liver oil contains EPA but may have too much vitamin A for some.

One can safely take up to 4,000 mgs of fish oil daily. Ideally you would like to have about 1,000 mgs of EPA per day. An enteric coated fish oil capsule is advantageous because it releases in the intestinal tract, not the stomach. This would ensure that you would be getting the maximum EPA into the intestinal tract. The stomach may degrade some of the EPA before it reaches the colon.

L-Glutamine

L-glutamine is a supplement that provides metabolic fuel for the intestinal cells. It helps to sustain the villi and absorptive surfaces of the intestinal tract lining. Vitamin C and B complex help to enhance the absorption of L-glutamine. Recommended dosage for adults is two to six grams per day with meals. There are no known side effects of L-glutamine.

High potency Multi vitamin

People who suffer from Crohn's disease are at risk for vitamin and mineral deficiencies. It is wise to take a daily multi vitamin in a liquid or capsule. These are easier to assimilate than a tablet. I usually don't recommend "one a day" types of vitamins because they contain so many vitamins and minerals, they are packed very tightly to enable one to swallow them. If they did not, people would choke on them. If your stomach acid and digestion are not good, you will not be able to properly break down the tablet. Take a liquid form or a multi that you have to take in divided doses throughout the day.

Probiotics

Every person has billions of bacteria in their intestinal tract. Most bacteria are beneficial and maintain health. A small percentage of bacteria in our intestines are harmful if they spread. If these bad bacteria overgrow it may have negative health consequences such as immune dysfunction, infections, constipation and/or diarrhea.

Good flora helps to maintain the immune system and displace the bad bacteria in the gut. They also help to sustain normal arrangement and function of the intestine's cells. The most popular beneficial bacteria are lactobacillus acidophilus and bifidobacteria. The lactobacilli can be found in fermented foods such as yogurt, miso, tempeh and kefir. However, the number of bacteria is not standardized. The bacteria may not be an active culture if they are not stored properly.

It is best to use a standardized capsule of probiotics. It should be stored in the refrigerator which helps ensure that it is a live culture. Follow the directions on the package. Typical dosage for a probiotic supplement is one to 10 billion cells per capsule. One to three capsules can be taken daily. There are no known side effects from probiotics.

Quercitin, Tumeric and Bromelain

These herbs are helpful for a number of reasons:
- they reduce inflammation
- they combat free radicals
- protect the liver against toxins
- decrease allergic reactions
- reduce platelets from sticking to each other which aids in circulation
- decrease cholesterol
- act as an antibiotic, anti-inflammatory and anti-cancer supplement

Take as directed on the individual package. These herbs may come together in one pill.

HOMEOPATHIC REMEDIES FOR CROHN'S DISEASE

There are many homeopathic remedies for Crohn's disease. Some of the more common remedies are listed with their symptoms here. For more information on how to self prescribe a homeopathic remedy, go to Chapter Two. If you cannot find a remedy suited to you, or find you are not improving or your symptoms get worse, seek the help of a professional homeopath or your medical doctor.

ALOE SOCOTRINA
Common indications include:
- distended abdomen after drinking water
- rumbling and gurgling gas
- urgent diarrhea after eating
- **urgent stools at 5:00 a.m.**
- **stools jelly-like that contain lumpy mucous** and blood
- anus is burning with itching hemorrhoids
- weakness of the anal sphincter
- **involuntary stool while urinating or passing gas**
- suited to beer drinkers who lead a sedentary life
- mental and physical work causes fatigue
- **hemorrhoids that are congested like a bunch of grapes, that are better with a cold bath**
- **hot sensation when passing gas**
- **early morning sudden diarrhea that drives one out of bed**
- pain felt in the stomach when walking and making a misstep
- pain radiates to the back and upwards with every belch
- aggravated by eating, heat, after eating
- relieved by passing gas with distension, drinking cold water, bending forward

> **Did you know?**
> At the turn of the century Thomas Lindsley Bradford, MD, wrote a book called "The Logic of Figures" where he documented statistics that compared the conventional therapeutics with homeopathic ones.
> These statistics included epidemics such as scarlet fever, yellow fever and typhoid for example. The homeopathic hospitals typically had 50 to 80% less deaths per 100 people, depending on the disease they were comparing.
> www.nationalcenterforhomeopathy.org

ARSENCIUM ALBUM
Common indications include:
- abdominal distension with a **burning sensation**
- painful inguinal glands
- **burning diarrhea after anxiety, cold drinks and fruits**
- burning rectum with stools and intense cutting pain
- **offensive and putrid discharges**
- fears they may die and it is useless to take medicine
- cold and clammy with the **feeling they can never get warm enough**

- desires hot drinks and applications despite burning sensation
- **great thirst yet only takes small sips of water**
- **tongue is discoloured white**
- canker sores in the mouth
- nausea after meals
- **mentally these types are restless, anxious and fearful of diseases**
- **worse after midnight**, after eating, cold, during rest
- **relieved by hot drinks, warmth**, motion and exercise

CAUSTICUM
Common indications include:
- chilly people who are affected at any change of weather
- burning in the rectum with piles
- **stool is covered with mucous**
- painful swelling of the abdomen
- stool is passed better whilst standing than sitting
- stools seem too slender from rectal cramps
- anxiety is felt after a stool
- colicky pains felt in the morning that extend to the back and chest
- **rectal fissures** and fistulas that are painful whilst walking
- pustules near the anus that discharge blood, pus and serum
- **constant desire to clear the throat and hoarseness**
- **these types tend to have rheumatic complaints**
- **aversion to sweets** and stomach pressure from eating bread
- thirst for cold drinks with a weak appetite
- **cravings for bacon, salt and smoked meats**
- **aggravated by cold**, change of weather, walking, sitting, suppressed skin disease, after eating the least amount of food, tight clothes
- relieved by standing, bending double

IGNATIA
Common indications include:
- **spasmodic, cramping pains**, painful urging for stool
- stools are pasty, bloody, mucous filled, burning
- sensation of a sharp instrument is in the rectum
- **constriction of the rectum** for one or two hours after a stool
- blind hemorrhoids that are aggravated whilst both sitting and standing
- prolapsed anus
- **these types have the sensation of a lump in their throat**
- fruit causes diarrhea
- diarrhea alternates with constipation
- **mentally these types are easily offended, have alternating moods and much grief**
- **may sigh or cough often**

- **aggravated by eating sweets, grief, unrequited love** and worries
- aggravated by tobacco, coffee, drug use, fruit, after grief
- relieved by walking

MERCURIUS CORROSIVUS
Common indications include:

- successfully treats dysentery
- bloody frequent bowel movements
- stool is green with mucous, scanty, pure blood, black, pasty, burning, slimy
- burning felt in the anus
- **urging for elimination**
- gums may be swollen, purple, spongy
- ulcers are corroding, acid and full of pus
- constriction in the throat with spasms
- **constant urging without remission on passing stools**
- great deal of perspiration and salivation
- complaints in the summer or from May to November
- aggravated by fats, acids, cold, during the summer
- relieved by rest, motion

NITRIC ACID
Common indications include:

- bright red hemorrhage from the bowel after stools
- straining as if stool has been left behind
- pain in the rectum for hours after a bowel movement
- stools are offensive, green and putrid
- breaks into a sweat during stool
- **tendency to rectal warts that bleed easily**
- glands are painful and swollen
- fissures and ulcers of the anus, mouth and throat
- **splinter-like pains, especially in the rectum**
- **these types desire fat and salt**
- raw ulcers that have zigzag edges
- **mentally these types are anxious, hypochondrical, irritable and hold a grudge**
- aggravated by milk

NUX VOMICA
Common indications include:

- said to treat dysentery
- constipation alternating with diarrhea with painful urging
- **spasmodic sharp cramps and flatulence**
- errors in diet aggravate these types
- enlarged liver and gallstone colic

- **urging to go to stool**
- pain felt two or three hours after eating
- **stomach pains worse from anger and tight clothes**
- sour, watery, bitter heartburn after meals
- painful ulcers in the mouth and throat
- bleeding piles with urging for stools
- nausea and vomiting in the morning or after meals
- **cravings for spices, alcohol, fat and coffee**
- suited to sedentary types who do a lot of mental work
- **suited to competitive, impatient, workaholic types who over indulge**
- **chilly types who seek the warmth**
- worse in the morning, mental overwork, alcohol, coffee, overeating and drugs
- **relieved by warmth**, rest and during damp weather

PHOSPHORUS
Common indications include:
- chronic diarrhea
- watery stools preceded by great rumbling noises
- watery stools expelled like a hose
- **tendency to hemorrhages, nose bleeds etc.**
- stools may be involuntary, watery, green, mucous-filled, bloody
- anus feels like it is wide open, stool easily escapes
- **easily dehydrated and debilitated**
- fistula that secretes a thin, foul smelling pus
- **hunger soon after eating**
- **very thirsty for cold drinks**
- distended, painful abdomen worse after dinner
- tearing and burning pain in the stomach, worse in morning
- sour and burning belching
- enlarged and/or cirrhosis of the liver
- **these types may have lung problems, bronchitis, infections, pneumonia, tickling coughs**
- **desires cold food and drinks, salt, spice, milk and wine**
- cold drinks vomited after they warm up in the stomach
- **emotionally these types are open, anxious, like company and fear thunderstorms or that something bad will happen**
- relieved by cold drinks or food
- **aggravated by fasting, warm foods, salt and spices**

Picture This….
You are in your first year of university and have been feeling really fatigued. You have been having frequent stools with bloody diarrhea. Your stomach gurgles and when you 'go', your stools are mixed with blood, water and mucous. You have been getting some leg cramps and heart palpitations as well. With all of the stress of university, these

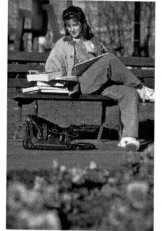

symptoms couldn't have come at a worse time. To top it off, you can't go far from the washroom because you are fearful you won't make it in time! Your anxiety has turned to desperation.

You go through some tests and are diagnosed with Crohn's disease. Your doctor starts you on a drug called Salfasalazine for now and recommend steroids if your condition doesn't improve. You decide to go to a local Homeopath who was recommended by a friend. The Homeopath recommends you take a high quality liquid multi-vitamin, vitamin B12, calcium, magnesium and acidophilus bifidus and lactobacillus. You are also to take one teaspoon of liquid fish oil with a good quantity of EPA. A homeopathic medicine called Aloe 6 CH is prescribed because of your urgency for stools. In school you had been eating a lot of take out and fried foods, which your Homeopath has since told you to avoid. You have started to eat low glycemic foods and avoid anything fried. You are tested for food sensitivities through an electrodermal screening test and find out that wheat and sugar are problematic. This is a bummer for you because you love bread! However, at this point you are willing to do whatever it takes to get better. After one month of following the Homeopath's recommendations, you feel an amazing improvement in energy. You have no more blood in the stools and diarrhea is down to once a week, instead of daily. Your heart palpitations and leg cramps disappear after the first week.

Detoxification for the Intestinal Tract, Liver and Gallbladder

According to some First Nations or indigenous people's traditions, detoxification or cleansing should be done every change of season. With the climate change comes a change in food supply, temperature and sun exposure. People tend to get sick at this time, which is due to the stress the body goes through to adjust to its environment. Given that we are harmonious creatures with nature, it would seem wise to cleanse during these seasonal shifts. I would recommend a whole body cleanse because as one organ system is worked on, it can create a rebound stress for other systems. When the organ systems work in harmony, it releases toxins more effectively. (Toxins are defined as a poisonous substance that may cause damage to the structure or function of the body's cells. They can accumulate in the body and cause harm.)

If one organ system is sluggish, it can cause a back up in toxins. For example, the intestine creates a toxic flow to the liver. If the intestines hold impacted fecal matter, candida, bacteria or parasites, it creates toxins because of the putrification process. The liver works to detoxify the body of both external and internal sources of toxins.

What is detoxification?

Detoxification or cleansing stimulates the organs of elimination to release toxic burdens which in turn aids in maintaining health. Organs of elimination are those that work to excrete poisons or toxins, such as the kidneys, liver, lymph, intestines, lungs and skin. Cleansing has been around since ancient Egyptian times and was carried out as a purification ritual. Detoxification can occur through diet, supplements or through other means such as saunas, epsom salt baths and exercise. Exercise stimulates the lymph to drain toxins. This is because the heart pumps fluids more vigorously through the body. The lungs also release toxins from the body through respiration from deep conscious breathing or exercise.

Why detoxify?
- The digestive system affects the health of the whole body. If you cannot digest certain foods and have poor elimination, detoxification and absorption, you will not feel well. Having better absorption of nutrients and excretion of waste promotes good health.
- Reduction of toxic burdens frees up energy for our organs to work more efficiently on other important functions. For example, women who need a liver detox may feel their menstrual cycles are smoother after they have cleansed. This is because the liver works to metabolize hormones in addition to hundreds of other functions.
- Detoxification aids in the removal of toxic substances from the body. It makes them less toxic through excretion or binding. It also helps with enzymes that are required to alter negative substances for excretion.
- With the release of toxic burdens, health is gained. The purer the cell, the more efficiently it functions.
- Clearer mental focus and improved emotional state often results from an effective cleanse. Even solutions for problems may seem clearer when your body is purified.
- Increased peristaltic motion means less transit time for waste to be eliminated from the body. This means less contact with putrefying fecal matter and less toxic byproducts. This eliminates a breeding terrain for bacteria, fungus and parasites. The cells and the blood are no longer poisoned from the intestinal tract.
- Improved nerve flow in the digestive tract also lessens back pain by acting on the nerves in the spinal column.
- Toxic accumulation may block receptor sites for various biochemical processes. For example, certain things can block the thyroid's receptor sites for thyroid hormone. These events result in hypothyroidism due to lack of absorption of the hormone.
- Weight loss is a natural occurrence of cleansing.
- The standard North American diet is full of acids, fats and proteins that cause health concerns.

What are the signs that I may need to detoxify?
- bad breath and/or body odour
- skin problems such as acne, rosacea, hives, eczema
- constipation
- nausea and poor appetite
- over or underweight
- gas and bloating
- hemorrhoids
- sinus trouble and headaches

- premenstrual syndrome
- vertigo and dizziness
- water retention
- brain fog
- chronic colds and flu
- food cravings
- irritability and mood disorders
- fatigue, tired in the morning or mid afternoon
- tired on sleeping a full night
- dry and hard stool
- bowel movements that take longer then 30 seconds to pass
- chronic diseases
- unexplained pains in the muscles or joints
- eating too many fats, animal proteins, alcohol and smoking
- lack of exercise

Who should not detoxify?

- If you have a serious health concern, seek proper medical counsel before you detoxify.
- If you are pregnant or breast feeding, do not detoxify. The toxins that may be stirred up in your system may affect the baby in utero or through the breast milk.
- Vegetarians who eat mainly whole grains, legumes and plenty of fruits and vegetables rarely need to cleanse. They naturally eliminate more often and have a very clean digestive tract.
- People who do heavy physical work should postpone cleansing until they have more time and energy. Cleansing can produce symptoms of fatigue which may hinder expending energy.
- If you suspect you have heavy metal toxicity, it is not a good idea to cleanse without supervision. You may release some damaging toxins into your system that would be better off hidden, until you are properly instructed how to cleanse.
- Diabetics should not partake in a fasting type of cleanse.

What is a healing crisis?

A healing crisis is a reaction whereby the body is trying to excrete toxins faster then the organs can handle. This can be frightening for those who are uninformed. It is a result of bringing toxins to the forefront to be excreted. It is highly beneficial to release them, which reduces the burden on the body and prevents disease. Typically, healing crisis symptoms only last a few days, usually three in total. Afterwards, the person feels much stronger then before. Most people who cleanse have no major reaction.

Symptoms of a healing crisis usually pertain to organ excretion. For example, one may urinate more; have more bowel movements, a slight headache, fatigue, a breakout and/or a rash. Sometimes people may feel more irritable or moody. A cold may pop up because the body's immune system was busy working on other things before. It now can focus on these bugs that previously have been left unattended. Usually these symptoms are just the body's way of expelling toxins and are not to be feared but embraced as a good sign. If for any reason you are not sure about cleansing, seek professional help or put it off until you are ready.

According to Hering's "Law of Cure," symptoms usually appear from inside out, up to down and from the reverse order that they appeared in. If you have eczema as a child and asthma in later life, your asthma would be cured first. Then your skin may flair up again. This is an example of "reverse order of appearance." Typically, suppressed skin symptoms drive the disease further into the lungs. Suppression occurs with the use of corticosteroids. The skin is a safer place for your body to release toxins than in the lung tissue. This is an example of "inside out." The skin will then clear up with proper treatment, hopefully without suppressive corticosteroids.

A disease crisis is different from a healing crisis. This is when a person's disease worsens. For example, a diabetic person developing a leg ulcer is a progression of the disease because the circulation and healing capability worsens. This is not related to cleansing, but a worsening of the symptoms of the disorder. Seek professional help if you have any serious disease.

WHAT DO I NEED TO DO TO DETOXIFY?

Choose your detoxification protocol

1. Dietary Detoxification
Some people chose to diet to do their cleansing. I have scoured many good books on detoxification diets. Here is some good advice for doing a dietary detox.
Avoid the following for 21 days:
   i.   Fruit juices contribute to yeast overgrowth and acidity because they have no fibre or solids in the liquid. They are empty calories.
   ii. Wheat, rye, spelt and barley contain gluten that can cause problems with digestion, the nervous system and energy.
   iii. Yeast, mould and fungi feed bad bacteria in the gut and are found in baked goods, wine, beer, whiskey, cheese, mushrooms.
   iv. Refined products such as sugar and white flour contribute to poor bowel function, blood sugar instability and feed microbes in the body (parasites, viruses, bacteria and fungus).
   v.   Artificial flavourings, colours and additives are chemicals that add toxins to the body.
   vi. Red meat, beef, pork and shellfish are all proteins that add to inflammation. Pork is said to have many microbes, parasites and viruses. Shellfish are bottom feeders and not appropriate for a cleansing diet.
   vii. Caffeinated drinks such as coffee, black tea and colas rob the body of nutrients and water. They also negatively affect the nervous system.
   viii. Condiments such as jam, jelly, ketchup, vinegar and sauces usually add to the bad bacteria in the gut. These things usually contain food colouring and sugar. Vinegar is fermented and contributes to allergic symptoms.
   ix. Dairy products such as cow milk and cheese can create mucous in the gastrointestinal tract which impedes digestion.
   x.   Alcoholic or carbonated beverages are empty calories.

Consume the following foods freely:

i. Plenty of organic vegetables and their juices. Organic foods decrease the toxic burden that pesticides cause.
ii. Cilantro, parsley, dark leafy greens help to bind up toxins, such as heavy metals, for excretion.
iii. Goat milk, yogurt and cheese are more readily digested than cow dairy products.
iv. Rice and soya milk are alternatives to goat or cow milk.
v. Cottage cheese and plain cow milk yogurt are acceptable.
vi. Oatmeal, buckwheat, quinoa and brown rice are healthy grains that do not contain gluten. Sometimes oatmeal is cross contaminated with wheat, which contains gluten. If you are a celiac, be careful with oats.
vii. Use seasonings such as olive oil, honey, Bragg's seasoning, sea salt and spices.
viii. Drink purified water, spring water, filtered water and green tea.
ix. Choose lean protein such as chicken turkey, fish, egg whites, tofu and legumes.
x. Drink eight to 10 glasses of filtered water per day.
xi. Vegetables and their juices are beneficial such as ginger, kale, carrots, dandelion greens, celery, wheat grass, garlic, cabbage, broccoli and beets.
xii. Sprouts are used as a garnish or a nice addition to salads.

2. Emotional Detoxification

Every thought and emotion has a direct impact on your physical body. Stress can affect your hormones. Have you ever felt energetic when you got good news? Did you get a cold after you were run ragged with work? Your mind can trigger hormones that affect your body's physiological processes.

Focus on what you want and not the opposite. The law of attraction will bring the negative or positive to you. Often people are a victim of themselves. Every choice has an outcome. Make choices for your higher good and release the burdens of your negative emotions. You have absolute control over what you put in your body, how you exercise and what you focus on.

People choose many ways to detoxify emotionally. They may seek out or partake in prayer, group meetings, talking to friends, attending church, spiritual counsel or through retreats. Some big decisions may need to be made in order to make the changes required. Consciously establish your intent to choose to heal while cleansing. If you are unwell now, you can meditate on an image of a vibrant and vital you.

3. Water Therapies

Water has many beneficial properties. Alternating hot and cold showers stimulates the circulation and lymph flow. Steam rooms and hot/dry saunas help the skin to eliminate toxins through perspiration. Epsom and sea salt baths help to draw toxins from the skin. Epsom salts in particular help to ease lactic acid build up in muscles which can make the body more alkaline.

4. Cleansing Using Supplements

Probiotics: Whilst cleansing, some toxins may be deposited into the intestinal tract for excretion. Maintaining a healthy intestinal flora is crucial in cleansing. Every person has billions of bacteria in their intestinal tract. Most bacteria are beneficial and maintain health. A small percentage of bacteria in our intestines are harmful if they spread. If these bad bacteria overgrow it may have negative health consequences such as immune dysfunction, infections, constipation and/or diarrhea. Good flora helps to maintain the immune system and displace the bad bacteria in the gut. They also help to sustain normal arrangement and function of the intestine's cells. The most popular beneficial bacteria are lactobacillus acidophilus and bifidobacteria. The lactobacilli can be found in fermented foods such as yogurt, miso, tempeh and kefir. However, the numbers of bacteria in these food products are not standardized. The bacteria may not be an active culture if they are not stored properly. It is best to use a standardized capsule of probiotics. It should be stored in the refrigerator which helps ensure that it is a live culture. Follow the directions on the package. Typical dosage for a probiotic supplement is one to 10 billion cells per capsule. One to three capsules can be taken daily. There are no known side effects from probiotics.

COLON CLEANSING

Colon cleansing helps remove toxic debris of impacted fecal matter from the intestinal tract. Our bowels are a holding tank for our body's waste. Our waste is not only what we eat and drink but our manufactured toxins such as hormones, acids, alcohols and cholesterol. Some environmental toxins that we absorb are pesticides, heavy metals and pollution. A popular revision of the old proverb is "We are what we eat and don't excrete."

Some colon hydrotherapists administer colonics using distilled water mixed with probiotics to flush out the intestinal tract. This is a helpful temporary solution for constipation. It is not suited to those with diverticulitis or the elderly.

Aloe Vera Juice

Aloe Vera juice is very healing to the lining of the gastrointestinal tract. It is said to be a tonic, laxative, stimulate bile flow, eliminate parasites and heal the stomach. Aloe works as a cathartic laxative which stimulates intestinal contractions that cause bowel movements. Typical dosage is three tablespoons to three ounces, one to three times daily. Start with the lowest dose and increase it until you find your comfort zone. If you take too much Aloe Vera, you may suffer from cramps and diarrhea. Take aloe vera three or more hours away from medication because it may reduce the absorption of some prescription drugs. This supplement is not suited to those who suffer from diarrhea, heavy periods, kidney disease and/or are pregnant.

Dandelion Extract

Dandelion (roots or leaves) is a bitter herb. It helps to support digestion and the function of the liver and gallbladder. It stimulates bile flow and removal of excess fluids in the body. Bile helps to break down fats and lubricates the intestinal tract. It helps the skin, anemia, reduces uric acid in the blood and helps with jaundice. It is also a laxative and reduces the risk of gallstones.

Some people eat dandelion greens as a salad which is very beneficial. Dandelion comes fresh or as a tea, capsules or tincture. This herb is best taken right before a meal to aid with digestion. Dosage varies depending on which form you purchase.

Digestive Enzymes

Digestive enzymes are a means for the body to break down foods and absorb their nutrients. Our body naturally makes digestive enzymes through the liver, the pancreas and stomach. If you do not have good digestion, digestive enzymes act as insurance for proper absorption. Partially or improperly digested foods cause many health issues, such as heartburn, food allergies and constipation.

Digestive enzymes usually include protease, which aids in protein digestion, lipase, which aids in fat digestion and amylase or cellulose which aids in carbohydrate digestion. Some digestive enzymes contain Betaine HCL, which helps with protein digestion. Take them as directed on the package. This supplement is not suited to those with high acidity, intestinal or stomach ulcers.

Psyllium

Psyllium is an inexpensive source of soluble fibre and a mild bulking agent. When mixed with water, psyllium expands and forms a gel in the intestinal tract. This expansion stimulates bowel movements. This bulk gently scrubs along the intestines and makes stools softer. Psyllium absorbs water so drink at least eight to 10 glasses of water per day. If you do not, expect to become more constipated.

In addition to its benefits for the bowels, psyllium is useful for diabetes. It helps to lower cholesterol, high blood pressure and reduces elevated blood sugar. Take psyllium away from meals with a large glass of water. If you have a spastic bowel, impacted feces or a narrowed intestinal tract avoid psyllium. Psyllium comes in powder or capsule form. Typical dosage is one teaspoon or five grams of psyllium husks, in 10 ounces of water, twice a day or as instructed on the label.

Vitamin C

Vitamin C has a colon flushing ability. Take 1,000 mgs of powdered ester or buffered vitamin C in a glass or water. Take this dose every half an hour. Record how many milligrams it takes to produce loose stools. Then reduce the dose by one spoonful every day, until a dose is found where the stools are a comfortable consistency. Alternatively, some people start with 500 mgs of vitamin C per day and work up to 5,000 mgs a day. Do not take vitamin C if you have inflammatory bowel disease, kidney stones, ulcers or are undergoing surgery.

Chlorella

This supplement works to bind toxins in the intestinal tract and aid in their excretion. Chlorella is also a good source of nutrients such as B12 and has an alkalinizing effect on the body.

LIVER AND GALLBLADDER CLEANSING

Choline and Inositol

Both these supplements help to support the liver and gallbladder. They help with the reduction of fat in the liver and metabolism of cholesterol. They are good for a fatty liver, aid in constipation and help with mood and sleep. Inositol is usually taken in 500 mg capsules.

N-Acetylcysteine (NAC)

NAC is a sulphur containing amino acid needed to produce glutathione, which is a substance that combats free radical damage and helps to maintain cellular health. This also aids in slowing the rate of aging. The liver uses NAC to detoxify pollutants and toxins like smoke and alcohol. This supplement is not for diabetics as it interferes with insulin.

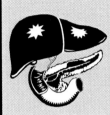

Did you know?
The liver is the biggest internal organ weighing in at 3 1/3 pounds. It has two blood supplies, one from the hepatic artery and one through the portal vein. Blood is cleaned and leaves the liver through the hepatic vein. The hepatic vein empties the blood into the inferior vena cava of the heart. The liver can usually re-grow or regenerate itself if a portion of it is removed and it is not injured beyond repair.

Dandelion

See the description in the colon cleansing section earlier.

Milk Thistle

Milk thistle is a herb that is useful for the liver because it can actually help the liver cells to regenerate. It is used to treat disorders such as hepatitis, cirrhosis and liver poisoning. It aids in fat digestion by aiding in bile production. Bile acts as a lubricant for the bowels. It helps to prevent free radical damage from environmental toxins and medications. It also aids in blood sugar stabilization, decreasing cholesterol and promotes excretion of toxins. It has been studied by researchers and found beneficial in some types of cancer, such as breast and prostate.

BLOOD CLEANSING

Juicing of vegetables is a good way to purify the blood. Typical vegetables used for juicing are carrots, garlic, tomato, celery, parsley, cilantro and kale. One may also use wheat grass, beet tops and roots, dandelion greens, chlorophyll and barley greens. There are many excellent combinations that can turn out quite tasty if you play around with the vegetables used.

Nettle Root

Nettle root is a herb that is useful to clear acid from the blood. This is good for those who suffer from gouty arthritis. It acts as a diuretic and also cleanses the kidneys. It is a good tonic for energy and contains many minerals. Nettle comes in capsules, tea or herb form. Capsules are usually 300 to 500 mgs. Follow the directions on the individual package.

Yellow Dock Root

Yellow dock is a blood cleanser and purifier. It also helps with colon and liver function. It is said to decrease inflammation in the sinuses and helps clear up skin disorders. Do not eat the leaves of yellow dock; only use the root. You can find this in a tincture or capsule form. Dosage of this herb is usually 400 to 500 mgs per capsule taken up to three times a day.

Red Clover

Red clover flowers purify the blood and help to fight infection. This herb is useful in liver and kidney disease, skin disorders and supports the immune system. Red clover doses are usually around 250 to 500 mgs per capsule. Follow the directions on the individual package. It is said to have a mild estrogenic effect so it is not suitable for those who have hormone dependent disorders like breast, uterine or ovarian cancer and endometriosis. Do not use if you are pregnant or breastfeeding.

KIDNEY CLEANSING

Remedies that are good for kidney cleansing are also good for the blood. This is because the kidneys filter the blood to remove wastes and they recycle the blood back into the circulation.

Dandelion Root and Leaves

See the description under liver and blood cleansing.

Nettle Root

See the description under blood cleansing.

Burdock Root

Burdock clears the blood of congestion in the circulation, lymph and urinary tract. It helps to release excess fluids and increases perspiration, which release toxins. Typical dosage for this herb would be one gram three times a day in a capsule form. This herb should not be used during pregnancy.

HOMEOPATHIC ORGAN CLEANSING

You can often order special blends of homeopathic remedies from your health food store. Certain Canadian companies will do special mixtures by request. There are also pre-made homeopathic remedies that are very efficient for drainage of organ systems.

Liver Homeopathic Combination

Order this special mixture as a tincture using equal parts of the following:
- Lycopodium 6 CH
- Chelidonium 6 CH
- Nux Vomica 6 CH
- Carduus Marinarus 6 CH
- Taraxicum 6 CH

Take 15 drops two to three times a day, in water or under the tongue. These should be taken between meals by at least half an hour.

Kidney Homeopathic Combination

Order this special mixture in a 30 mls size, using equal parts of the following:

- Taraxicum Officinalis 6 CH
- Solidago Virga 6 CH
- Berberis Vulgaris 6 CH
- Cantharis 6 CH
- Sarsaparilla Officinalis 6 CH
- Equisitum Hymale 6 CH

Take 15 drops two to three times a day, in water or under the tongue. These should be taken between meals by at least half an hour.

Lymphatic and Blood Combination:

Order this special mixture using equal parts of the following:

- Trifolium Pratense 6 CH
- Urtica Urens 6 CH
- Taraxicum 6 CH
- Echinacea Purpurea 6 CH
- Scrophularia Nodosa 6 CH
- Phytolacca 6 CH

Take 15 drops two to three times a day, in water or under the tongue. These should be taken between meals by at least half an hour. If you decide to use all three tinctures, separate the liver combination from the others by 10 to 15 minutes.

Diarrhea

Diarrhea is not a disease but a symptom. It may be a sign of an underlying disorder or infection. Conditions that have a tendency to produce diarrhea are food poisoning, allergies, bacterial, viral and/or fungal infection. Some chronic diseases that manifest symptoms of diarrhea are celiac disease, irritable bowel syndrome, Crohn's disease, diverticulitis and colitis. Those who have had bowel surgery usually suffer from diarrhea until their intestines heal.

Certain foods or supplements may cause diarrhea such as coffee, tea, chocolate, black licorice, prunes, excess fibre, antibiotics, laxatives, vitamin C and magnesium. Cut back on these products if your bowels are loose.

Symptoms of Diarrhea

Diarrhea symptoms usually consist of frequent, loose and liquid stools. Some may suffer from cramps, vomiting and stomach aches. Typically, symptoms clear up after a few days. If it is persistent and severe, one may become dehydrated. Weakness and lethargy may ensue. Seek medical attention if you feel exhausted or your diarrhea has lasted more than a few days.

DIETARY MEASURES FOR DIARRHEA

To give your bowels a chance to heal, try fasting for a day and drink water only. Drink plenty of fluids to replace water lost. This is not recommended if you have blood sugar troubles, such as diabetes or hypoglycemia. If you do eat, adhere to a bland diet. Stay away from hot spices, acids, citrus fruits, deep fried or fatty foods, caffeine, sugar and alcohol. Dairy products may aggravate diarrhea, so avoid them until your diarrhea improves. Eat smaller meals with fresh fruits and vegetables, lean meat, fish and whole grains. To stay healthy, eat foods from column one listed in the chart in Chapter Three. These foods are lower fat and low glycemic. Foods high in saturated fat enhance inflammatory proteins in the body. This means that high fat foods cause inflammation in the body, including the bowels. The glycemic index is how quickly a food turns into a sugar in the blood. Sugar is high glycemic. Sugars in the blood tend to feed microbes such as bacteria, fungus, parasites or viruses that may cause diarrhea. Thus, low glycemic foods do not feed the bad bacteria the way that high glycemic foods do.

If your diarrhea is severe, high fibre foods may aggravate you. If you have chronic diarrhea, you may do better on cooked vegetables and fruits. However, it is better to find your underlying cause and treat it accordingly. Fresh fruits and vegetables have enzymes that are beneficial to health.

SUPPLEMENTS FOR DIARRHEA

Essential Fatty Acids (EFAs)

Essential fatty acids, mainly flax and fish oil, are good for symptoms such as pain, inflammation, dry skin, gas, bloating, gastrointestinal function and secretion, and immune system deficiency. EFAs can also help with other problems such as depression, concentration, joint pains, inflammation, skin eruptions and cardiovascular disease.

Eicosapentaenoic acid (EPA) found in fish oil is most beneficial for inflammatory bowel disease and diarrhea. It acts to heal the lining of the intestinal tract. EPA can be found in cold water fish such as herring, trout, salmon and mackerel. It increases a type of prostaglandin that actually decreases inflammatory proteins. Take about 1,000 mgs of EPA per day. An enteric coated fish oil capsule is advantageous because it releases in the intestinal tract, not the stomach. This would ensure that you would be getting the maximum EPA into the intestinal tract which is where its anti-inflammatory properties are needed. Be sure to keep your EFAs in the fridge to prevent them from spoiling. Do not use your EFA liquid for cooking. Once it is heated, it releases free radicals that cause damage to cells.

Probiotics

Every person has billions of bacteria in their intestinal tract. Most bacteria are beneficial and maintain health. A small percentage of bacteria in our intestines are harmful if they spread. If these bad bacteria overgrow it may have negative health consequences such as immune dysfunction, infections, constipation and/or diarrhea.

Good flora helps to maintain the immune system and displace the bad bacteria in the gut. They also help to sustain normal arrangement and function of the intestine's cells. The most popular beneficial bacteria are lactobacillus acidophilus and bifidobacteria. The lactobacilli can be found in fermented foods such as yogurt, miso, tempeh and kefir. However, the number of bacteria is not standardized. The bacteria may not be an active culture if they are not stored properly.

It is best to use a standardized capsule of probiotics. It should be stored in the refrigerator which helps ensure that it is a live culture. Follow the directions on the package. Typical dosage for a probiotic supplement is one to 10 billion cells per capsule. One to three capsules can be taken daily. There are no known side effects from probiotics.

Digestive Enzymes

If you suffer from undigested food in the stool and your diarrhea is a result of poor digestion, digestive enzymes may be an answer. Digestive aids that contain pancreatic enzymes (protease, lipase, and amylase) aid in digestion and help the body to absorb nutrients from food. Protease helps one to digest protein, lipase for fats and amylase for carbohydrates. Supplementing with enzymes is particularly helpful for diarrhea caused by food allergy and nutritional malabsorption disorders. Take as directed on the label.

L-Glutamine

L-glutamine is a supplement that provides metabolic fuel for the intestinal cells. It helps to sustain the villi and absorptive surfaces of the intestinal tract lining. Vitamin C and B complex help to enhance the absorption of L-glutamine. Recommended dosage for adults is two to six grams per day with meals. There are no known side effects of L-glutamine.

HOMEOPATHIC REMEDIES FOR DIARRHEA

There are many homeopathic remedies for diarrhea. Some of the more common remedies are listed with their symptoms herein. For more information on how to self prescribe a homeopathic remedy, go to Chapter Two. If you cannot find a remedy suited to you, or find you are not improving or your symptoms get worse, seek the help of a professional homeopath or your medical doctor.

ALOE SOCOTRINA
Common indications include:
- distended abdomen after drinking water
- rumbling and gurgling gas
- urgent diarrhea after eating
- **jelly-like stools that contain mucous** and/or blood
- anus is burning with itching hemorrhoids
- weakness of the anal sphincter
- **involuntary stool while urinating or passing gas**
- **urgent stools at 5:00 a.m.**
- suited to beer drinkers who lead a sedentary life
- mental and physical work causes fatigue
- **lumpy stool mixed with liquid**
- **early morning diarrhea that drives one out of bed**
- pain felt in the stomach when walking and making a misstep
- pain radiates to the back and upwards with every belch
- **hemorrhoids that are congested, like grapes and better with cold bathing**

- aggravated by eating, heat, after eating
- relieved by passing gas with distension, drinking cold water, bending forward

ARSENICUM ALBUM

Common indications include:

- abdominal distension with a burning sensation
- may have both vomiting and diarrhea
- painful glands in the groin or inguinal area
- burning rectum with stools and intense cutting pain
- watery, painful diarrhea
- useful for traveler's diarrhea
- **anxiety, restlessness with exhaustion**
- cold and clammy with the feeling they can never get warm enough
- **desires hot drinks and applications despite burning sensation**
- **great thirst yet only takes small sips of water**
- nausea after meals
- **worse after midnight**, after eating, cold, during rest
- **relieved by hot drinks, warmth, motion** and exercise

Treatment of Acute Childhood Diarrhea with Homeopathic Medicine: A Randomized Clinical Trial in Nicaragua; J. Jacobs, L. Jimenez, S. Gloyd,
May 1, 1994 by J. Jacobs
Pediatrics, May 1994, 93,5:719-25.

This was the first study on homeopathy to be printed in an American medical journal. The study compared individualized high potency homeopathic preparations against a placebo in 81 children with acute diarrhea. The treatment group benefited from a statistically significant 15% decrease in duration. The authors noted that the clinical significance would extend to decreasing dehydration and post diarrhea malnutrition and a significant reduction in morbidity.

Source: nationalcenterforhomeopathy.org

MERCURIUS CORROSIVUS

Common indications include:

- successfully treats **dysentery**
- bloody frequent motions
- stool are green with mucous, scanty, pure blood, black, pasty, burning, slimy
- burning felt in the anus
- **painful urging not helped by passing stool**
- gums may be swollen, purple, spongy
- constriction in the throat with spasms
- great deal of perspiration and salivation
- complaints in the summer or from May to November
- aggravated by fats, acids, cold, during the summer
- relieved by rest, motion

NUX VOMICA
Common indications include:

- said to treat dysentery
- constipation and diarrhea with painful urging
- **spasmodic cramps** and flatulence
- errors in diet aggravate these types
- enlarged liver and gallstone colic
- pain felt two or three hours after eating
- **stomach pains worse from anger and tight clothes**
- sour, watery, bitter heartburn after meals
- painful ulcers in the mouth and throat
- bleeding piles with urging for stools
- nausea and vomiting in the morning or after meals
- **mentally these types are irritable, ambitious and impatient**
- suited to sedentary types who do a lot of mental work
- **chilly types who seek the warmth**
- **cravings for alcohol, spices, coffee and fat**
- **aggravated by overindulgence, alcohol**, in the morning, mental overwork, coffee, overeating and drugs
- **relieved by warmth**, rest and damp weather

PHOSPHORUS
Common indications include:

- watery stools preceded by great rumbling noises and expelled like a hose
- stools may be involuntary, watery, green, mucous-filled, bloody
- anus feels like it is wide open, stool easily escapes
- loss of appetite and hunger soon after eating
- **tendency to hemorrhages**
- distended, painful abdomen worse after dinner
- tearing and burning pain in the stomach, worse in morning
- sour and burning belching
- **these types may suffer from lung problems such as asthma or bronchitis**
- enlarged and/or cirrhosis of the liver
- desires cold food and drinks
- **cold drinks vomited after they warm up in the stomach**
- **cravings for cold food, spices, salt, milk, wine and chocolate**
- **mentally these types are open, anxious and like company**
- **relieved by eating, cold drinks or food**
- **aggravated by spices, warm food and sat**

PODOPHYLLUM
Common indications include:

- this remedy acts on the liver and digestive tract especially the duodenum and rectum

- **rumbling and gurgling in the abdomen before a stool**
- **stools are sputtering and mixed with air**
- green sour stools in the mornings
- diarrhea typically in the morning and better in the evening
- exhaustion from stools
- **explosive diarrhea**
- **profuse watery and offensive**, pours out like a hydrant
- undigested food in stool, jelly-like, green and watery
- **stool can be yellow, pasty, mucous filled or bloody**
- liver area in right side under rib feels swollen and sensitive
- thirsty for large quantities of cold water
- desires sour foods
- **anxious sinking sensation after a bowel movement**
- **worse in morning at 5:00 a.m.**, hot weather, whilst teething, during stools and from motion
- relieved by bending double, external warmth, lying on the stomach and rubbing the liver

SULPHUR
Common indications include:
- diarrhea with stools that contain undigested food
- **sour smelling diarrhea that lingers on the person**
- **stool drives one out of bed in the morning (5:00 a.m.)**
- parts around the anus becomes red and excoriated
- pulsation in the anus after a stool
- feeling hot and sweaty
- **redness of the margins of the skin (lips, anus and eyes)**
- burning sensation anywhere in the body
- **skin eruptions are common in these types**
- **itching and burning of the rectum**
- **hemorrhoids**
- feels very weak with the diarrhea, hates standing
- **craving for sweets, fat, spices, beer or whiskey**
- **aversion to eggs**
- **these types tend to be messy, lazy and intellectual**
- **aggravated by warmth of bed, whilst standing, at 11a.m., suppressed discharges**, change of weather, milk products or alcoholic beverages
- relieved by lying down on the right side and in open air

Picture this….
You had been working a lot of extra hours at the office and in addition to that you had a few assignments. You managed to keep your young family in order. Needless to say, if you could have cloned yourself you would! Lately you have had no time for your usual exercise. If you had an hour after the kids went to bed, you would turn on the tube, have a

glass of wine and some sweets. This was a nice relaxant for you, although you would get pretty tired afterwards and through to the next day.

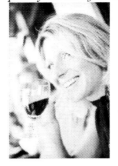

Unfortunately your schedule didn't let up and your digestion was becoming angry. After a weekend of overdoing the food and drink, your bowel movements became more frequent and loose. You started to get some nasty painful cramps long before your bowels passed stool. Because you took a weekend course at the Homeopathic College, you felt you needed a dose of Nux Vomica. (This remedy is good for sedentary types who over indulge in alcohol, food or drugs.) You took one dose of 200 CH of Nux Vomica and your bowels started to behave after two days. You decided that drinking and eating to relax only made the problem worse, so you limited your wine intake to once a week.

Diverticulitis

Diverticulitis is a disorder of the elderly and typically affects those aged 50 and up. It is characterized by infection, inflammation and in serious cases perforation of diverticula of the intestines. Diverticula are small pockets in the large intestine that are weakened areas that protrude from the intestinal wall. Diverticula themselves do not cause symptoms but an infection does. Infections may be a result of eating foods that are poorly digested. Waste remains in an intestinal pocket and bacteria overgrows. This creates pain, fever and inflammation.

THE CAUSES OF DIVERTICULITIS

The causes of this disorder are low fibre diets, a weakened intestinal wall and aging. Chronic constipation and straining with hard stools weaken the intestine wall over time. People who smoke, are obese, stressed, have cardiovascular or gallbladder disease tend to have a greater incidence of diverticulitis.

THE SYMPTOMS OF DIVERTICULITIS

Diverticulitis has several symptoms, such as:
- abdominal cramps
- bloating
- constipation
- pain and cramps in the lower abdomen
- sore and tender abdomen
- a change in bowel habits
- constipation or diarrhea
- fever
- nausea and/or vomiting
- bloody stool
- tender in the left side of the abdomen

THE COMPLICATIONS OF DIVERTICULITIS

Complications of diverticulitis are unusual. In severe cases the intestine may split open and leak bacteria and stool into the abdominal cavity. This causes severe inflammation and requires immediate medical attention and most likely surgery.

Medical Diagnosis and Treatment of Diverticulitis

Diagnosis of diverticulitis includes a barium swallow, colonoscopy or a sigmoidoscopy. Medical treatments are antibiotics, surgery and a high fibre diet. This diet is crucial in preventing stool from becoming stuck in the diverticula and forming bacteria.

DIETARY MEASURES FOR DIVERTICULITIS

Diet is crucial for health of the intestinal tract and preventing a flair up of diverticulitis. Be sure to drink at least eight to 10 glasses of water per day. See Chapter Three on eating a healthy diet which it also decreases the prevalence of many other diseases such as heart disease, diabetes, cancer and hormone imbalances.

Foods to Limit and/or Avoid

Sugar, alcohol and refined carbohydrates feed bad bacteria in the gut that cause constipation. These foods do not contain fibre or nutrients. Refined carbohydrates are white flour, white rice and sugar. Honey, stevia or pure maple syrup may be used to sweeten things without negative consequences. Eating excessive animal protein and fat can cause inflammation and constipation.

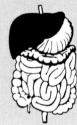

Did you know?
Our large and small intestines are about four to five times our height. The intestinal tract is approximately 25 feet long. The small intestine makes and receives enzymes which aid in digestion. It absorbs nutrients into the blood stream. The large intestine is bigger than the small intestine. It absorbs water and propels waste out of the body.

Beneficial Foods for Diverticulitis

Foods that are high fibre help with constipation. Increase your fibre slowly every day. Some people experience cramps or diarrhea if they have a steep increase in fibre at once. Examples of high fibre foods are:
- Vegetables: beets, brussel sprouts, cabbage, carrots, cauliflower, celery, green beans, kale, okra, potato skins
- Fruits: apples, apricots, blackberry, citrus fruits, cranberry, figs, peaches and prunes, pears
- Beans: cooked legumes such as adzuki beans, garbanzo beans, kidney beans, lentils, lima beans, navy beans, split pea
- Whole grains that are high in fibre are brown rice, bulgur, millet, oat bran, slow cooked oatmeal, quinoa, whole wheat and wheat bran

GENERAL SUPPLEMENTS FOR DIVERTICULITIS

Aloe Vera Juice

Aloe vera juice is very healing to the lining of the gastrointestinal tract. It is said to be a tonic, laxative, stimulate bile flow, eliminates parasites and heal the stomach. Aloe works as a cathartic laxative which stimulates intestinal contractions that cause bowel movements.

Typical dosage is three tablespoons to three ounces, one to three times daily. Start with the lowest dose and increase it until you find your comfort zone. If you take too much aloe vera, you may suffer from cramps and diarrhea. Take aloe vera three or more hours away from medication because it may reduce the absorption of some prescription drugs. This supplement is not suited to those who suffer from diarrhea, heavy periods, kidney disease and/or are pregnant.

Digestive Enzymes

Digestive enzymes are a means for the body to break down foods and absorb their nutrients. Our body naturally makes digestive enzymes through the liver, the pancreas and stomach. If you have diverticulitis, you need to be sure you have adequate digestion for absorption and to prevent fermentation of undigested foods in the intestinal tract. Improperly digested food may lead to constipation and fermentation in the bowels which can trigger diverticulitis.

Digestive enzymes usually include protease, which aids in protein digestion, lipase, which aids in fat digestion and amylase or cellulose which aids in carbohydrate digestion. Some digestive enzymes contain Betaine HCL, which helps with protein digestion. Take it as directed on the package. This supplement is not suited to those with high acidity, intestinal or stomach ulcers. Follow the directions on the individual package.

L-Glutamine

L-glutamine is a supplement that provides metabolic fuel for the intestinal cells. It helps to sustain the villi and absorptive surfaces of the intestinal tract lining. Vitamin C and B complex help to enhance the absorption of L-glutamine. Recommended dosage for adults is two to six grams per day with meals. There are no known side effects of L-glutamine.

Probiotics

Every person has billions of bacteria in their intestinal tract. Some bacteria are beneficial and some are pathogenic. If the bad bacteria are given the opportunity, they will overgrow and cause an infection, fever, constipation and/or diarrhea. Probiotics are essential for intestinal health in those with diverticulitis. They are supplements that help to replenish the good bacteria and displace the bad. The most popular beneficial bacteria are lactobacillus acidophilus and bifidobacteria. The lactobacilli can be found in fermented foods such as yogurt, miso, tempeh and kefir. However, the number of bacteria in food is not standardized. The bacteria may not be an active culture if they are not stored properly.

Antibiotics wipe out both the bad and good bacteria from the intestinal tract, which may leave one open to more infections. Probiotics replenish the good flora that is wiped out by these drugs. Use a standardized capsule of probiotics that is stored in the refrigerator. Keeping the probiotics cool helps to ensure that the culture is live rather then dead. Follow the directions on the package. Typical dosage for a probiotic supplement is one to 10 billion cells per capsule. One to three capsules can be taken daily. There are no known side effects from probiotics.

Psyllium

Psyllium is an inexpensive source of soluble fibre and a mild bulking agent. When mixed with water, psyllium expands and forms a gel in the intestinal tract. This expansion stimulates bowel movements. This bulk gently scrubs along the intestines and makes stools softer. It also improves the consistency of the stool and reduces straining during bowel movements. Psyllium absorbs water, so drink at least eight to 10 glasses of water per day. If you do not, expect to become more constipated.

In addition to its benefits for the bowels, psyllium is useful for diabetes. It helps to lower cholesterol, high blood pressure and reduces elevated blood sugar. Take psyllium away from meals with a large glass of water. If you have a spastic bowel, impacted feces or a narrowed intestinal tract avoid psyllium. Psyllium comes in powder or capsule form. Typical dosage is one teaspoon or five grams of psyllium husks in 10 ounces of water, twice a day or as instructed on the label.

Vitamin A and C

Vitamin A and C have a healing affect on the mucous membranes of the intestines. Take 10,000 IU of vitamin A and 1,000 to 2,000 mgs of buffered vitamin C. Alternatively some people start with 500 mgs of vitamin C per day and work up to 2,000 mgs a day. Do not take vitamin C if you have inflammatory bowel disease, kidney stones, ulcers or are undergoing surgery.

Natural Antibiotics

Peppermint oil is useful to reduce abdominal pain and spasms. It has a mild antimicrobial effect on the intestines. Olive leaf extract, oregano oil and grapefruit seed extract help to maintain proper intestinal health, fights bacteria, fungi, viruses and parasites. Follow the directions on the individual labels.

HOMEOPATHIC REMEDIES FOR DIVERTICULITIS

There are many homeopathic remedies for diverticulitis. Some of the more common remedies are listed with their symptoms here. For more information on how to self-prescribe a homeopathic remedy, go to Chapter Two. If you cannot find a remedy suited to you, or find you are not improving or your symptoms get worse, seek the help of a professional homeopath or your medical doctor.

ALUMINA
Common indications include:
- even soft stools are expelled with great difficulty
- stools are dry and hard
- **no desire to have a bowel movement**
- **stools are so stubborn the fingers may be used to assist passing stool**
- wants to eat indigestible things like starches, tea or coffee grounds

- **dryness of the mucous membranes**
- long lasting pain in the rectum after a bowel movement
- left sided abdominal pains
- blood is passed with stools and may be profuse and clotted
- suited to elderly people with a sedentary habit
- **mentally these types may be dull, slow in answering or confused**
- **aggravated by an aversion to potatoes, in the morning on waking**, soups, alternate days or in cold air
- relieved by warm drinks, while eating, evening, open air, moderate exercise and alternate days

ARSENICUM ALBUM
Common indications include:
- distension of the abdomen
- bowel troubles such as constipation or diarrhea
- **watery burning, diarrhea that smells putrid**
- peritonitis
- burning pains anywhere in the body, intestines, rectum or stomach
- cold and clammy
- **these types cannot seem to feel warm enough**
- **thirsty for small sips of water and hot drinks**
- weakness after stools
- **mentally these types are anxious, restless and fear disease**
- **aggravated by cold, fruits, cold drinks, after midnight**, after eating and drinking and dairy products
- **relieved by warmth, motion and hot drinks**

BRYONIA
Common indications include:
- colic pains causing one to lie completely still
- peritonitis with stinging and burning pains
- abdomen very sore to touch
- **thirsty for large quantities of water**
- these types cannot stand to be touched or fussed over
- **constipation with dryness of the mucous membranes**
- **tongue is coated white or brownish**
- stitching pains aggravated by motion
- **stools are dry and hard**, large and look burnt
- morning diarrhea
- **rheumatism that is worse from motion,** joints may be sore and swollen
- irritability when sick
- stools contain undigested food and are watery and burning
- **mentally these types are irritable and want to be left alone and quiet**
- **aggravated by motion, fruits, at 9:00p.m.,** morning and from touch

- **relieved by lying, rest, pressure** and cold drinks

CHINA
Common indications include:
- debility from loss of fluids, diarrhea, bleeding or sweating
- loss of appetite
- **excessive flatulence, fermentation, belching and grumbling**
- longs for acidic foods
- extreme hunger at night
- **stomach full and distended, feels packed full and not relieved by belching or passing gas**
- diarrhea of watery undigested food which is worse at night
- sweats profusely if covered in bed
- **these types may be irritable, fear animals and sensitive**
- **aggravated by loss of fluids, light touch, autumn,** milk, at night, after eating and drinking and from motion
- **relieved by hard pressure**, bending double and lying down

HYDRASTIS
Common indications include:
- stools are mixed with mucous
- diarrhea alternates with constipation
- constipation after use of drugs
- pain in the rectum after stool
- **thick yellow discharges**
- profuse sweating
- heat alternates with coldness
- aggravated by wine, drugs, after stool and alternate days, all foods upset the stomach
- relieved by warm covering and pressure

KALI CARBONICUM
Common indications include:
- stitching pain over the abdomen
- abdomen is tight like a drum
- these types are easily startled when touched
- abdominal muscles are painful to touch
- swelling of the lymph glands
- water retention in the extremities
- suited to weak, anemic types who are easily tired and startled easily
- constipation
- dyspepsia of the elderly
- stitching pains an hour before stools
- lots of gas and intestinal distension

- fatigue after meals
- **desires sweets**
- aggravated by exertion and after eating
- relieved by belching, warmth and being in the open air

Picture this....

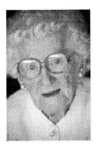

You are an elderly lady who had been diagnosed with diverticulitis about 20 years ago. Lately you have felt a strange pain in the left side of your abdomen. Along with it was a bubbling sensation as if there was something moving in there. You wondered if you had parasites. You tended to suffer from constipation and took psyllium daily to keep regular. At your local health food store, you were advised to take digestive enzymes and aloe vera juice for constipation. It was helpful, but the strange bubbling sensation was still there. In the store, they had a Homeopath who told you to try four pellets of Kali carbonicum 30 CH per week until you saw a change. After a few months, your left-sided pain was completely gone and the bubbling was better. What a relief! No more thoughts of bugs!

Dyspepsia

Dyspepsia is also known as indigestion. It is an older term that is not used frequently. It is not typically a serious disorder but an uncomfortable one and is usually related to other conditions. Dyspepsia is a disorder of the function of the gastrointestinal tract. It is characterized by pains in the upper abdominal area, bloating, belching, nausea and loss of appetite. It is considered to be a condition related to the muscles of the digestive tract, nervous system, poor diet choices and food sensitivities. Typical medical treatments of dyspepsia include antacids and other digestive medications as needed. Antacids render the stomach acid ineffective and actually cause the problems they are meant to treat. They hinder the body from digesting nutrients. Some people are actually low acid and show the same symptoms as high acid.

Quick Home Test for Acid:
To establish if you lack hydrochloric acid (HCL), try this simple test. When you have indigestion, take a tablespoon of apple cider vinegar. If this alleviates your heartburn or digestive troubles then you need more HCL. If it aggravates it, you are too acidic and should avoid betaine HCL and vinegar. Drink a large glass of water if this is the case. If you are low acid take betaine HCL or apple cider vinegar in water with your meals.

What are the Symptoms of Dyspepsia?
- upper abdominal pain
- bloating/distension
- burning after meals
- bitter taste in the mouth
- bowel symptoms such as constipation, diarrhea or soft stools
- gurgling and rumbling
- sensation as if something is lodged in the throat

- belching
- fullness after eating very little
- nausea and/or vomiting
- eating aggravates most symptoms

What Causes Dyspepsia?

- Diet is key in treating dyspepsia. An overfilled stomach can cause digestive problems because gastric contents are pushed up into the esophagus. Too short an interval between meals can also cause problems. Foods that may aggravate heartburn are also those that cause indigestion. They are fried foods, fat, spices, salt, coffee, tea, sugar, vinegar, carbonated drinks, dried meats, alcoholic beverages, citrus fruits, tomatoes, chocolate and bread. Do not try your digestion beyond its capacity. Drinking with meals is said to be inadvisable as it dilutes the stomach acid. Cold water supposedly renders enzymes less effective for adequate digestion.
- Digestive insufficiencies, such as a lack of hydrochloric acid (HCL), bile and enzymes, can cause digestive problems. Digestive enzymes are made by the pancreas and liver. Bile is made by the liver and stored in the gallbladder. Bile helps to emulsify fats. If you don't make enough bile, you don't digest fats as well. Many people who have their gallbladder removed do well taking digestive enzymes that include bile salts.
- Hydrochloric acid is manufactured by the stomach and helps to break down proteins. Low stomach acid causes gas, bloating and heartburn. Sometimes low stomach acid has the same symptoms as high stomach acid. Excessive HCL can cause heartburn.
- Drug use and stimulants increase the risk of indigestion. This would include substances such as alcohol, tobacco, immuran, cortisone, iron, aspirin, antibiotics and pain killers.
- Eating too fast may cause dyspepsia. This can be due to rushing whilst eating or not chewing due to pain in the teeth. Chewing your food not only breaks it down into smaller pieces but it also improves the digestion of starches. Saliva mixes with foods and produces an enzyme that helps to pre-digest starches before they enter the stomach.
- Hormone imbalances (premenstrual syndrome, endometriosis and menopause) seem to influence the gastrointestinal tract.
- Inflammation of the gallbladder or gallstones can cause bloating, pains and belching.
- Injuries to the spine and abdomen may contribute to indigestion.
- Lack of friendly bacteria in the gut adds to indigestion because the bad bacteria is able to overgrow without being put in check by the good bacteria.
- Nervous conditions such as anxiety, depression and stress can cause dyspepsia. When we have chronic stress, our blood supply travels to our extremities. This is because we have an evolutionary fight or flight response. This is to help us run when we are fearful of impending danger. Thus, the blood supply travels away from the stomach and impacts our digestion. Our nervous system is tightly connected to our digestion.

Other Diseases Linked to Dyspepsia
- alcoholism
- anxiety
- Crohn's disease and colitis
- depression
- diabetes
- drug abuse
- food sensitivities
- gallstones
- gastroesophageal reflux
- heartburn
- infections (bacterial, fungal, viral and parasitic)
- irritable bowel syndrome
- kidney disease
- obesity
- thyroid disease
- ulcers

How to Prevent a Dyspeptic Attack
- chew your food well
- reduce stress levels
- take your time eating and do not swallow too much air
- avoid tight belts that compress the stomach contents upwards
- cut back on caffeine, alcohol, fats and sugar
- exercise before meals, not after
- ask your doctor about cutting back on medications that may be causing your symptoms
- sleep with your head elevated to prevent food from rising up and aggravating you at night

DIETARY MEASURES FOR DYSPEPSIA

Dyspepsia sufferers should avoid sugar, tea, pop, spicy foods, coffee, fats, grease, pastries, tomatoes, citrus and alcohol. Eat smaller meals every four hours and do not eat three hours before bed. Include fresh fruits, vegetables, lean meat, fish and whole grains in your diet. Some foods have healing properties. For example, papaya and pineapple have natural enzymes that aid in digestion. Raw potato and cabbage juice are said to heal the lining of the stomach and reduce acid. Eat foods mostly from column one from the chart in Chapter Two. These foods are lower fat and low glycemic which help keep you healthy overall. Avoid foods that trigger indigestion even if they are in column one. Food sensitivities may be an issue for you. For more information on, them go to Chapter Three.

SUPPLEMENTS FOR DYSPEPSIA

Aloe Vera Juice

Aloe vera juice is very healing to the gastrointestinal tract. Aloe is said to be a tonic, laxative, to stimulate bile flow, eliminate parasites and heal the stomach. Typical dosage is one tablespoon to three ounces, one to three times daily. Start with the lowest dose until you find your comfort zone. If you take too much aloe vera, you may suffer with diarrhea. This supplement is not suited to those who suffer from diarrhea, heavy periods, pregnancy and/or kidney disease.

Apple Cider Vinegar

Hippocrates touted vinegar as an antibiotic. It was used in the war to cure stomach disorders. There is a lot of promotion about the healing wonders of apple cider vinegar. It is an acidic substance that, when taken internally, aids in digestion. Typical dosage is one to two tablespoons in a glass of water, up to three times a day before a meal. This supplement is not suited to those with high acidity.

Calcium and Magnesium, 2:1 ratio

Take a 2:1 ratio of calcium to magnesium. It is an alkalinizing mineral that helps to absorb the stomach acid. Take in between meals. Typical daily dosage would be 800 to 1200 mgs of calcium and 400 to 600 mgs of magnesium. It is best to split this into two or three doses throughout the day.

Did you know?

Homeopathy Most Popular Alternative Therapy in Italy, New Study Shows
Reported by Dr. Elvira Draga, **Global Insight***, August 30, 2007*
Results from a healthcare study involving 60,000 families in Italy, found that homeopathy is the most popular alternative therapy in the country, with around 7% of Italians having been treated homeopathically. Women are more likely to have tried alternative therapy, with 15.8% of women having tried at least one form of alternative medicine, compared to 11.2% of men. The second most popular alternative therapy is osteopathy and chiropractic treatments with 6.4%, followed by phytotherapy at 3.7% and acupuncture at 1.8%.

Source: www.nationalcenterforhomeopathy.org

Deglycyrrhizinated Licorice (DGL)

DGL is an excellent remedy for heartburn and healing the stomach and esophagus. It has been known since ancient Greek and Egyptian times. It is said to help heal ulcers of the gastrointestinal tract. It has anti-inflammatory, antiviral, antimicrobial, mucoprotective and expectorant properties. Typical dosage is 500 mgs half an hour before each meal, up to three times a day. Licorice decreases potassium which increases sodium in the body. This is why licorice is not suitable to those who have high blood pressure. Avoid licorice if you have low potassium, during pregnancy, liver disease, kidney disease and heart failure. Avoid licorice if you are taking diuretics or prednisone like drugs.

Digestive Enzymes and HCL

Digestive enzymes are a means for the body to break down foods and absorb their nutrients. Our body naturally makes digestive enzymes through the liver, the pancreas and stomach. If you do not have good digestion, digestive enzymes act as insurance for proper absorption. Partially or improperly digested foods cause many health issues, such as indigestion, heartburn, food allergies, constipation and the like.

Digestive enzymes usually include protease, which aids in protein digestion, lipase, which aids in fat digestion and amylases or cellulose which aids in carbohydrate digestion. Use a digestive enzyme that includes Betaine HCL. Take as directed on the package. This supplement is not suited to those with high acidity.

Garlic

Garlic is a great anti-microbial, which means it is effective in killing yeast, viruses and bacteria. It may be helpful in inhibiting the growth of bacteria that causes ulcers. Garlic is medicinal to the GI tract because it has antimicrobial, anti-dyspepsia and beneficial digestive properties. Note: Avoid garlic if you take blood thinners, prior to surgery and/or have hypoglycemia.

Papaya and Pineapple

You can consume these fruits. They contain beneficial enzymes that help with heartburn and digestion. Some people take a digestive supplement that contains bromelain and papain which are made from pineapple and papaya, respectively.

Probiotics

Probiotics such as acidophilus and bifidobacterium are beneficial bacteria. They help re-colonize the beneficial bacteria in the GI tract. You always have bad and good bacteria in your gut. If these bad and good floras become imbalanced, your gastrointestinal lining may become irritated. Bifidobacterium has also been shown to suppress Helicobacter pylori. The bacterium, Helicobacter pylori, causes peptic ulcers, anemia and gastric cancer. Products that are not refrigerated may be a dead culture, which does not help the beneficial flora to grow. Take as directed on the label.

HOMEOPATHIC REMEDIES FOR DYSPEPSIA

There are many homeopathic remedies for dyspepsia. Some of the more common remedies are listed with their symptoms here. For more information on how to self prescribe a homeopathic remedy, go to Chapter Two. If you cannot find a remedy suited to you, or find you are not improving or your symptoms get worse, seek the help of a professional homeopath or your medical doctor.

ABIES NIGRA

Common indications include:
- stomach pain
- heart palpitations after eating
- acid belching
- **sensation of a lump in the upper abdomen, as if one swallowed a rock or an egg**
- chronic indigestion of the elderly
- indigestion may be accompanied with heart palpitations

- pain not improved by avoiding food
- constriction felt above the pit of the stomach
- aggravated by eating a hearty meal, tea or smoking

ALUMINA
Common indications include:
- dyspepsia in the elderly from decreased gastric juices
- heartburn with dry mouth and throat
- bitter belching
- dryness and constriction of the stomach extending up to esophagus and throat
- difficulty swallowing food
- these types tend to be chilly and sedentary
- **dryness of the mucous membranes** (dry throat, stools, mouth etc.)
- food is felt traveling all the way down the esophagus
- **tendency to severe constipation without an urge to pass stools**
- **evacuations are so stubborn they use fingers to help it pass**
- heartburn accompanied by excessive saliva
- after meals blood rushes to the face
- **these types may have mental dullness, slow to answer questions and seem unsure of their identity**
- dislikes meat and beer
- cravings for acids, chalk, charcoal, dry food, fruit and vegetables, tea grounds
- **aggravated by an aversion to potatoes, the morning** and soup

ANTIMONIUM CRUDUM
Common indications include:
- **white, thick and milky coating on tongue**
- burning in the pit of the stomach
- stomach always feels overloaded
- **these types are hot-blooded and worse from heat**
- overeating causes digestive distress
- heartburn, nausea, vomiting
- **weak digestion that is easily disturbed**
- rising of fluid tastes like food that was eaten
- constant belching and flatulence
- vomiting continues long after nausea is gone
- sensation of something lodged in throat which makes him swallow
- milk becomes curdled in the stomach
- vomits as soon as eats
- **suited to types who are irritable and cannot bear to be touched or even looked at**
- **cravings for pickles, acids, vinegar and wine**
- aggravated by fats, acids, sweets, vinegar, pork and alcohol

ARGENTUM NITRICUM
Common indications include:
- heartbeat may be affected by digestion
- **craving for sugar which aggravates the stomach**
- much flatulence and belching
- food lodges in the throat
- expelling gas relieves symptoms
- pain in the stomach pit that radiates in all directions
- bending double relieves the pains
- pains increase and decrease gradually
- **loud belching**
- tendency to stomach ulcers
- **these types tend to be hot-blooded**
- ameliorated by warm drinks and alcohol
- **these types tend to be anxious, especially for events, test and health, impulses to jump from a height**
- **craving for salt and sweets**
- **aggravated by sweets**, pressure, any food, cold food and drinks
- worse one hour or immediately after eating

ARSENICUM ALBUM
Common indications include:
- watery belching
- **burning pains** like fire in the stomach
- these types are cold and weak
- nausea with a low appetite
- **desire to sip hot drinks**
- heartburn feels like a fire, as if hot coals are against the affected parts
- chronic digestive disturbance
- **easily exhausted**
- irritation of the mucous membrane of the stomach
- red tongue with thin white silvery coating, may have red raised taste buds
- stomach ulcers
- **no desire to eat**
- dry mouth with intense thirst
- cold water sits in the stomach like a stone
- **suited to chilly, restless and anxious types**
- **these types tend to be worried about health, tidy and fearful**
- improved by drinking small sips of hot drinks despite suffering burning heat
- worse by changing of weather, cold and damp, lying with the head low
- **relieved by heat and hot drinks**
- **worse after midnight**, by ice, cold drinks, spoiled meat, alcohol, lobster and salad

BRYONIA
Common indications include:

- bitter taste in mouth from belching
- food and drink tastes bitter
- watery belching
- **tendency towards constipation with dryness of the rectum**
- sensation of a stone in the pit of the stomach
- rheumatism may alternate with indigestion
- better after burping
- **dryness of all mucous membranes**
- **great thirst for large quantities of cold water with dry mouth**
- sharp pains after eating that may extend to the shoulders
- **white or brown coating on tongue**
- heartburn from drinking cold water when the person is overheated
- **tendency to headaches, especially the left side**
- stomach sensitive to touch and lying still improves their symptoms
- **rheumatic complaints worse with motion**
- **suited to irritable types who want to be left alone and quiet**
- craving for coffee and wine
- **worse at 9:00 p.m., motion,** after eating and from vegetables, sauerkraut, cabbage, potatoes, acids, warm drinks

CALCAREA CARBONICA
Common indications include:

- acid sour risings and loud belching
- excessive stomach acid with burning
- rawness with a bitter taste in the throat
- stricture of the esophagus, food will not go down
- throat seems to contract on swallowing
- food tastes sour
- **may be constipated without urging for stool**
- these types are cold and clammy
- bloated abdomen requires loose clothing around the waist
- may have sour perspiration and **perspire a lot on the head**
- **these types tend to be heavy set, hard working and responsible people**
- **can be stubborn and be anxious about their health**
- **craving for eggs and sweets**
- **aggravated by from cold and damp weather,** many foods, milk products, beans, sugar, pastries, oil and fats, cold drinks, vegetables and hard and dry foods
- aggravated during and after eating

CARBO VEGETABILIS
Common indications include:

- sour belching and risings

- violent burning stomach with external chilliness
- sluggish digestion
- bloated upper abdomen with much loud belching
- **shortness of breath from overeating**
- **feels better with a breeze or fanning**
- weak and slow digestion
- sensation as if all food sits and putrefies before digesting
- gas with cramps and chest pains
- **stomach full and distended**
- sensation as if the stomach would burst
- **fainting from indigestion**
- may be suited to sluggish constitutions
- **belching offers temporary relief**
- desires fanning, open air or windows
- desires whisky, brandy, coffee
- aggravated by overeating, milk products, fat, tainted meats, fish, oysters and ice cream
- aggravated by lying down and warm sultry weather

HYDRASTIS
Common indications include:
- chronic heartburn
- weak digestion with hard bloating in the abdomen
- frequent sour belching
- vomits sour mucous
- **thick, ropey, discharges from the sinuses**
- struggles to swallow
- regurgitates food by the mouthful
- shortness of breath from digestive disturbance
- all foods turn into gas
- sharp pains in the stomach
- abuse of antacid mixtures
- tongue large, flabby and has a burnt sensation
- sore and ulcerous mouth
- aggravated by breads, alcohol, vegetables, excess wine and drugs

LYCOPODIUM
Common indications include:
- sensation of fullness from the stomach up to throat
- food may be regurgitated through the nose
- food may taste sour
- water brash
- sour belching with or without regurgitation
- difficulty swallowing liquids, feels as if pharynx is closed

- sensation that a ball rises into the throat and esophagus is clutched
- **distended and full after least amount of food**
- **heartburn and sour belching** with white tongue
- flatulence and constipation
- **may be suited to types with low self-esteem, anger from contradiction, fear of public speaking**
- **craving for sweets**, alcohol, warm drinks and food
- **aggravated by cold drinks, form 4:00 till 8:00 p.m.,** milk, cabbage, wheat, beans, onions, wine, rye and beer
- **relieved with open air**
- least pressure of clothes bothersome

NATRUM PHOSPHORICUM
Common indications include:

- stomach pains
- heartburn, water brash
- trouble swallowing
- acid stomach and belching
- regurgitates fluid that is as sour as vinegar
- **yellow coating of the tongue**
- vomiting sour, acid fluids
- liquids are not tolerated as well as solid food
- fullness after eating very little
- high uric acid in blood
- **cravings for fried eggs, salt**, beer, fried fish and spices
- worse two hours after eating, sugar, milk, bitter and fatty foods

NUX VOMICA
Common indications include:

- bitter acid and watery belching
- sour taste in the morning after eating
- heartburn may occur before breakfast
- pain in the stomach like a weight or pressure, two or three hours after meals
- bloating and distension
- putrid bitter taste in the mouth
- back of tongue is coated brown
- squeezing stomach aches, tender stomach
- aversion to food with nausea
- reverse peristalsis, spasms from disordered peristalsis, pain when food passes down into the pyloric sphincter
- acute indigestion of improper foods
- tightness of the abdomen after eating, must loosen pants
- altered sense of taste for milk, coffee, water and beer
- digestive complaints with accompanying headaches

- may be suited to zealous, impatient, fiery temperaments who overindulge and overwork
- cravings for fats and tolerates them well
- cravings for tea, coffee, alcohol and spicy
- relieved by warmth
- aggravated by anger, overeating, eating, drug use, tobacco poisoning, overindulgence, alcohol, spices, stimulants, tea and coffee

PULSATILLA
Common indications include:
- water brash and heartburn
- sour, bitter, putrid belching
- thick, white, coated tongue, flat taste in mouth
- nothing tastes good, aversion to food
- sensation of a lump in mid sternum, food seems stuck there
- bowels are loose and have a different consistency each time
- mucous sensation in mouth
- thirstless with a dry mouth
- may be suited to fair skinned people who are gentle and weepy by nature
- emotionally these types are timid, weepy and moody
- cravings for butter, cream, cheese and ice cream
- relieved with open air, cool and crisp weather, breezes
- worse one hour after eating
- aggravated by rich fat foods, pork, ice cream and pastry

SEPIA
Common indications include:
- water brash
- heartburn extends to the throat
- belching may be sour, milky, bitter, rancid, foamy
- belching tastes like rotten eggs or manure
- stomach pain after simple foods
- sour or salty taste after eating
- tendency to left sided headaches
- pressure in the stomach like a stone
- thirstless and nauseated at the thought of food
- twisting in the stomach, rises into the throat
- empty feeling in the stomach that is not helped by eating
- cravings for acids, vinegar, pickles, sweets and wine
- sores on tongue
- these types may be chilly and worse for cold
- may be suited to women who are irritable, exhausted and prone to hormonal troubles

- **hormonal troubles include symptoms since pregnancy, menopause or childbirth and low libido**
- these types may be fatigued but feel better with vigorous exercise
- vomiting helps improve heartburn symptoms
- aggravated by over lifting, smoking, fat, meat, milk and bread
- **improved by violent exercise despite being exhausted**

SULPHUR

Common indications include:

- **burning pains are common** in this remedy, burning may travel into the throat with sour belching
- pressure in the throat like a lump, splinter or hair
- throat feels swollen like a ball that rises and closes the pharynx
- regurgitation of food tastes acid shortly after a meal
- water brash and saliva after eating
- feels full after eating a little
- **hearty appetite**, must eat simply as most foods turn sour, does well on soup
- tendency to eat too quickly and not chew food well
- sinking sensation in epigastrum
- **hungry feelings at 11:00 a.m.**
- taste in mouth like rotten eggs
- **tendency to soft stools that drive one out of bed**
- **stools tend to be very offensive**
- loss of appetite
- **very thirsty for cold drinks**
- may be worse in spring and fall
- gastric complaints may alternate with skin conditions
- **may be suited to lazy, intellectual and/or slovenly types**
- **skin eruptions are common in this remedy**
- **cravings for sweets, fats, alcohol, spices, beer and whiskey**
- **worse in the morning at 11:00 a.m.**, after eating, eggs, milk products, sweets, alcohol
- worse before the menstrual flow

Picture this….

Your husband has been suffering with a terrible pressure in his upper abdomen with pains as if he had been kicked in the stomach. He has a worried facial expression and feels like he is going to die. He is restless and cannot relax. Belching is not relieving any of the pressure. He suffers with night sweats, sour belching and is restless. You call your Homeopath with the hope that she would be working late that night. Luckily she answered. She noted that your husband didn't fit into the Calcarea Carbonica or Arsenicum Album profile but that he did have properties of both. She recommended a combination remedy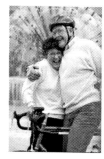

called Calcarea Arsenicum. He took a 30 CH potency. Within one hour, it worked to relieve his suffering. He takes it from time to time whenever he gets indigestion.

Dysphagia

Dysphagia is a term that means difficulty swallowing. It becomes troublesome to swallow saliva, liquids and/or solids. The most common symptom is a sensation of food being stuck in your throat or chest. This condition dampens the joy of eating and drinking which causes weight loss. Food may accidentally be inhaled into the lungs and an infection may occur.

In the act of swallowing, the muscles and nerves work in synergy to move food from the mouth into the stomach. The tongue pushes on the back of the mouth to elicit a swallowing reflex. Breathing temporarily stops to swallow food. Difficulty swallowing happens when any one of these steps becomes uncoordinated or impeded.

It is important to have a thorough check-up from your medical doctor to determine the underlying cause of dysphagia. They may do laboratory tests such as an endoscopy, ultrasound, X ray or barium swallow. Medical treatments include prescription drugs, surgery or procedures to open up the esophagus. People may be required to do certain exercises to strengthen the muscles of the face and improve co-ordination. Some may have to eat in a certain position to enhance their swallowing.

Symptoms of dysphagia
- belching
- difficulty in swallowing
- choking or inhaling food or saliva into the lungs while swallowing
- coughing when swallowing
- feeble voice
- painful swallowing
- pressure in the sternum or mid chest
- regurgitating fluids through the nose
- sensation of food stuck in the throat
- sore throat
- weight loss

What Causes Dysphagia?
Dysphagia can occur for a number of reasons.

A stricture or Barrett's Esophagus may cause difficulty swallowing. This is when the lining of the esophagus (the tube that runs from the mouth into the stomach) becomes irregular and may thicken.

Esophageal irritated by injury or infection may cause dysphagia. The trouble swallowing may be from pain or from swollen tissues.

Benign and/or cancerous growths or tumours may cause dysphagia.

Neuromuscular conditions can cause weak muscles of the tongue, cheek and throat. Normally these muscles are working in tandem to move food from the mouth into the stomach. Nervous system disorders can cause the nerves and muscles that usually work in the simple act of swallowing to be uncoordinated. These diseases are Parkinson's disease, multiple sclerosis, myasthenia gravis, ALS and cerebral palsy. People who have had a stroke or head injury may also have difficulty swallowing. There are many factors to consider in dysphagia.

Excessive alcohol or nicotine use and/or prescription drugs may cause dysphagia.

DIETARY MEASURES FOR DYSPHAGIA

A healthy diet is crucial for healing from any disorder. Follow the guidelines for a healthy diet outlined in Chapter Three. Eat mostly from column one and some from column two. These foods are low to medium glycemic and fat. These foods are healthier than high fat and high glycemic foods which cause inflammatory reactions and many other disorders. If your dysphagia is caused by other disorders such as acidity or heartburn and barrett's esophagus, cross reference the treatment guidelines for these disorders. Sugar, tea, pop, spicy foods, coffee, fats, grease, pastries, tomatoes, citrus and alcohol usually aggravate heartburn and may aggravate dysphagia. Chew your food well and eat smaller meals every four hours and do not eat three hours before bed.

Depending on whether the problem is with swallowing liquids or solids, one may have to compensate by pureeing food or thickening drinks. Drinking whilst eating may help to flush the food down. Others may find this not helpful.

GENERAL SUPPLEMENTS FOR DYSPHAGIA

Aloe Vera Juice

Aloe vera juice is very healing to the lining of the gastrointestinal tract and the esophagus. It is said to be a tonic, laxative, stimulate bile flow, eliminates parasites and heal the gastrointestinal tract.

Typical dosage is one tablespoon to three ounces, one to three times daily. Start with the lowest dose and increase it until you find your comfort zone. If you take too much Aloe Vera, you may suffer from cramps and diarrhea. Take aloe vera three or more hours away from medication because it may reduce the absorption of some prescription drugs. This supplement is not suited to those who suffer from diarrhea, heavy periods and kidney disease or are pregnant.

Deglycyrrhizinated licorice (DGL)

DGL is an excellent remedy for heartburn and healing the stomach and esophagus. It is very soothing to the esophageal lining. It is also useful for stomach ulcers. Typical dosage is 500 mgs half hour before each meal, up to three times a day. Take this in the form of a lozenge. Avoid licorice if you have low potassium, during pregnancy, liver disease, kidney disease and heart failure. It is not compatible with diuretics or prednisone like drugs.

Marshmallow Root

Marshmallow root contains mucilage, which coats and soothes esophageal lining. Typical dosage is 300 to 450 mgs taken one to three times daily with meals. Teas and tinctures are available. Avoid tincture that contains alcohol because it may further irritate the throat. Do not take marshmallow root if you have hypoglycemia, diabetes or are pregnant and nursing.

Slippery Elm

Slippery elm is a herbal remedy that is used to soothe and heal the throat. The inside of the bark contains mucilage, which is a gel-like substance that expands with water. This gel is what coats and soothes the throat. Slippery elm can be purchased in lozenge format which soothes the esophageal lining on the way to the stomach. The typical dosage for this remedy is 500 to 600 mgs, one to three times a day. This remedy has no known side effects.

HOMEOPATHIC REMEDIES FOR DYSPHAGIA

There are many homeopathic remedies for dysphagia. Some of the more common remedies are listed with their symptoms herein. For more information on how to self prescribe a homeopathic remedy, go to Chapter Two. If you cannot find a remedy suited to you, or find you are not improving or your symptoms get worse, seek the help of a professional homeopath or your medical doctor.

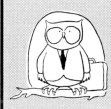

Did you know?
Studies that show people who are higher educated and socioeconomic status are more likely to use homeopathic medicines?

Note to self: People who use homeopathy are smart, educated and influential!
Source: www.nationalcenterforhomeopathy.org

ALUMINA
Common indications include:
- food gets lodged in the throat
- sensation of a splinter or plug in the throat
- throat stings as if it is full of sticks
- **constriction of the pharynx and/or stomach**
- esophagus is contracted and food cannot pass
- swallowing food is easier with drinks
- **dryness of all mucous membranes, like the throat and intestinal tract**
- **stubborn constipation without an urge to stool**
- **the person may use the fingers to assist the removal of stool**
- swelling of the esophagus
- **these types may be elderly, mentally dull and slow to answer**
- **aggravated by potatoes,** swallowing solids and soup
- relieved by warm drinks, drinking with food and empty swallowing

BAPTISIA
Common indications include:

- difficulty swallowing solids with gagging
- paralytic weakness of the throat muscle
- **mouth is terribly offensive (also stool and perspiration)**
- liquids may be tolerated well, but dislikes them
- food is forced through the nose rather then down the esophagus
- **red and inflamed throat without pain**
- useful in cases of diphtheria
- **stupor with facial expression is confused**
- **these types may suffer from a sore body**
- aggravated by swallowing solids
- ameliorated by drinking liquids

BARYTA CARBONICUM
Common indications include:
- **difficulty swallowing with large tonsils**
- spasm of the esophagus when food enters
- gagging and choking when swallowing
- **hard swelling of the cervical glands**
- feeling like food pieces have to move over a sore spot in the throat
- sensation as if a plug is in the throat when swallowing solids
- sensation as if the thyroid gland is pressing inwards
- tongue feels paralyzed
- pain whilst swallowing
- these types can only swallow liquids
- **mentally these types can lack self confidence, be passive and have difficulty making decisions**
- **some of these types ,may have delayed physical or emotional growth**
- aggravated by swallowing solids
- relieved by cold food

BRYONIA
Common indications include:
- stitching pains when swallowing
- throat is dry and raw on empty swallowing
- needle like pains in the throat
- **dryness of the throat and all mucous membranes**
- spasm or contraction of the throat that causes choking pains
- sensation of a hard object is in the throat
- **these types suffer from constipation with dryness of the rectum**
- pressure in esophagus from overloaded stomach
- pain behind the adam's apple
- **great thirst for large quantities of water**
- **may tend to have rheumatic complaints that are better with rest and worse for motion**

- **these types tend to be irritable, want to be left alone and quiet**
- **aggravated by motion, at 9:00 p.m.**, eating, warm food and weather, vegetables, acids
- **improved with pressure**, cold food and drinks

CAUSTICUM
Common indications include:
- difficulty swallowing with paralysis of the throat/esophagus
- **mouth and throat are incessantly dry**
- sensation as if a ball were rising in the throat
- sensation as if the throat were too narrow due to a swelling
- **choking sensation**
- **unable to hawk up mucous must swallow it**
- throat worse from stooping
- feeling like food gets lodged in the throat
- **incessant swallowing**
- **jaw pain when opening the mouth**
- swallows things the wrong way and goes down the wrong pipe
- food comes through the nose
- loss of voice may be related to paralyzed sensation in the throat
- **cravings for smoked meat**
- **aggravated by inhaling cold air**, coffee, swallowing solids
- **relieved by cold drinks**

HYOSCYAMUS
Common indications include:
- spasmodic constriction of the throat and/or tongue, worse swallowing liquids
- **cannot swallow liquids**
- dry, burning, shooting and pricking in the throat
- food taken through mouth comes up through the nose
- constriction muscles of tongue and throat
- **choking when swallowing**
- **marked fear of choking**
- paralyzed sensation in the throat and esophagus
- fears to eat or drink
- **sensation of an elongated uvula**
- **swallowing difficult**
- swallowing liquids may cause hiccoughs, nausea and stiff neck
- may fear they are being poisoned
- **sight or sound of water aggravates** and may produce spasmodic constriction of esophagus
- **aggravated by drinking liquids**
- relieved by swallowing warm and solid foods

IGNATIA

Common indications include:

- spasmodic constriction of the throat
- **sensation of a lump or plug in the throat** that cannot be swallowed
- **choking sensation** from the stomach to the throat
- **sharp or stitching pains in the throat**
- food feels lodged over the stomach opening and cannot go down
- **dryness of the mouth**
- hysterical spasm of the throat from grief
- **these types tend to yawn and sigh**
- **these types tend to have ailments from grief, are easily offended and moods alternate**
- **aggravated by sweets, grief and trauma, spasm of the throat**
- improved with swallowing and drinking

KALI CARBONICUM

Common indications include:

- **desire to swallow but chokes on swallowing**
- food gets stuck half way down
- **stitching pains**
- gagging, vomiting with stricture of the esophagus
- particles of food go into windpipe
- **throat pain on becoming cold**
- throat feels squeezed
- **contraction and choking feeling in the esophagus**
- **throat feels as if it has a splinter or fishbone in it**
- **much hawking of mucous**
- sensation as if the lungs are squeezed into the throat
- sensation of something hard in the throat
- **pain from empty swallowing**
- **these types tend to be conservative and stick to the rules**
- these types tend to have a lot of post nasal drip, mucous in the throat and sinus
- **desires sweets**
- neck feels as though it is too large and collars are tight
- **worse from 2:00 to 4:00 a.m.**, from solid food

LACHESIS MUTA

Common indications include:

- **swallowing is difficult for liquids, empty swallowing and better for solids**
- empty swallowing hurts
- sensation of a lump in the left side of the throat
- **constriction, choking when swallowing**
- sensation of constriction around the neck, in the throat area
- constriction sensation is less when eating solids

- **throat tissues may be purple**
- **dry throat on waking and at night**
- sensation of a ball rising in the throat
- **throat is sensitive to touch, cannot tolerate collars, necklaces or turtlenecks**
- **left sided symptoms**
- throat feels stiff and paralyzed
- liquids are regurgitated through the nose
- cannot cough up a lump in the throat
- **these types tend to be extroverted and/or chatty, jealous and hyper-sexual**
- aggravated by bread, hot drinks, drinking liquids
- relieved by eating

MERCURIUS CORROSIVUS
Common indications include:
- **burning pain in esophagus**
- **choking sensation**
- swallowing even a drop of liquid causes spasms of the throat
- **swollen uvula and ulcers**
- swollen glands and painful throat
- **raw, burning pain from pressure**
- prickling pain as if from needles when swallowing
- constriction with difficulty swallowing
- **constant desire to swallow**
- **swallowing worse with liquid and better for solids**
- sensation of something stuck in the lower esophagus
- spasm of the glottis, esophagus and stomach
- ulcers in the throat
- fluid is regurgitated through the nose
- very thirsty for cold drinks

NITRIC ACID
Common indications include:
- choking whilst eating
- pressure in the throat from swallowing
- **ulcers in the throat**
- **sharp pain on swallowing that extends to the ear**
- **sensation of crumbs in the throat**
- smarting pain in the tongue from even soft food
- **food sticks in the pharynx when swallowing**
- **esophagus and tonsils seem swollen and inflamed**
- pains in the cardiac orifice when swallowing
- suited to angry types
- **cravings for fat and salt**

- confusion of muscular action of throat causes food to stop in throat with choking sticking in throat like a splinter on swallowing
- **mentally these types can be irritable, anxious about health and pessimistic**

SULPHUR

Common indications include:

- throat feels a pressure as from a lump
- **swelling tonsils**
- sensation of a splinter of hair in the throat
- **choking constriction of the throat**
- empty swallowing feels like a piece of meat is in the throat
- **stitching pain on swallowing**
- **dry throat**
- **elongated uvula**
- **burning pain** in the throat
- may be suited to hot people or those with skin conditions
- sensation of a ball rising and closing over the pharynx
- **these types have a tendency towards skin conditions**
- **tendency to be hot and worse from heat**
- **mentally these types tend to be lazy, messy and intellectual**
- **cravings for sweets, fat, spices and alcohol**
- **worse at 11:00 a.m.**, from empty swallowing
- improved by drinking liquids

Picture this....

Your grandmother was overly concerned about food becoming stuck in her throat. She had a history of hypertension, cataracts and arthritis. She had been on antacids for years. She ate a lot of fried foods and meat such as pork. The past night she had a frightful experience when a piece of food got stuck half way down her throat. She feared she would choke and gagged. She drank a lot of water which pushed the food down. After this experience, she had the sensation of a small sharp stick in her throat.

She searched some alternative health books and started to eat low glycemic foods and leaner meats. She started to really take her time chewing. You were surprised that your grandmother was so hip; she was even taking a broad spectrum digestive enzyme with each meal and a high potency multi vitamin with antioxidants for her cataracts. Every day she took 3,000 mgs of vitamin C and 800 mgs of a 1:1 ratio of calcium to magnesium for her hypertension. She also took four pellets twice a day of the homeopathic remedy Kali carbonicum 30CH..

You were shocked that after one month she did very well! Not only did your grandmother successfully prescribe for herself, she actually stuck with it! She had much less trouble swallowing and her energy improved. Her blood pressure was going down and although not yet normal, it was improving considerably. Her dysphagia was gone and her arthritis only bothered her occasionally. She continued to take her supplements and the occasional dose of Kali carbonicum

Eructations

Cross Reference Belching

Fissures, Anal

An anal fissure is split skin on the anal opening and can cause cutting pains when moving the bowels. Diagnosis is usually done by symptoms and visual inspection of the area. Fissures are very common and many people do not seek medical treatment for them. Often they heal in time, but can linger for quite some time. They can be a recent occurrence or chronic. Recent fissures look like a cut and older fissure may have some whitish fibrous tissue exposing the internal sphincter and may have built up or thickened tissue around the tear. Fissures typically occur at the back of the anus and occasionally appear elsewhere. Fissures are different from hemorrhoids. Hemorrhoids are painful, swollen and/or bleeding varicose veins in the anal area.

Most often, fissures do not cause damage to the underlying tissues. However, in some instances if an anal fissure is left, it may deepen and reach the tissues underneath such as the anal sphincter. This is the circular band of muscles that surround the anus. These muscles expand and contract to pass stool or flatus. With chronic irritation, skin tags, scar tissue or papilla may form. These changes in tissue may affect the passage of stool. Your medical doctor may recommend surgery if this becomes a problem. Medical treatments also include topical treatments, botox injections to paralyze the muscles of the anus, cortisone and laxatives. It is important to get it checked as it could be a sign of an underlying disease.

Symptoms Associated with Anal Fissures
- pain when having a bowel movement or remaining long afterwards
- pain may be sharp and cutting and may hinder sitting comfortably
- rectal bleeding
- itching and swelling of the rectum
- anal discharge
- anal skin tags and growth like papilla

What Causes Anal Fissures?
- Constipation and diarrhea
- A low fibre diet contributes to many diseases such as constipation, hemorrhoids, high cholesterol, colon, breast and prostate cancer. Fibre binds up toxins, negative hormones and cholesterol and excretes them via the intestinal tract. Constipation allows a build up of toxins that can cause headaches, bloating and flatulence.
- Medications, such as pain killers, may cause constipation.
- Physical inactivity causes poor bowel movements. A lack of exercise contributes to constipation. Exercise has been shown to help with constipation in a number of ways. Motion helps to move food along which stimulates muscle contractions. Hormones that are released during exercise help to relax the nervous system. This relaxation of the nervous system helps the intestinal tract. Stress can be a trigger

for constipation. Exercise also helps with elimination of toxins through lymphatic drainage and increased circulation.

- Dehydration causes hard stools. We require water to have a normal soft consistency to the stools. If we are dehydrated, our stools become hard and difficult to pass. Water is the best liquid to hydrate your body. Drinking eight to 10 glasses of pure water a day is often enough to stimulate a normal bowel movement. It also helps to flush toxins out through the kidneys.
- Hemorrhoid surgery using a rubber band ligation of the enlarged vein
- Straining on hard stools may tear the anal skin
- Spasm of the anal sphincter during stools makes it difficult to pass stools
- Other disease such as Crohn's disease, colitis, irritable bowel disease, herpes or tuberculosis

DIETARY MEASURES FOR ANAL FISSURES

Diet is crucial for health and proper digestion. Drink eight to 10 glasses of water per day. Consume low glycemic and healthy fats, found in column one of the chart in Chapter Three. Eat plenty of fresh fruits and vegetables and whole grains. These foods are higher in fibre and decrease the prevalence of many other diseases such as heart disease, diabetes, cancer and hormone imbalances. Foods that are high fibre help with constipation. Increase your fibre slowly every day. Some people experience cramps or diarrhea if they have a steep increase in fibre at once. Examples of high fibre foods are Brussels sprouts, kale, cabbage, cooked legumes, ground flaxseed and whole grains. Whole grains that are high in fibre are brown rice, bulgur, millet, oat bran, slow cooked oatmeal, quinoa, whole wheat and wheat bran. Eat plenty of fruits and vegetables.

GENERAL SUPPLEMENTS FOR ANAL FISSURES

Aloe Vera Juice
Aloe vera juice is very healing to the lining of the gastrointestinal tract. It is said to be a tonic, laxative, stimulate bile flow, eliminates parasites and heal the stomach. Aloe works as a cathartic laxative which stimulates intestinal contractions that cause bowel movements.

Typical dosage is one tablespoon to three ounces, one to three times daily. Start with the lowest dose and increase it until you find your comfort zone. If you take too much Aloe Vera, you may suffer from cramps and diarrhea. Take aloe vera three or more hours away from medication because it may reduce the absorption of some prescription drugs. This supplement is not suited to those who suffer from diarrhea, heavy periods, kidney disease and/or are pregnant.

Digestive Enzymes
Digestive enzymes are a means for the body to break down foods and absorb their nutrients. Our body naturally makes digestive enzymes through the liver, the pancreas and stomach. If you do not have good digestion, digestive enzymes act as insurance for proper absorption. Partially or improperly digested foods cause many health issues, such as heartburn, food allergies and constipation.

Digestive enzymes usually include protease, which aids in protein digestion, lipase, which aids in fat digestion and amylase or cellulose which aids in carbohydrate digestion. Some digestive enzymes contain Betaine HCL, which helps with protein digestion. Take it as directed on the package. This supplement is not suited to those with high acidity, intestinal or stomach ulcers.

Probiotics

Every person has billions of bacteria in their intestinal tract. Most bacteria are beneficial and maintain health. A small percentage of bacteria in our intestines are harmful if they spread. If these bad bacteria overgrow it may have negative health consequences such as immune dysfunction, infections, constipation and/or diarrhea.

Good flora helps to maintain the immune system and displace the bad bacteria in the gut. It also helps to sustain normal arrangement and function of the intestine's cells. The most popular beneficial bacteria are lactobacillus acidophilus and bifidobacteria. The lactobacilli can be found in fermented foods such as yogurt, miso, tempeh and kefir. However, the number of bacteria is not standardized. The bacteria may not be an active culture if they are not stored properly.

It is best to use a standardized capsule of probiotics. It should be stored in the refrigerator which helps ensure that it is a live culture. Follow the directions on the package. Typical dosage for a probiotic supplement is one to 10 billion cells per capsule. One to three capsules can be taken daily. There are no known side effects from probiotics.

Psyllium

Psyllium is an inexpensive source of soluble fibre and a mild bulking agent. When mixed with water, psyllium expands and forms a gel in the intestinal tract. This expansion stimulates bowel movements. This bulk gently scrubs along the intestines and makes stools softer. Psyllium absorbs water so drink at least eight to 10 glasses of water per day. If you do not, expect to become more constipated.

In addition to its benefits for the bowels, psyllium is useful for diabetes. It helps to lower cholesterol and high blood pressure, and reduces elevated blood sugar. Take psyllium away from meals with a large glass of water. If you have a spastic bowel, impacted feces or a narrowed intestinal tract, avoid psyllium. Psyllium comes in powder or capsule form. Typical dosage is one teaspoon or five grams of psyllium husks in 10 ounces of water twice a day or as instructed on the label.

Vitamin A and C

Vitamins A and C have healing properties. Take 1,000 mgs of powdered ester or buffered vitamin C and 10,000 IU of vitamin A. Do not take vitamin C if you have inflammatory bowel disease, kidney stones, ulcers or are undergoing surgery. Do not exceed the recommended dosage of vitamin A.

HOMEOPATHIC REMEDIES FOR ANAL FISSURES

There are many homeopathic remedies for anal fissures. Some of the more common remedies are listed with their symptoms here. For more information on how to self prescribe a homeopathic remedy, go to Chapter Two. If you cannot find a remedy suited to you, or find you are not improving or your symptoms get worse, seek the help of a professional homeopath or your medical doctor.

GRAPHITES
Common indications include:
- **burning fissures** caused by large and hard stools
- **excoriated rectum**
- hard feces covered with mucous or mucous threads
- mucous remains in the anus after stool has passed
- **constipated with a sore anus**
- **constipation during menses**
- **stools seem to remain in the rectum for a period of time**
- **suited to people who are inclined to be overweight and chilly**
- **flatulence**
- those who suffer from habitual constipation
- **moist rectum with itching and bleeding**
- stool has an unbearable odour
- **aggravated by suppressed discharges** and after stools

> **Did you know?**
> The Townsend Letter for Doctors and Patients, May 2006
> A study by Alan R. Gaby found that in a small study of 18 people, applying L-Arginine gel to the fissure five times a day for 18 weeks healed fissures in eight of the participants. This is a small study, however fissures tend to be difficult to heal. This information is very promising.
> Source: www.findarticles.com

NITRIC ACID
Common indications include:
- pain and oozing of foul discharges
- **urging for stool**
- diarrhea comes off and on
- **sticking pains as if from a splinter**
- **profuse bleeding after a bowel movement**
- these types crave fat and salt
- pains are felt with great intensity
- **constipation with ineffectual urging**
- **burning and cutting pains**
- rectal pain lasting for hours after stool
- **constipation alternating with diarrhea**
- **stools hard and like balls**
- **blood streaked stools**
- **these types are described as anxious, irritable and spiteful**

- pains so intense that one becomes restless and breaks into a sweat
- aggravated by the least touch, milk, after stools

PAEONIA
Common indications include:
- **burning and cutting pains after stool, lasts for hours**
- itching and swelling of the anus
- these types may suffer from pasty sudden stools
- **rectal pains**
- chills felt after stools
- constipation or diarrhea
- extreme pain after stool
- person may have to lie for a time with buttocks separate to prevent touching the painful area
- **aggravated by touching the rectum**

PETROLEUM
Common indications include:
- diarrhea in the daytime
- watery and gushing stools
- **itching of the anus, rubs it until it is raw**
- cracks in the skin along the rectum
- **pressing pain in the rectum**
- skin may be rough and dry
- **stitching pain in the rectum when standing upright**
- fissures bleed easily
- burning and greenish crusts
- aggravated by car rides, gentle motion and eating

RATHANIA
Common indications include:
- rectal fissures with aching pains
- **burning and pains after a bowel movement** for minutes to hours
- **sensation of a splinter** or broken glass in the rectum
- constricted sensation of the rectum
- **cutting pain while sitting**
- chapped rectal area with oozing
- **sticking pain after stools**
- stools are thin, loose and burning
- aggravated by passing a hard stool and from touch
- relieved by cold bathing, walking slowly or lying

THUJA OCCIDENTALIS
Common indications include:

- fissure and tags at the anus
- diarrhea felt in the mornings
- **burning pains**
- onions tend to upset these types
- flatulence and bloating
- **constipation with ineffectual urging**
- fissures are painful to touch
- **tendency to warts or growths**
- growths around the anus like skin tags, polyps or warts
- sensation of something moving in the abdomen as if alive
- **these types tends to have low self-esteem, feelings of being unattractive or worthless.**
- **aggravated by onion**, touch, after fat, coffee and breakfast

Picture this….

You have a long history of constipation, dry chapped skin, anal fissures and a low libido. You are fed up with taking laxatives and want to try a natural approach, so you go to your local Homeopath. Whilst being new to natural medicine, you decided to give a whole hearted effort to clean up your diet by eating a low glycemic and low fat diet. You drink one quarter cup of aloe vera juice per day. You take a homeopathic remedy called Graphites 30 CH and an antioxidant formula that contains 10,000 IU of vitamin A and 1,000 mgs of vitamin C. You are told that these remedies will help to heal the skin and mucous membranes of the intestinal tract. Although it takes three months for your fissure to finally heal, you no longer need to use laxatives and your skin continues to improve.

Fistula, Anal

Fistulas are essentially a small tunnel or tract that runs from the inside of the anal canal to the outside of the rectum. It is a channel with an opening at either end of it. Anal fistulas may occur in those who have had an anal abscess. This abscess fills with pus and drains through the fistula. The fistula may heal and the abscess without an outlet will fill up again. Fistulas can be recurring. However, a fistula can heal if properly treated. They are usually more of an annoyance due to the pus draining from the tunnel. They typically do not hurt and medical intervention is not always necessary.

Anal fistulas can be treated through natural means, although the treatment can take quite a while compared to surgical intervention. Typically a healthy diet and the appropriate homeopathic remedies can heal the tract over time. Several of the classic texts on homeopathy do not recommend sealing the outlet through surgery. They see this as a suppressive treatment which blocks the pathway for expelling toxins. Typically lung problems are said to come on after the suppression of the drainage route.

Medical Doctors diagnose fistulas through inspection and anoscopy. An anoscope is a viewing instrument for the anal canal and lower rectum. Typical medical treatments are antibiotics, surgery and a fibrin glue to plug the tract. Fibrin glue injection is a new method of treatment with varied success. It entails injecting the fistula with biodegradable glue which closes the fistula from the inside out. This is thought to help the area heal.

Symptoms of Anal Fistula
- pain and swelling
- bloody or pustular discharge
- rectal itching
- redness and discharge may be seen
- thickening of the lesion due to chronic infection
- infections cause fever, chills and fatigue

Other Diseases Related to the Formation of Anal Fistulas
- abscesses of the appendix
- abscesses of the diverticula
- abscesses of the anus
- Crohn's disease
- colitis
- AIDS and cancer

DIETARY MEASURES FOR ANAL FISTULAS

Fistulas may be related to an underlying health condition and people who suffer from them also have a great deal of individuality. Typically, a healthy diet would involve eating healthy fats and low-glycemic foods as outlined in Chapter Three. It is particularly beneficial in fistula treatment because it reduces inflammation, dysbiosis and prevents many other diseases. Any food on the list that has a "#" sign beside it should be avoided. These foods contribute to intestinal dysbiosis, which is an inappropriate balance of bad and good bacteria in the intestinal tract.

Food sensitivities may be a factor in chronic anal fistulas. Try the food challenge test as outlined in chapter three or be tested by a professional for food sensitivities. With either method, you will have more knowledge to control your symptoms. Typical offenders are wheat, dairy, citrus, gluten, peanuts, corn, soya or sugar. In practice, wheat and dairy are the top two culprits because people tend to over eat them which creates sensitivity. For more information about food sensitivities see Chapter Three.

If your anal fistula is related to inflammatory bowel disease (IBD), refer to the appropriate disorder for more information on natural treatments of your disease (see Crohn's, colitis and irritable bowel disease).

SUPPLEMENTS FOR ANAL FISTULAS

Aloe Vera Juice

Aloe vera juice is very healing to the lining of the gastrointestinal tract. It is said to be a tonic, laxative, stimulates bile flow, eliminates parasites and heals the stomach. Aloe works as a cathartic laxative which stimulates intestinal contractions that cause bowel movements.

Typical dosage is one tablespoon to three ounces, one to three times daily. Start with the lowest dose and increase it until you find your comfort zone. If you take too much Aloe Vera, you may suffer from cramps and diarrhea. Take aloe vera three or more hours away from medication because it may reduce the absorption of some prescription drugs. This supplement is not suited to those who suffer from diarrhea, heavy periods, kidney disease and/or are pregnant.

Berberis Vulgaris

Berberis vulgaris is a herb that is useful for healing digestive upsets such as diarrhea, anal fissures and hemorrhoids. It is good for liver dysfunction, urinary tract infections and heartburn. It has been used since ancient Egyptian times.

Typical dosage of this herb is 250 to 500 mgs per day up to three times a day for an acute infection. It may also be made as an ointment for topical application. This supplement is not recommended during pregnancy, breast feeding or for children.

Digestive Enzymes

Digestive enzymes are a means for the body to break down foods and absorb their nutrients. Our body naturally makes digestive enzymes through the liver, the pancreas and stomach. If you do not have good digestion, digestive enzymes act as insurance for proper absorption. Partially or improperly digested foods cause many health issues, such as heartburn, diarrhea, food allergies and constipation.

Digestive enzymes usually include protease, which aids in protein digestion; lipase, which aids in fat digestion; and amylase or cellulose which aids in carbohydrate digestion. Some digestive enzymes contain betaine HCL, which helps absorption of protein. Take it as directed on the package. This supplement is not suited to those with high acidity, intestinal or stomach ulcers.

Probiotics

Every person has billions of bacteria in their intestinal tract. Most bacteria are beneficial and maintain health. A small percentage of bacteria in our intestines are harmful if they spread. If these bad bacteria overgrow it may have negative health consequences such as immune dysfunction, infections, constipation and/or diarrhea.

Good flora helps to maintain the immune system and displace the bad bacteria in the gut. It also helps to sustain normal arrangement and function of the intestine's cells. The most popular beneficial bacteria are lactobacillus acidophilus and bifidobacteria. The lactobacilli can be found in fermented foods such as yogurt, miso, tempeh and kefir. However, the number of bacteria is not standardized. The bacteria may not be an active culture if they are not stored properly.

It is best to use a standardized capsule of probiotics. It should be stored in the refrigerator which helps ensure that it is a live culture. Follow the directions on the package. Typical dosage for a probiotic supplement is one to 10 billion cells per capsule. One to three capsules can be taken daily. There are no known side effects from probiotics.

Vitamin A and C

Vitamin A and C have healing properties. Take 1,000 mgs of powdered ester or buffered vitamin C and 10,000 IU of vitamin A. Do not take vitamin C if you have inflammatory bowel disease, kidney stones, ulcers or are undergoing surgery. Do not exceed the recommended dosage of vitamin A.

HOMEOPATHIC REMEDIES FOR ANAL FISTULAS

There are many homeopathic remedies for anal fistulas. Some of the more common remedies are listed with their symptoms here. For more information on how to self prescribe a homeopathic remedy, go to Chapter Two. If you cannot find a remedy suited to you, or find you are not improving or your symptoms get worse, seek the help of a professional homeopath or your medical doctor.

CALCAREA PHOSPHORICA
Common indications include:
- **fistulas** in those with a history of lung problems
- fistulas may alternate with lung problems
- bleeding after a hard stool
- colic and pain around the belly button
- these types tend to have headaches and be irritable
- stomach pains in school children
- **tendency to headaches**
- **these types crave smoked meat, bacon, hot dogs, salami etc.**
- **may be chilly and sensitive to cold or change of weather and drafts**
- **emotionally, these types may be irritable, complaining, easily bored, sigh often and love to travel**
- aggravated during puberty, fruits, cider and mental exertion
- relieved by lying down

CAUSTICUM
Common indications include:
- constipation that is improved whilst standing
- **burning pain after stools**
- **chronic constipation**
- stool covered with mucous
- **rectal pain while walking**
- **excoriation of the rectal area**
- **stools are difficult to pass with much ineffectual straining**
- **fistulas and large piles**
- **stitching pains**
- **constricted sensation of the rectum**
- rectum burns and itches
- **these types are chilly and dislike the cold but are happy in wet or damp weather**
- **mentally these types are sympathetic, idealists, they may be political or seek to fight injustice**
- **cravings for salt, smoked meats and bacon**
- **these types are averse to sweets** and tend to have joint problems
- **aggravated by cold**, motion and sitting

- relieved by standing

NITRIC ACID
Common indications include:
- pain and oozing of foul discharges
- **urging for stool**
- diarrhea comes off and on
- **sticking pains as if from a splinter**
- **profuse bleeding after a bowel movement**
- these types crave fat and salt
- pains are felt with great intensity
- **constipation with ineffectual urging**
- **burning and cutting pains**
- rectal pain lasting for hours after stool
- **constipation alternating with diarrhea**
- **stools hard and like balls**
- **blood streaked stools**
- **these types are described as anxious, irritable and spiteful**
- pains so intense that one becomes restless and breaks into a sweat
- aggravated by the least touch, milk, after stools

PAEONIA
Common indications include:
- **burning and cutting pains after stool, lasts for hours**
- itching and swelling of the anus
- these types may suffer from pasty sudden stools
- **rectal pains**
- chills felt after stools
- constipation or diarrhea
- extreme pain after stool
- person may have to lie for a time with buttocks separate to prevent touching the painful area
- **aggravated by touch of the rectum**

SILICEA
Common indications include:
- constipation without urging
- **stools may recede**
- rectal fissures, hemorrhoids, fistulas and abscesses
- **fistulas with ulcers**
- **burning, cutting and stitching pains during and after stools**
- this remedy helps the abscess to discharge its contents to heal
- **constriction of the rectum during stools**
- rectum stings and feels closed on passing stools

- **constipation**
- diarrhea with a decaying smell
- **these types are chilly**, tend to have low physical stamina and tend to get infections often
- **sweaty head during sleep**
- worse before the menses
- relieved by warmth

Flatulence

Flatulence is defined as an excess of gas in the intestinal tract which is caused from swallowing air, digestion of certain foods and bacteria. It is hard to distinguish what is a normal frequency of gas. The average person passes gas 14 times every 24 hours. The passage of gas moves through the anus. Its release is controlled by the anal sphincter muscles. Depending on the position of the sphincter and buttocks, gas may be loud or quiet. Flatus is composed of nitrogen, carbon dioxide, methane, oxygen and hydrogen. The odour of stools comes from sulphur compounds and additional stench comes from indole and skatole. The more bacteria in your gut, the more gas you make. If you eat a lot of sulphur-containing foods, you make more odour. Foods like cauliflower, broccoli, meat and eggs typically are offenders. Legumes produce quite a lot of gas in some.

One question asked by many is why do some people not expel gas? It is a fact that everyone has this bodily function. It is socially inappropriate, but a fact of life. It is not true that men pass more gas than women. It is more acceptable or humorous to men, so they have their moment of glory. According to Wikipedia (www.wikipedia.org), the Emperor Claudius passed a law legalizing passing flatus at banquets. He saw it as a health benefit. People of his times (10 B.C.) saw it as a public poisoning.

WHAT ARE THE CAUSES OF EXCESSIVE FLATULENCE?

Diet
Certain foods naturally produce gas in our system. They are foods such as beans, lentils, dairy products, corn, potatoes, onions, garlic, scallions, leeks, radishes, sweet potatoes, cashews, oats, wheat, yeast and cruciferous vegetables (cauliflower, broccoli, cabbage). Most of these foods are healthy and contain more fibre than other foods. Eating too much animal proteins and fats may cause foul smelling gas.

Swallowing Air
Swallowing air naturally causes a bit of gas to form in our intestinal tract. It usually affects those who are anxious or eat too quickly.

Other Diseases
Certain underlying diseases may cause excessive flatulence. They are constipation, diarrhea, Crohn's disease, colitis, irritable bowel syndrome and celiac disease.

Bacterial Dysbiosis
Excess bad bacteria such as candida albicans, parasites, bacterial or viral infections can cause gas and fermentation in the intestinal tract. Dysbiosis is characterized by an

imbalance of the gut flora as discussed. Dysbiosis can lead to leaky gut syndrome. It also creates dysfunction by not properly protecting the gastrointestinal lining that provides a safe barrier between the environment and your internal organs. Treating the underlying dysbiosis is crucial for eliminating excessive gas.

Poor Digestion

Poor digestion may be linked to poor food choices or a lack of digestive enzymes required for absorbing and breaking down food. If you eat too much of a particular food, you may not have enough enzymes to digest all of it. Thus it may be excreted in the large intestine partially undigested. This causes gas and fermentation. As we age, we do not make as many enzymes and hydrochloric acid, which are necessary for digestion of protein, carbohydrates and fats.

DIETARY MEASURES FOR EXCESSIVE FLATULENCE

If you have a specific disorder that is causing your flatulence, see the appropriate chapter on its treatment. For excessive flatulence there are a number of dietary measures that may prove useful. Drink a few tablespoons of lemon juice or vinegar in water before meals. It may help to break down proteins better, by stimulating stomach acid. Chew your food well and take your time eating. Consume a healthy diet, outlined in Chapter Three. Eat foods from column one that are low glycemic and fat foods. Eat a proper balance of proteins, carbohydrates and fats. Usually a healthy ratio of these foods is 30:40:30. Most people eat too much fat and starchy carbohydrates. Cut back on gas producing foods such as cabbage, broccoli, cauliflower, legumes, beer, onions, garlic, dairy products and yeast. They can cause excessive gas. However, these foods are healthy to eat. Usually it is only one or two foods causing the problem. Try to ascertain which foods are bothersome and avoid them. If your gas is a new phenomenon, you can likely have those foods again once your excessive gas is gone.

Food Combining for Optimum Digestion

Food combining is described in the first chapter on healthy eating. In a nutshell, it helps people to optimize their natural ability to digest and absorb nutrients from their foods. Combining certain foods utilize our digestive chemistry to the fullest. This is a particularly good idea for those who suffer with bloating, gas, constipation and diarrhea. Eat fruit alone and at least a half hour or more away from other foods. Combine starches with vegetables and combine protein or fat with vegetables. Do not eat fruit with any other food and don't combine protein or fat with starches.

Fruits are a simple carbohydrate. They are digested very quickly if you eat them on an empty stomach. If you combine them with any other complex carbohydrate or fat you may find that you have a lot of gas, bloating and pains. This is because the fruit that is normally digested and absorbed very quickly ferments when it is mixed with other types of foods. It creates a gassy soup of bacteria which ferments and turns into alcohols, acetic acids and vinegars.

Starches are things like potatoes, rice, bread, pasta and crackers. Proteins are fish, meats and legumes. Legumes also fall into the starch category. They are best to be combined with grains to get all of the amino acids required. Usually these amino acids are found in meat and in combination with legumes and grains. Fats are things like nuts, seeds, oils and animal fats.

SUPPLEMENTS FOR FLATULENCE

Chlorella

Chlorella is a good source of nutrients such as B12 and has an alkalinizing effect on the body. Take as directed on the package. It is not irritating to the stomach or intestinal tract.

Digestive Enzymes

Digestive enzymes are a means for the body to break down foods and absorb their nutrients. Our body naturally makes digestive enzymes through the liver, the pancreas and stomach. If you do not have good digestion, enzymes act as insurance for proper absorption. Partially or improperly digested foods cause many health issues, such as heartburn, diarrhea, food allergies and constipation.

Digestive enzymes usually include protease, which aids in protein digestion, lipase, which aids in fat digestion and amylase or cellulose which aids in carbohydrate digestion. Some digestive enzymes contain Betaine HCL, which helps absorption of protein. Take it as directed on the package. This supplement is not suited to those with high acidity, intestinal or stomach ulcers.

Fennel Tea or Fennel Seed

Half a teaspoon of fennel seed or a fennel tea after eating can prevent excessive flatulence. Fennel should not be used in women who are pregnant or have estrogen dependent disorders such as endometriosis, breast cancer or fibroids. It increases the body's natural estrogen. Separate fennel from antibiotics by a few hours. It can interfere with its absorption.

Papaya and Pineapple

You can consume these fruits. They contain beneficial enzymes that help with heartburn and digestion. Some people take a digestive supplement that contains bromelain and papain which are made from pineapple and papaya, respectively. Papain helps to dissolve protein. It helps with heartburn, appetite and ulcers. Papain is not suitable to those who use anti-coagulant drugs and have cystic fibrosis. Bromelain is a protein digesting enzyme that is useful for other conditions such as an anti-inflammatory, irritable bowel syndrome, gout and parasites. Typical dosage is 500 mgs with each meal. However, both bromelain and papain may be purchased together in one pill. As with most herbs, do not take them during pregnancy or breast feeding.

Probiotics

Every person has billions of bacteria in their intestinal tract. Most bacteria are beneficial and maintain health. A small percentage of bacteria in our intestines are harmful if they spread. If these bad bacteria overgrow it may have negative health consequences such as flatulence, immune dysfunction, infections, constipation and/or diarrhea.

Good flora helps to maintain the immune system and displace the bad bacteria in the gut. It also helps to sustain normal arrangement and function of the intestine's cells. The most popular beneficial bacteria are lactobacillus acidophilus and bifidobacteria. The lactobacilli can be found in fermented foods such as yogurt, miso, tempeh and kefir. However, the number of bacteria is not standardized. The bacteria may not be an active culture if they are not stored properly.

It is best to use a standardized capsule of probiotics. It should be stored in the refrigerator which helps ensure that it is a live culture. Follow the directions on the package. Typical dosage for a probiotic supplement is one to 10 billion cells per capsule. One to three capsules can be taken daily. There are no known side effects from probiotics.

HOMEOPATHIC REMEDIES FOR FLATULENCE

There are many homeopathic remedies for flatulence. Some of the more common remedies are listed with their symptoms here. For more information on how to self prescribe a homeopathic remedy, go to Chapter Two. If you cannot find a remedy suited to you, or find you are not improving or your symptoms get worse, seek the help of a professional homeopath or your medical doctor.

CARBO VEGETABILIS
Common indications include:
- excessive formation of gas
- **passing gas helps relieve discomfort**
- **foul smelling gas**
- weak digestion
- simple foods aggravate
- **frequent belching which helps the stomach**
- belching and flatulence with colicky pains
- **tremendous bloating and indigestion**
- unceasing passing of flatus
- **heartburn, belching and flatulence**
- **shortness of breath from gas or overeating**
- cannot bear anything around the waist
- **bloating and gas felt under the ribs**
- **abdominal pains may extend to the legs**
- **desire to be fanned or have open air**
- weak and tired people with slow thinking
- aggravated by butter, warmth and tight clothes
- **relieved by belching, being fanned** and loosening the clothing

COLOCYNTHIS
Common indications include:
- colicky pains with gas
- **pains come on after an anger-causing event**

- **sharp pains as if being cut with a knife**
- **stitching pains in the sides or around the belly button**
- abdominal pains that drive one to lean into something hard
- pain as if the bowels were pressed between two rocks
- **restlessness during the pains**
- these types may suffer form diarrhea, sciatica or ovarian pains
- **mentally these types may be impatient and easily angered**
- **aggravated by anger**, after eating, drinking and motion
- **relieved by bending double, lying on the abdomen, putting pressure on the abdomen, heat,** coffee, passing gas and from coffee

LYCOPODIUM
Common indications include:
- these types are intellectually strong but physically weak
- palpitations during digestion
- **flatulent after eating**
- loud grumbling and flatulence
- **full after eating very little**
- **distended abdomen which is better by passing gas and worse after eating**
- constipation
- **cravings for sweets and olives**
- **heavy sensation in the stomach after eating**
- **right sided complaints**
- canine hunger, the more one eats, the more one craves
- **mentally these types have low self esteem, fear public speaking or can be dominating**
- **aggravated by missing a meal, oysters**, in the afternoon, evening, **from 4:00 to 8:00 p.m** and lying down
- relieved by belching, warm food and drinks, loosening the clothes and in open air

SILICEA
Common indications include:
- **abdomen is distended, hard and tight**
- **constipation with stools that recede**
- stools are very offensive
- **stitching pains felt under the ribs**
- **sensation of trapped flatulence**
- **cramping pains that may extend from under the ribs to the back**
- these types may tend to have hemorrhoids, fistulas or fissures
- **sweating of the head**
- aversion to a lot of food especially cooked, boiled and animal proteins
- gas is expelled with great force
- worse during the menses, night, full moon and from motion
- **improved by warmth**

SULPHUR

Common indications include:

- rumbling of the bowels
- **cravings for alcohol, chocolate, fat, spices and sweets**
- abdomen is painful to touch
- **thirsty for ice cold drinks**
- constipation alternates with diarrhea
- **offensive smelling gas and stools**
- **tendency to have loose stools that get one out of bed early**
- pain in the anus after stools
- **hungry around 11:00 a.m.**
- **hot blooded types who are worse for heat**
- **tendency to have skin problems such as acne, eczema and rashes**
- **mentally these types can be lazy, messy and intellectual**
- **aversion to eggs**
- aggravated by milk, alcohol and in the evening
- relieved by lying on the right side, moving and in the open air

Picture this....

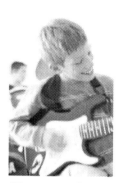

Your 12 year-old son has been terribly flatulent. Being a boy of that age, he tends to think of it as funny; however, you are a bit more civilized and worried that there may be a problem! He eats a lot of sweets. For example, you would be surprised to get home from work and find that he has eaten almost a whole box of cookies or some other sweets after school. He has one heavy duty sweet tooth! He has a good intellect but does not partake in any sports. He seems to fear getting hurt or exerting himself. At your direction, he takes Lycopodium 30 CH, four pellets twice a day for a few days based on his symptoms. His first day he has a lot of gas but by the second day he is back to normal. He responds very quickly to homeopathy, as do most children.

Food Cravings

Food cravings are defined as a strong desire to eat something. Often food cravings are not related to nutrient deficiencies but to a sensation of deprivation, an addiction or other underlying issues such as food allergies, adrenal gland stress, candida or hypoglycemia.

Some cravings are out of the norm. One type of craving is called "pica" and is defined as an appetite for non-food substances such as chalk, paper, coal or dirt. Some people eat foods that are not appropriate such as flour, uncooked potatoes, starch and raw meat. Pica happens in all ages but typically during pregnancy and in children. It sometimes occurs in those who have parasites such as pinworms. Some people who suffer from emotional disturbances or developmental delay may eat things that are unusual such as hair, skin, feces, paint or wallpaper. It is certainly disturbing to witness. Some worries with consumption of these things are parasites, intestinal blockage and poisoning with lead or glue.

CAUSES OF FOOD CRAVINGS

WHAT YOU THINK ABOUT EXPANDS

Some people who are trying to restrict their intake of fats, fried foods, salt, sugar or chocolate may desire these foods more. This could be due to the common principle that what you think about expands. Knowing you cannot have it fixes your mind on having it. Cement in your mind that you are someone in control that can eat one chocolate or one small piece of cake. Rather than thinking about what you cannot have, treat yourself to a normal portion and savour it. Do not beat yourself up over eating taboo foods. If you eat 21 meals per week and you mess one up, you are normal! It is what you do the majority of the time that counts. It is actually good to treat yourself on occasion than to completely deny yourself. It is only food, not a criminal act!

Lets eat some grub, literally…..
Many cultures eat bugs as a source of protein. Among the top bugs are grasshoppers, earthworms, caterpillars, grubs, crickets, ants and termites. Grasshoppers are eaten in Japan and China and served with rice!

FOOD SENSITIVITIES

Some people actually crave the foods that they are sensitive to. See chapter five for more information on food allergies and intolerance. People may feel well temporarily when they eat the food they are sensitive to. They get a slight rush afterwards. Then they feel worse again and would like another hit of it. Food sensitivities cause other symptoms such as headaches, joint pains, irritability, hives, acne and bloating.

CANDIDA ALBICANS

If you have candida albicans, hypoglycemia or diabetes you may tend to crave sugars and carbohydrates more than other people. (See the candida section for a more detailed treatment.) Candida is a fungus that is naturally occurring in the body. It is found in the skin, respiratory, digestive and genitourinary tract. It will overgrow if given the right conditions, such as a highly acid environment, eating high amounts of carbohydrates, sweets and after antibiotic use. When candida dies, off it makes toxic byproducts and people tend to feel sluggish and crave sweets. Eating them keeps the yeast growing. However, these bad feelings are transient and pass after one week or less. By avoiding yeast, sugar, mould and refined carbohydrates, you can keep these bad bacteria in check.

HYPOGLYCEMIA

Hypoglycemia is a condition where the blood sugar drops too low. This is a precursor to diabetes. If you have hypoglycemia, eat a protein with each meal. Also eat low glycemic foods that contain high fibre, such as those outlined in the table in Chapter Two. Low glycemic foods are listed mostly in column one. High fibre foods and proteins take longer to break down and keep the blood sugar constant and stable. If you eat sweets to balance your blood sugar, it will raise it and then drop it. It becomes an up and down cycle. Low blood sugar signals to your brain to eat foods that will supply a quick rush of glucose. This can be prevented by adding in protein, fibre and eating healthy snacks in between meals.

The supplement chromium is helpful to balance the blood sugar. It is an essential trace element and balances the blood sugar. Typical dosage is 200 to 400 mgs per day with meals.

DIABETES

Diabetics have high blood sugar and are insulin resistant. This means insulin is not absorbed in the cells. The cells do not absorb the glucose they need and they signal the brain that more carbohydrates and sugar are needed. Most diabetics do very well by eating low glycemic foods (outlined in Chapter Three, column one of the chart). Be sure to have a lean protein with each meal. Eat healthy snacks between meals, such as nuts, yogurt, low fat cheese or fresh cut vegetables. This keeps cravings away because when the blood sugar is stable, you don't need to have sugar or carbohydrates to boost your energy and feed your brain.

Did you know....
According to John Hopkins researchers, lowering blood sugar in those with and without diabetes decreases the risk for heart disease and diabetes.

Source: Selvin E, Coresh J, Golden SH, Brancati FL, Folsom AR, Steffes MW. Glycemic control and coronary heart disease risk in persons with and without diabetes: the atherosclerosis risk in communities study. Arch Intern Med. 2005 Sep 12;165(16):1910-6.

Supplements for Diabetes

Keep an eye on your blood sugar when you take any of these remedies with insulin because they may decrease your need for it. Seek professional help if you have concerns regarding your medications and these remedies. There are many useful supplements for diabetics. However, mainly chromium, vanadium, fish oil and gymnema act to stabilize blood sugar and indirectly help with cravings.

- Chromium is often deficient in people with diabetes, low blood sugar and obesity. It helps decrease insulin resistance, aids in weight loss and sugar cravings. It is also said to reduce cholesterol and triglycerides in patients with diabetes. Typical dosage of chromium is 200 to 800 mgs per day with meals.
- Vanadium is a trace element that helps improve blood glucose levels in both type 1 and 2 diabetics. It is a little studied mineral; however it is gaining more popularity and research interest. Vanadyl sulfate is the type of vanadium that lowers the blood glucose levels. Typical dosage is 30 to 300 mcgs per day. It is usually found in combination with chromium supplements.
- Gymnema is an Indian herb useful for diabetes because it reduces blood sugar, helps with weight loss and acts on the beta cells in the pancreas. It acts as a mild appetite suppressant. These cells produce insulin. Typical dosage is 200 to 400 mgs per day.
- Fish oil is a useful supplement to help keep the blood sugar stable. It is a source of essential fatty acids, mainly EPA and DHA. EPA is an anti-inflammatory and

useful for the cardiovascular system. DHA is good brain food that increases your mood. One thousand to 4,000 mgs of fish oil can be taken daily with meals.

LACK OF SLEEP

A lack of sleep may make you pack on the pounds. For some interesting studies on sleep and other natural remedies, go to the Life Extension Foundation (LEF) online at www.lef.org. This group is manned with many medical doctors who research natural supplements and disease. They have many studies and commentary on a wide variety of disorders. LEF wrote an interesting article on sleep and obesity. Sleep and insulin interact between leptin, which tells the brain there's no need for food, and ghrelin, which tells the brain it's time to eat. According to researchers, these two hormones start to misfire with reduced sleep. In a study, test subjects slept only four hours a night. After only two nights, the hormones malfunctioned and leptin production decreased by 18% and ghrelin production increased by 28%. Studies found that participants, healthy male college students, started to eat much more. They reported craving more high calorie, high density and carbohydrate foods. They had a 24% increase in appetite for candy, cookies, chips, nuts and starchy foods such as bread and pasta. After just one week into the experiment, blood tests showed a poor insulin response that mimicked diabetes. A lack of sleep also increased the production of cortisol, a hormone associated with increased belly fat. The researchers concluded that sleep deprivation boosted appetite. Increased appetite caused overeating. This, in turn, caused weight gain.

Some supplements that help with relaxing are those such as passionflower, hops, valerian, magnesium, GABA or melatonin. Take these as directed on the label.

ADRENAL FATIGUE

The adrenal glands are small glands which sit on top of our kidneys. They excrete hormones that help with stress, sleep, sex hormones, blood pressure, cholesterol and menstrual cycles. They are small glands with a mighty job. Certain diets, lifestyle and situations may leave the adrenal glands sluggish.

What causes adrenal fatigue?
- Drugs such as cortisone, prednisone, steroids and inhalers
- Foods such as coffee and tea
- Overwork
- Poor sleeping habits
- Stress that is prolonged and even self-induced

What are signs of adrenal fatigue?
- Cravings for salt, sugar, coffee, tea and/or carbohydrates
- Low energy especially in the morning or right after lunch
- Vertigo or light headedness
- Excessive sweating
- Recurrent infections
- Heart palpitations
- Night sweats
- Low blood sugar

- A desire for snacking needed around 11:00 a.m. or 2:00 p.m.
- Increased irritability or emotions that are not typical
- Significant event that you have never felt well since

How do I fix my adrenal fatigue?

- Skip the caffeinated beverages. They suck the energy out of the adrenal glands and deplete the body of minerals such as calcium and magnesium. They also can keep people awake.
- Diet: Eat foods that are low glycemic as outlined in Chapter Two. Have a healthy snack between meals to keep your blood sugar stable. These foods are whole grains, lean protein and fish, fruits and vegetables.
- Reduce emotional stress by working on your lifestyle. Reduce your workload. Work on your family and relationships in a positive and loving way. Find ways to reduce your financial worries by taking steps for debt repayment.
- Get a good night's sleep. The most restorative sleep happens when you fall asleep around 10:00 p.m. If you have sleep troubles, try some relaxing supplements such as passionflower, hops, valerian, magnesium, GABA or melatonin.
- Get some exercise and have some fun! Many of us forget that we are meant to move our bodies. If you are stuck in the office for an extra long day, you can feel very cooped up. Exercise is a very good way to keep healthy both psychologically and emotionally.
- Take a good quality multi vitamin and extra vitamin C. Take an adrenal gland extract as this helps to support your adrenal. It is not suited to those with Addison's disease or high blood pressure. The B vitamin, pantothenic acid or B5 is very good for adrenal gland stress. Typical dosage is 50 to 250 mgs per day. It works well to take when taking a regular B complex 50 mgs per day as well. If you take the B vitamins, take them in the morning. Licorice extract is said to be nourishing for the adrenal glands, however it is not suitable for those with high blood pressure.

DEPRESSION

Many people turn to food in times of stress. Usually the foods include chips, breads, pastries, sugar or chocolate. If depression is longstanding, carbohydrate cravings are a sign of decreased serotonin levels. Serotonin is believed to be instrumental in the regulation of mood such as anger, anxiety, depression and sleep. Many people learn to eat carbohydrates in order to control mood, sleep and pain. However, the byproduct of such eating is weight gain and further cravings. These types tend to get obese during times of stress. People who suffer with Seasonal Affective Disorder may also crave carbohydrates to naturally increase serotonin.

Supplements for Depression and Food Cravings

- Exercise daily because it increases the feel good hormones.
- Get outdoors during the daylight. Natural sunlight exposure stimulates your pineal gland which controls your sleep and waking cycles, seasonal affective disorder (the winter blues) and improves your mood.
- Seek the support of a trusted friend, counsellor or your church.

- Take 5HTP or 5-hydroxytryptophan. This is a precursor to serotonin and helps mood and carbohydrate cravings. This is not suitable for those taking antidepressants.
- B complex helps with stress, mood and the nervous system. Typical dosage is 50 mgs per day. You can increase B6 by 100 mgs per day. It is useful for mood, sleep, immune system and hormone balance. Take these supplements with breakfast because they can increase your energy and keep you awake at night.
- St. John's Wort is a good remedy for mild cases of depression. If you take this, you would not also use 5-HTP. This is not suited to those taking antidepressants.
- Fish oil is a good mood support. Take 1,000 to 3,000 mgs per day with meals. DHA in fish oil is good brain food. It is useful for depression, ADHD, nervous conditions and schizophrenia.

NUTRIENT DEFICIENCIES

Some people think that food cravings are related to nutrient deficiencies. Most often it is not the case but more of a hormonal problem such as blood sugar instability or emotional stress. The simplest way to combat food cravings is to eat a well-balanced diet and use a good quality multiple vitamin.

Some Food Cravings and Their Suspected Cause

- Chocolate = magnesium deficiency, depression, desiring feel good hormones
- Alcohol = hypoglycemia, depression
- Baked goods = depression, wheat allergies, candida
- Red Meat = iron
- Acid foods = low stomach acid, candida
- Caffeine = adrenal exhaustion, addiction
- Chalk or plaster = calcium
- Salt = sodium deficiency, adrenal gland exhaustion

HOW TO CONTROL CRAVINGS

See your specific cause of food cravings for individualized advice on what action to take. Always eat a healthy diet. This would involve eating a wide variety of colours of fruits and vegetables, lean proteins and fish, legume and whole grains. Eating foods outlined in Chapter Two that are low glycemic are the best insurance for health. Be sure to eat at regular intervals. It is okay to have a snack in between meals. Make sure it is a healthy choice, like nuts, yogurt or fresh cut vegetables. Exercising is a good way to boost your feel good hormones and prevents stress eating. Be sure to get a good night's sleep because not doing so will increase your food cravings.

HOMEOPATHIC REMEDIES FOR FOOD CRAVINGS

Because there are so many homeopathic remedies for food cravings, there are a few main remedies beside each food. If you try these remedies, take a 30CH potency, four pellets once or twice a day for one week. You may want to try to look them up in a Materia Medica (see bibliography) to see which one fits you the most.

ACIDS: abies canadensis, antimonium crudum, antimonium tartaricum, apis, arnica, arsenicum album, borax, bromium, bryonia, calcarea carbonica, carbo vegetabilis, chamomilla, china, conium, corallum rubrum, hepar sulphur, sepia, sulphur, veratrum album

ALCOHOL: arsenicum album, asarum, aurum metallicum, capsicum, crotalis horridus, hepar sulphur, lachesis muta, nux vomica, sulphur, sulphuric acid

BEER: aconite, nux vomica, sulphur

BITTER FOOD: aconite, digitalis, natrum muriaticum

CHOCOLATE: argentum nitricum, calcarea carbonica, carcinosinum, chocolate, lycopodium, lyssin, phosphorus, sepia, sulphur

COFFEE: alumina, angustera, arsenicum album, aurum, bryonia, capsicum, carbo vegetabilis, china, mezerium, nux moschata, nux vomica, selenium

EGGS: calcarea carbonica, carcinosinum, hydrastis, natrum phosphoricum, oleum animale, pulsatilla

FAT: arsenicum album, hepar sulphur, nitric acid, nux vomica, sulphur

HAM: calcarea phosphorica, mezereum, sanicula, tuberculinum

ICE: arsenicum album, calcarea carbonica, elaps, medorrhinum, mercurius corrosivis, natrum, phosphorus, veratrum album

LARD: arsenicum album, nitric acid

LEMONS: arsenicum album, belladonna, benzoic acid, mercurius, sabadilla, sepia, tarentula, veratrum album

MEAT: abies canadensis, aloe, aurum metallicum, cantharis, cyclamen, ferrum metallicum, graphites, helleborus, iodum, kreosotum, lilium tigrinum, magnesia carbonica, menynathes, mercurius, natrum muriaticum, sabadilla, sanicula, sulphur, tuberculinum

MILK: apis, arsenicum, aurum metallicum, bryonia, calcarea carbonica, carcinosinum, chelidonium, elaps, lac caninum, mercurius, natrum muriaticum, nux vomica, phosphoric acid, rhus toxicodendron, sabadilla, silicea, staphysagria, strontium, tuberculinum

ONIONS RAW: allium cepa, cubeba, sabadilla, thuja occidentalis

PASTRIES/DAINTIES: aurum metallicum, calcarea carbonica, china, ipecacuana, pulsatilla, rhus tox, sabadilla, spongia, tuberculinum

PEANUT BUTTER: pulsatilla

PICA (INDIGESTIBLES): alumina, calcarea carbonica, cicuta, ferrum met., natrum muriaticum, nitric acid, nux vomica

- Ashes: calcarea carbonica, silicea, tarentula

- Dirt, sand or mud: calcarea carbonica, silicea, tarentula

- Paper: lac felinum

- Pencils: calcarea carbonica

PICKLES: antimonium crudum, lachesis muta, sepia, sulphur, sulphur iodatum

PORK: crotalis horridus, radium bromide, tuberculinum

RAW FOODS: sulphur

- Raw potatoes: calcarea carbonica

SALT: aloe, argentum nitricum, calcarea carbonica, calcarea phosphorica, carbo vegetabilis, conium, natrum muriaticum, nitric acid, phosphorus, plumbum, sanicula, tarentula, veratrum

SMOKED FOODS: calcarea phosphorica, causticum, kreosotum, pulsatilla

SOUR: antimonium crudum, antimonium tartaricum, apis, arnica, arsenicum album, borax, bromium, bryonia, calcarea carbonica, carbo vegetabilis, chamomilla, cistus canedensis, conium, corallium rubrum, ferrum, fluoric acid, hepar sulphur, ignatia, kali arsenicosum, kali carbonicum, lachesis muta, magnesia carbonica, medorrhinum, natrum muriaticum, phosphorus, podophyllum, pulsatilla, sabadilla, sabina, secale, sepia, squilla, stramonium, sulphur, veratrum

SPICES: china, fluoric acid, hepar sulphur, lac caninum, nux vomica, phosphorus, pulsatilla, sanguinaria, sepia, sulphur, tarentula

SUGAR: argentum nitricum, calcarea carbonica, kali carbonicum, phosphorus, saccharum off., secale

SWEETS: ammonium carbonicum, argentum nitricum, bryonia, calcarea carbonica, calcarea sulphurica, cannibis indica, carbo vegetabilis, china, elaps, ipecacuana, kali carbonicum, kali sulph., lycopodium, magnesium muriaticum, medorrhinum, natrum carbonicum, plumbum, rheum, rhus toxicodendron, sabadilla, secale, sepia, staphysagria, sulphur, tuberculinum

TEA: alumina, asterias rubens, calcarea sulphurica, china, hepar sulphur, hydrastis, pulsatilla, thea

VINEGAR: bacillinum, hepar sulphur, kali muriaticum, natrum muriaticum, sepia

WARM FOODS: arsenicum album, chelidonium, ferrum metallicum, lycopodium, phosphoric acid, sabadilla

Gallstones and Gallbladder Colic

The gallbladder is a small pouch found under the liver on the right hand side. This pouch holds bile which is made by the liver to digest fats. Bile is excreted into the small intestine through a duct from the gallbladder. Gallstones are made of cholesterol and bilirubin. They happen when liquid bile crystallizes and forms stones. Excessive cholesterol in the bile tends to harden as gallstones. Stones can range in size from a sand particle to a golf ball. Some people have hundreds of small stones and/or a few large ones. These stones can become lodged in the bile ducts and cause pain. Some stones are smooth and others are jagged. This may influence the amount of pain that is felt.

Gallstones may block the normal flow of bile into the small intestine. Many people have gallstones, up to 20% of the population is thought to have them and only one to 3% of people are thought to experience symptoms.

Some people have pains in their gallbladder with the absence of any stones. These people have what is called "gallbladder colic." The gallbladder can actually become infected and/or spasm if it is irritated. Usually people experience this dull or cramping pain under the right rib. Often people are left to suffer with their symptoms or have their gallbladder removed. If the gallbladder is not diseased, there are many natural remedies to help with the pains.

What are the Symptoms of Gallstones?
- Pain in the right abdomen happening after meals
- Pain in the right shoulder blade or between the shoulder blades
- Pain in the upper abdomen across the diaphragm
- For any symptoms that are listed here, seek medical attention: Pain that lasts more than a few hours, nausea and vomiting, fever and chills, yellow skin or eyes or pale stools

When gallstones travel into the bile ducts and create a blockage, symptoms may occur. However, many people have gallstones and don't know it. They are symptom free. If you are symptom free, the best course of treatment is to leave well enough alone.

Who is at Risk for Gallstones?
- People who suffer from diabetes, hypoglycemia and insulin resistance tend to develop more kidney and gallstones. This is likely because they tend to have higher cholesterol and eat too many fats and refined carbohydrates.
- The elderly tend to develop gallstones more so than other people.
- Women are two times more likely to develop gallstones. Too much estrogen is thought to contribute to increased cholesterol and decreased gallbladder movement. Too much estrogen may occur in those who take birth control pills, are pregnant or suffer with endometriosis.
- Gallstones are thought to run in families. However, diet often runs in families as well. It is hard to say there is a true genetic or environmental factor in gallstone development.
- High fat diets are linked to gallstones. This makes the liver make more bile to break down fats. People who then do not eat as much fat are still producing quite a bit of bile. It is stored in the gallbladder and can then crystallize there. This is why many people on yo-yo diets tend to develop gallstones.
- Poor digestion and a sluggish liver increase the tendency to make gallstones or have gallbladder colic.
- Certain ethnic groups have a higher tendency to develop gallstones such as Mexicans and North American indigenous people.
- Cholesterol lowering drugs increase the risk for gallstones.

How are gallstones diagnosed?
- An ultrasound may be useful to detect gallstones

- Some doctors inject a dye into your veins and X-ray the gallbladder. This shows the stones more clearly
- A simple test for gallbladder or liver inflammation is as follows. Have the person breathe out. Put a hand with steady pressure under the right ribcage. This may cause pain. This is called "Murphy's sign". This is not a true diagnosis, but may lead to further appropriate testing.

How are they treated?

Gallstones do not always need treatment. If you do not suffer from symptoms they are better left alone. Some doctors will recommend removing the gallbladder if one has pains and/or stones. This does remove the pain of the gallbladder but since removing the gallbladder takes away a source of bile to break down fats, this leaves only the liver to make bile to digest fats.

If there is a fear of the stone becoming lodged in a duct, surgery may be recommended as well. Laser surgery is another avenue that is open through the medical route. Most doctors simply remove the whole gallbladder. There are many natural methods of treating gallbladder colic and stones that will be discussed here.

DIETARY TREATMENT FOR GALLBLADDER COLIC AND STONES

People who tend to form gallstones and kidney stones have a tendency to be overweight and/or insulin resistant. Therefore, the best diet for those who suffer with gallbladder troubles is a low fat and low glycemic diet. Low glycemic foods flip into a sugar less quickly in the blood. Sugar and white bread are high glycemic and turn into a sugar very fast after digestion. High fat foods increase cholesterol which creates more gallstones. The low glycemic and low fat diet is a very sensible diet for anyone who wants to stay healthy and lose weight. For a listing of low, medium and high glycemic foods and fats, go to the chart in Chapter Three. Limit the intake of fried foods and animal fats if you have gallbladder trouble as they tend to increase cholesterol and gallstone formation. Fats and oils that are acceptable are nuts, flax, walnut and olive oil. These fats are said to help the gallbladder make bile to flush out gallstones. Anything that stimulates bile flow helps. Bitter foods such as artichokes, rhubarb, bitters, dandelion greens, lemon, lettuce and chicory are very good.

Eat a high fibre diet because it binds up cholesterol and expels it through the gastrointestinal tract. High fibre foods are oat bran, whole wheat, beans and many fruits and vegetables. See the section on constipation in this chapter for a more extensive list of high fibre foods.

Certain foods may cause allergic reactions that lead to gallbladder inflammation, spasms and colic. They are typically those such as eggs, pork, onion, milk, coffee and citrus fruits. Do not overeat as this causes undue stress on the gallbladder by making it pump out too much bile. It then slows down when you eat normally and gallstones can become worse. Drink plenty of water, at least six glasses per day. This keeps the body hydrated and may help with flushing toxins from the gallbladder.

SUPPLEMENTS FOR GALLBLADDER COLIC AND STONES

Bile Salts

Ox bile is often used as a digestive aid. This supplement is useful for those who lack bile, have had their gallbladder removed or other liver disorders. Bile salts may be included in digestive enzymes. Enzyme supplements usually include protease, which aids in protein digestion, lipase, which aids in fat digestion, and amylase or cellulose which aids in carbohydrate digestion. Typical dosage is 250 to 500 mgs with meals.

Lecithin

Lecithin is a type of fat made from soya beans that is needed by every human cell. It is composed mostly of Choline, which is a B vitamin, linoleic acid and inositol. It aids the liver and helps to reduce cholesterol. This is beneficial in gallstones because gallstones are made up of cholesterol. It helps to protect the liver from damage caused by alcohol, toxins, viruses and disease. It binds to cholesterol and reduces it in the blood stream. Studies have shown that lecithin is protective of liver diseases like fibrosis and cirrhosis in groups of rats that were fed a lot of alcohol. Typical dosage is one to three grams per day. There is no reported toxicity with lecithin use.

Dandelion

Dandelion is a bitter herb that supports the digestion and function of the liver and gallbladder. It stimulates bile flow and aids in fat digestion. It also acts as a tonic for the intestines which helps alleviate the symptoms of constipation. Stimulating bile flow can help to flush out gallstones and cholesterol from the gallbladder.

Some people eat dandelion greens as a salad which is very beneficial. Dosage varies depending on which form you purchase. Dandelion comes fresh or as a tea, capsules or tincture. This herb is best taken right before a meal to aid in digestion.

Goldenseal

Goldenseal is a gentle, bitter herb. It improves the digestion, increases bile flow and tones the gallbladder. Goldenseal is also a useful anti-microbial that kills candida and other bacteria that cause stomach and gastrointestinal disorders. Typical dosage of goldenseal is 300 to 450 mgs taken three times a day.

Because goldenseal has mild anti-bacterial properties, it may deplete your body of the beneficial bacteria in the gut. Take probiotics when you take goldenseal to maintain healthy gut flora. Do not take goldenseal for longer then two weeks at a time. Goldenseal is contraindicated during pregnancy, if you take blood thinners or have a peptic ulcer.

Milk Thistle

Milk thistle is a fabulous herb that is known to protect, cleanse and stimulate the liver to release toxins and manufacture bile. Any herb that aids in bile flow helps to flush out gallstones. This herb has a detoxifying affect and is often used for jaundice, cirrhosis or hepatitis. It is better used in the early stages of cirrhosis than late stages of liver failure. Typical dosage is 200 to 250 mgs per day with each meal. Drink lots of water whilst using milk thistle to flush your system of toxins.

Swedish Bitters

Bitters preparations are made by an infusion and/or distillation process using aromatic herbs, bark, roots and/or fruit. Bitters may contain herbs like aloe, myrrh, saffron, orange peel, gentian, quinine, angostura bark, cassia, senna leaves, camphor, angelica roots, manna, rhubarb roots, goldenseal, artichoke leaf, blessed thistle, wormwood and yarrow flowers.

Historically, bitters were taken as a dinnertime aperitif to stimulate the digestive juices. Swedish bitters are useful to aid in digestion, settle a stomach before eating and good to ward off the ill effects of alcohol. The help the liver and gallbladder to stimulate bile flow. They were used as a tonic and taken in a shot glass. The liquor variety of bitters has a high percentage of alcohol. Purchase your bitters from a health food store, not the liquor store. Typical dosage is one tablespoon before meals. Follow the directions on the individual package.

Vitamin C
Vitamin C is required to convert cholesterol into bile. This helps to prevent gallstone formation. Typical dosage of vitamin C is 500 mgs to 3,000 mgs per day with meals.

Gallbladder Flushes
Some people claim to do a gallbladder flush and many little stones are passed in their stool. It usually involves drinking one cup of olive oil and lemon juice in equal parts. I had a pathology professor say that they x-rayed someone before and after doing a flush. They said they passed small greenish particles and assumed they were stones. However, their x-ray still showed the same stones. Some people have told me that it works and others have tried with no success. I suppose it is like most things; it may work for some and not others. I have had people in the clinic pass small stones. However, if your stones are large, it can get lodged in the bile duct. Emergency surgery may be required. If your stones are small you may try a gallbladder flush. If they are larger, it would be inadvisable trying to pass them.

HOMEOPATHIC REMEDIES FOR GALLBLADDER COLIC AND STONES

There are many homeopathic remedies for gallstones. Some of the more common remedies are listed with their symptoms here. For more information on how to self prescribe a homeopathic remedy, go to Chapter Two. If you cannot find a remedy suited to you, or find you are not improving or your symptoms get worse, seek the help of a professional homeopath or your medical doctor.

BELLADONNA
Common indications include:
- spasmodic pain in the upper abdomen
- **severe pains that extend to the back and shoulder blades**
- **pains feel as if beaten**
- **clawing pain under the right ribcage**
- cutting and clutching pains as if being squeezed
- clutching pains
- **right sided pains**

- **thirstless**
- **cravings for lemon or lemonade**
- **intense heat felt**
- **worse at 3:00 p.m.**
- aggravated by jarring, motion or pressure, touch, slightest touch by linens of the bed
- **relieved by pressure**, bending backwards

BERBERIS VULGARIS
Common indications include:
- biliary and gallbladder colic
- **sudden, sharp and stitching pains**
- **pains radiate outwards or downward**
- **colicky pains in the gallbladder and liver area**
- these types are sleepy after eating
- pains in the lumbar region, gallbladder and liver
- pains transient, stitching and radiate
- stools are hard, round, tough and may be watery
- gouty and rheumatic complaints
- these types who are easily mentally and physically fatigued
- suited to fleshy people

CHELIDONIUM
Common indications include:
- this remedy decreases inflammation in the common bile duct
- **a good remedy for jaundice**, gallbladder pains from stones or infection
- yellow eyes, face, urine and stool with liver disturbance such as jaundice
- needs to lie down after eating
- **colicky pains**
- **cramping pain that extends into the back and shoulder blade (especially the right)**
- **pains may travel transversely**
- **burning pain under the right ribcage**
- constipation with hard, small and round stools
- diarrhea that is slimy, light grey, yellow, white or pasty
- **tongue may be coated yellow and show teeth marks**
- **food and saliva may taste bitter**
- **cravings for cheese, milk and hot drinks**
- **relief from pains when lying on the left side with the legs pulled up, after eating**, with warmth, hot drinks, pressure and bending backwards, walking
- **worse on the right side**, 4:00 a.m. or p.m., change of weather

CHINA
Common indications include:

- colic from gallstones and bile duct obstruction
- **liver and gallbladder colic and disease**
- weight felt after eating a small amount of food
- pain comes on alternating days
- painful liver **sensitive to light touch but better by hard pressure**
- **distension and flatulence a long time after eating**
- eating at night causes food not to digest at all
- **cutting pains**
- diarrhea can be watery and containing undigested food
- involuntary stool with fruits
- loosens the belt after eating
- **craving for sweets**
- relieved with hard pressure on the abdomen, bending double
- **aggravated by from loss of bodily fluids (perspiration, diarrhea, urination or blood) , light touch** and eating late
- aggravated by eating fruits, diarrhea, milk, night, fish, tea

CHIONANTHES VIRGINICA
Common indications include:
- this remedy is good for the liver, spleen and gallbladder
- it is said to be useful in jaundice
- **skin discoloured yellow**
- helps to prevent the formation of gallstones
- promotes the expulsion of gallstones

LYCOPODIUM
Common indications include:
- liver affections, right-sided pains
- **fullness after eating very little**
- sensitive to touch in the region of the liver
- always hungry and headaches if not appeased
- inactivity of the gastrointestinal tract
- **much rumbling of gas**
- sleepy after eating
- **abdominal pains extending from the right to left side**
- **pain in the right side that may extend to the back**
- **colicky pains with gallstones**
- bitter taste in the mouth on waking
- bloated with a **sensitivity to tight pants or belts**
- **cravings for sweets**
- distention with much gas and fermentation in the bowels
- **mentally these types may have low self-esteem, fear public speaking and may be domineering**
- these types are tired, annoyed easily, weak physically, sensitive

- relieved by warm foods and drinks, loosening pants
- **worse on the right side, from 4:00 to 8:00 p.m.**, heavy meals

NUX VOMICA
Common indications include:
- **ailments from over indulgence** (food, alcohol, coffee, tea, drugs)
- digestion easily disturbed
- **these types are easily angered, irritable and impatient**
- **mentally they can be workaholics and competitive**
- painful constipation with **colicky pains**
- **cramps and spasms** of the gallbladder
- enlarged liver, cirrhosis of alcoholics
- nauseated in the morning on waking
- constipation with colicky pains
- fatty foods seem to be tolerated well
- nervous dyspepsia with mental work
- **relieved by warmth** and hot drinks
- **aggravated by overindulgence**, bread, sour foods, alcohol, drugs, tobacco
- aggravated by high living, **morning**, sedentary habits

Picture this....

Your friend who is 35 is complaining of pains under his ribs. They don't seem to come on after meals. It seems more like painful bloating to him. He took some common gas remedies for one month. They did not relieve his symptoms. An ultrasound revealed that he has gallstones. He works in a factory and does a lot of manual labour so he didn't want to have surgery and couldn't manage to take time off work. Since you have had training in natural medicine, you recommended that your friend eat a lower fat diet and take 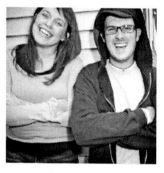 *the remedy Berberis 3CH; four pellets twice daily. After one month he had no pains under his ribs. He didn't have any further symptoms of gallstones. There was no indication that he passed them but since he had no symptoms, he could continue on with his work uninterrupted.*

Gastritis

Gastritis is a condition that is characterized by an inflammation of the lining of the stomach. Usually this lining is strong enough to withstand acids and bacteria. If the integrity of the lining is weakened, gastritis may result. Gastritis can be acute or chronic.

Symptoms of Gastritis

Symptoms of gastritis include abdominal pain, fever, fatigue, nausea, anorexia, bleeding, vomiting and discomfort after eating.

Tests for Gastritis

A medical doctor would usually order a test where one would swallow a type of liquid that would allow the lining of the stomach lining to be seen under X-ray. Using this test the doctor can rule out ulcers. They may do a biopsy to rule out cancer. Other blood or stool tests may be required to determine if there is a parasitic or bacterial infection. Treatment of gastritis by a medical doctor includes proton pump inhibitors, antacids, steroids, antibiotics, surgery and/or stopping medications that cause gastritis.

Causes of Acute Gastritis

Acute gastritis can be caused by:
- Drugs such as non-steroidal anti-inflammatories, aspirin and corticosteroids which can weaken and damage the lining of the gastrointestinal system.
- Foods in excess can irritate the lining of the stomach such as caffeine, alcohol and spices.
- Burns from radiation treatment cause inflammation in the stomach lining.
- Bacteria, such as H.pylori, cause ulcers and gastritis. It can be tested by your Medical Doctor through a stool sample or a blood test. Typical treatment for this would be antibiotics. Other microbes like viruses and fungus can cause problems in those with a compromised immune system. Those with AIDS, the elderly and prolonged debilitating illness like cancer may be more susceptible to viruses or fungal infections.

Causes of Chronic Gastritis

Chronic gastritis is usually related to an underlying condition like peptic ulcers, stomach cancer and/or Crohn's disease.

DIETARY TREAMENTS FOR GASTRITIS

People who suffer with gastritis should eat a plain diet. They should avoid sugar, tea, pop, spicy foods, coffee, fats, grease, pastries, tomatoes, citrus and alcohol. Eat a healthy diet that includes fresh fruits, vegetables, lean meat, fish and whole grains in your diet. Some foods have healing properties. For example, papaya and pineapple have natural enzymes that aid in digestion. Raw potato and cabbage juice are said to heal the lining of the stomach and reduce acid. Eat foods mostly from column one from the chart in Chapter Three. These foods are lower fat and low glycemic which help keep you healthy overall. Avoid foods that trigger indigestion even if they are in column one. Food sensitivities may be an issue for you. For more information go to Chapter Four.

SUPPLEMENTS FOR GASTRITIS

Aloe Vera Juice

Aloe vera juice is very healing to the gastrointestinal tract. Aloe is said to be a tonic, laxative, to stimulate bile flow, eliminate parasites and heal the stomach. Typical dosage is one tablespoon to three ounces, one to three times daily. Start with the lowest dose until you find your comfort zone. If you take too much aloe vera, you may suffer with diarrhea. This supplement is not suited to those who suffer from diarrhea, heavy periods, pregnancy and/or kidney disease.

Calcium and Magnesium, 2:1 ratio

Take a 2:1 ratio of calcium to magnesium. It is an alkalinizing mineral that helps to absorb the stomach acid. Take in between meals. Typical daily dosage would be 800 to 1200 mgs of calcium and 400 to 600 mgs of magnesium. It is best to split this into two or three doses throughout the day.

Deglycyrrhizinated Licorice (DGL)

DGL is an excellent remedy for heartburn and healing the stomach and esophagus. It has been known since ancient Greek and Egyptian times. It is said to help heal ulcers of the gastrointestinal tract. It has anti-inflammatory, antiviral, antimicrobial, mucoprotective and expectorant properties. Typical dosage is 500 mgs half hour before each meal, up to three times a day. Licorice decreases potassium which increases sodium in the body. This is why licorice is not suitable to those who have high blood pressure. Avoid licorice if you have low potassium, during pregnancy, liver disease, kidney disease and heart failure. Avoid licorice if you are taking diuretics or prednisone like drugs.

Garlic

Garlic is a great anti-microbial, which means it is effective in killing yeast, viruses and bacteria. It may be helpful in inhibiting the growth of bacteria that causes ulcers. Garlic is medicinal to the GI tract because it has antimicrobial, anti-dyspepsia and beneficial digestive properties. Note: Avoid garlic if you take blood thinners, prior to surgery and/or have hypoglycemia.

Ginger

Ginger is a root that has been used for centuries for digestion and a poor appetite. It acts as an anti spasmodic and stimulates the gastrointestinal tract. Ginger is thought to have a mild antibiotic effect against various bacteria. It also has some anti inflammatory properties. Ginger is not well tolerated by those with a sensitive stomach as it is a hot herb. Typical dosage is 500 mgs two to three times a day or taken fresh with hot water.

Probiotics

Probiotics such as acidophilus and bifidobacterium are beneficial bacteria. They help re-colonize the beneficial bacteria in the GI tract. You always have bad and good bacteria in your gut. If these bad and good floras become imbalanced, your gastrointestinal lining may become irritated. Bifidobacterium has also been shown to suppress Helicobacter pylori. The bacterium, Helicobacter pylori, causes peptic ulcers, anemia and gastric cancer. Products that are not refrigerated may be a dead culture, which does not help the beneficial flora to grow. Take as directed on the label.

Zinc

Zinc is a mineral that is useful for a number of functions in the body. It helps to keep the immune system running well, it aids in healing and acts on the sex organs. Zinc carnosine is particularly useful in healing the lining of the stomach. Zinc carnosine aids in ulcers by increasing the mucoprotective layer of the stomach lining. It inhibits the growth of the Helicobacter pylori bacteria that causes ulcers. Typical dosage of zinc carnosine for ulcers is 150 mgs per day. Note: Do not use if you are pregnant or nursing.

HOMEOPATHIC REMEDIES FOR GASTRITIS

There are many homeopathic remedies for gastritis. Some of the more common remedies are listed with their symptoms here. For more information on how to self prescribe a homeopathic remedy, go to Chapter Two. If you cannot find a remedy suited to you, or find you are not improving or your symptoms get worse, seek the help of a professional homeopath or your medical doctor.

ACONITE
Common indications include:
- pains are terrible and agonizing
- person is full of fears
- **symptoms come on suddenly**
- **high fever and dry heat**
- burning in the stomach that travels all the way up to the mouth
- **intense thirst** for cold water
- **heart palpitations**
- **profuse perspiration**
- **cutting, burning and sore pains**
- weight in the stomach as a stone
- **red face or one cheek looks red and the other looks pale**
- vomiting of bile, mucous and/or blood
- **ailments from shock or fright**
- **inflammation and pain after eating or drinking cold things**
- **mentally these types are restless and anxious**
- **panic attacks, fear of death, flying and crowds**
- **desires cold drinks**
- **aggravated by from exposure to cold air or wind**, at night, in bed, warm room and from shock
- relieved by open air, drinking and rest

ARGENTUM NITRICUM
Common indications include:
- **craving for sugar which aggravates the stomach**
- **loud belching**
- food lodges in the throat
- expelling gas relieves symptoms
- pain in the stomach pit that radiates in all directions
- bending double relieves the pains
- pains increase and decrease gradually
- **faint with gastric problems**
- tendency to stomach ulcers
- **very hot-blooded types and worse for heat**
- **these types have ailments from anticipation**
- **fear of being late, alone and of heights**

- **relieved by belching**, by warm drinks and alcohol
- aggravated by pressure, any food, especially sweets, cold food and drinks
- worse one hour or immediately after eating

ARSENICUM ALBUM
Common indications include:
- watery belching
- **burning in the stomach like fire**
- these types are cold and weak
- nausea with a **low appetite**
- heartburn feels like a fire, as if hot coals are against the affected parts
- chronic digestive disturbance
- irritation of the mucous membrane of the stomach
- **white tongue**
- red tongue with thin white silvery coating, may have red raised taste buds
- stomach ulcers
- dry mouth with intense thirst
- cold water sits in the stomach like a stone
- **suited to chilly, restless and anxious types**
- **improved by drinking small sips of hot drinks despite suffering burning heat**
- worsened by changing of weather, cold and damp, lying with the head low
- **worse after midnight, from ice, cold drinks**, spoiled meat, alcohol, lobster and salad

BRYONIA
Common indications include:
- bitter taste in mouth from belching
- food and drink tastes bitter
- watery belching
- **dryness of all mucous membranes, such as the mouth and throat**
- sensation of a stone in the pit of the stomach
- **rheumatism** may alternate with indigestion
- better after burping
- **great thirst for cold water with dry mouth**
- sharp pains after eating that may extend to the shoulders
- **white or brown coating on tongue**
- heartburn from drinking cold water when the person is overheated
- stomach sensitive to touch and lying still improves their symptoms
- **suited to irritable types who want to be left alone and still**
- craving for coffee and wine
- **relieved by pressure**
- **worse at 9:00 p.m.**, after eating and from vegetables, sauerkraut, cabbage, potatoes, acids, warm drinks

LYCOPODIUM

Common indications include:

- sensation of fullness from the stomach up to throat
- food may be regurgitated through the nose
- food may taste sour
- water brash
- **sour belching with or without regurgitation**
- difficulty swallowing liquids, feels as if pharynx is closed
- **distended and full after least amount of food**
- heartburn with white tongue
- **least pressure of clothes bothersome**
- flatulence and constipation
- **may be suited to types with low self esteem, anger from contradiction, fear of public speaking**
- **craving for sweets**, alcohol, warm drinks and food
- **aggravated by cold drinks**, milk, cabbage, wheat, beans, onions, wine, rye and beer

MERCURIUS CORROSIVUS

Common indications include:

- increased saliva
- extreme weakness
- tendency to ulcers
- **feels as if beaten or sore, stitching and burning pain**
- distension of the stomach
- **green and bilious vomit**
- cold perspiration
- vomit that can be stringy, blood tinged or look like coffee grounds
- coffee ground vomit (could be a sign of bleeding in the stomach)
- anxiety
- **extreme thirst and a desire for cold drinks**
- **aggravated by drinking milk**, acids, fats, after stool, swallowing and motion
- improved with rest

NUX VOMICA

Common indications include:

- **sour, bitter acid and watery belching and vomiting**
- sour taste in the morning after eating
- **ailments after drinking too much**
- heartburn may occur before breakfast
- pain in the stomach like a weight or pressure, two or three hours after meals
- **bloating and distension**
- putrid bitter taste in the mouth

- **pressing, beaten pains**
- **unproductive retching and/or stool**
- squeezing stomachaches, tender stomach
- aversion to food with nausea
- **stone sensation in the stomach**
- reverse peristalsis, spasms from disordered peristalsis, pain when food passes down into the pyloric sphincter
- acute indigestion of improper foods
- **tightness of the abdomen after eating, must loosen pants**
- altered sense of taste for milk, coffee, water and beer
- **may be suited to zealous, fiery temperaments who overindulge and overwork**
- cravings for fats and tolerates them well
- **cravings for tea, coffee, alcohol and spicy**
- worse after eating, drug use, tobacco poisoning, **overeating, overindulgence, alcohol, spices, stimulants, tea and coffee**

SULPHUR
Common indications include:

- **burning into the throat with sour belching**
- **burning stomach pains**
- regurgitation of food tastes acid shortly after a meal
- water brash and saliva after eating
- **sour, vomiting after eating**
- feels full after eating a little
- **heavy after eating**
- **hearty appetite**, must eat simply as most foods turn sour, does well on soup
- **hunger at 11:00 a.m.**
- tendency to eat too quickly and not chew food well
- sinking sensation in epigastrum
- taste in mouth like rotten eggs
- loss of appetite
- may be worse in spring and fall
- gastric complaints may alternate with skin conditions
- **may be suited to lazy, intellectual and/or slovenly types**
- **skin eruptions are common in this remedy**
- **cravings for sweets, fats, spices, alcohol, beer and ale**
- aggravated in the morning, after eating, eggs, milk products, sweets, honey, alcohol
- worse before the menstrual flow

Gastroparesis

Gastroparesis is an unusual condition where the stomach takes a long time to empty its contents. This condition is one that is not common so there are very few remedies for this condition. The stomach is under the ribs and is about the size of a small melon. It can expand to a gallon of liquid. The stomach normally contracts and pushes food down into the small intestine using various muscles. The stomach normally takes about three hours to empty depending on what types of food have been eaten. A nerve called the vagus nerve is in control of the movement of food through the gastrointestinal tract. This nerve reaches from the brainstem to the colon. It helps to conduct signals to the digestive tract when to contract and move food along. This condition is thought to occur when the vagus nerve, stomach muscles or intestines do not function properly. Food moves slowly or not at all.

What is the Cause of Gastroparesis?

- Diabetes is a common cause of gastroparesis. People who have diabetes usually have high blood sugar which over time damages the blood vessels. This may cut off the blood, oxygen and nutrient supply to certain nerves. The vagus nerve may be damaged by diabetes which in turn causes poor gastric emptying.
- Any surgeries that involve the esophagus, stomach or small intestine may damage the vagus nerve.
- Anorexia or bulimia may cause gastroparesis because vomiting and starvation alters the metabolism and nerve conduction.
- Medication such as anti-depressants, calcium channel blockers, chemotherapy, lithium and narcotics may interfere with the vagus nerve.
- Diseases such as Parkinson's disease, hypothyroidism and multiple sclerosis.
- Medical tests may find no known reason for this disturbance.

What are the Symptoms of Gastroparesis?

- Feeling of fullness after eating very little
- Pain or spasms in the upper abdomen
- Nausea and vomiting of undigested food even hours after a meal
- Weight loss due to poor digestion of nutrients and low caloric intake
- Distension of the abdomen
- Fluctuating blood sugar levels

What are the Complications of Gastroparesis?

- Bacterial overgrowth may happen in the stomach when food sits and ferments.
- Food can harden in the stomach and solidify. These masses are called bezoars. These masses can cause an obstruction in the stomach which leads to nausea and vomiting.
- Gastroparesis can make blood sugar levels unstable and hard to manage. This is because food has been delayed going into the small intestine. The delivery of food may seem as though it has been consumed much later then it has, causing lows in blood sugar.
- Depression may be a consequence of this disorder. Many who have it can suffer from many gastrointestinal symptoms and not absorb nutrients that help with energy and a healthy mood.

How is Gastroparesis Diagnosed?

- Your medical doctor will try to rule out an intestinal blockage through various tests.
- Various tools are used to detect this disorder. An upper endoscopy checks the stomach by using a scope. An ultrasound of the abdomen may be performed to detect any other abnormalities such as gallbladder stones or pancreatic abnormalities. A barium x-ray is used to detect food still in the stomach even 12 hours after fasting. The barium is a thick liquid that lines the stomach so it is visible on an x-ray.
- A gastric emptying scintigraphy is a test that involves one eating something that contains a radioisotope that is detected on the scans. This can measure the rate at which the stomach empties at different intervals. There is a breath test as well that is said to measure the presence of food in the stomach. There are many other tests that can detect the way the stomach empties such as an MRI or electrogastrogram.

What Treatments are Used for Gastroparesis?

There are a few medications that doctors may use to treat this disorder. If one has a damaged vagus nerve from injury or surgery, a feeding tube may be required. This tube bypasses the stomach and puts food directly into the small intestine. Most drugs work to stimulate gastric contractions and help empty the stomach. Antibiotics may be prescribed to kill the bacteria. Antacids, anti-nausea and laxatives may be used. Check with your doctor to see what medication would be most appropriate for you.

DIETARY TREATMENTS FOR GASTROPARESIS

Changing your eating habits is crucial for those with gastroparesis. Eat small meals more frequently rather than three large meals. Some people puree food and may do well with it. Eating a low glycemic diet is very beneficial. Foods that are low glycemic flip into a sugar much less quickly in the bloodstream. High glycemic foods make blood sugar unstable and can lead to diabetic tendencies. As mentioned earlier, this can damage the vagus nerve which signals for the stomach to empty its contents.

Some authorities say that fibre is hard to digest for people with gastroparesis. It takes longer to break down. Food combining is described in the third chapter on healthy eating. In a nutshell, it helps people to optimize their natural ability to digest and absorb nutrients from their foods. Combining certain foods helps one to utilize one's digestive chemistry to the fullest. Eat fruit alone and at least a half hour or more away from other foods. Combine starches with vegetables and combine protein or fat with vegetables. Do not eat fruit with any other food and don't combine protein or fat with starches.

Fruit is a simple carbohydrate. They are digested very quickly if you eat them on an empty stomach. If you combine them with any other complex carbohydrate or fat you may find that you have a lot of gas, bloating and pains. This is because the fruit that is normally digested and absorbed very quickly ferments when it is mixed with other types of foods. It creates a gassy soup of bacteria which ferments and turns into alcohols, acetic acids and vinegars.

Starches are things like potatoes, rice, bread, pasta and crackers. Proteins are fish, meats and legumes. Legumes also fall into the starch category. They are best combined with grains to get all the required amino acids. Usually these amino acids are found in meat and in combination with legumes and grains. Fats are things like nuts, seeds, oils and animal fats.

The bright side of being shot!

Back in 1822, a fur trapper named Alexis St. Martin accidentally shot himself in the side and left a permanent opening into his stomach. Ouch! A U.S. Army surgeon Dr. William Beaumont carried a series of experiments out on Alexis over 11 years. He dangled different food stuffs into the opening to see how long they took to digest.

In 1833 Beaumont published his findings with great praise.

Source: *Body; An Amazing Tour of the Human Body,* by Richard Walker (see bibliography).

SUPPLEMENTS FOR GASTROPARESIS

Aloe Vera Juice

Aloe vera juice is very healing to the lining of the gastrointestinal tract. It is said to be a tonic, laxative, stimulate bile flow, eliminates parasites and heal the stomach. Aloe works as a cathartic laxative which stimulates intestinal contractions that cause bowel movements.

Typical dosage is one tablespoon to three ounces, one to three times daily. Start with the lowest dose and increase it until you find your comfort zone. If you take too much Aloe Vera, you may suffer from cramps and diarrhea. Take aloe vera three or more hours away from medication because it may reduce the absorption of some prescription drugs. This supplement is not suited to those who suffer from diarrhea, heavy periods, kidney disease and/or are pregnant.

B12

Vitamin B12 is a nutrient that is often deficient in those with gastroparesis. There are various other nutrients that are low in these types. Iron and calcium may also be low because they are one of the most difficult nutrients to digest and absorb. Typical dosage of B12 is 1,000 micromilligrams (mcgs) per day.

Digestive Enzymes

Digestive enzymes are a means for the body to break down foods and absorb their nutrients. Our body naturally makes digestive enzymes through the liver, the pancreas and stomach. If you do not have good digestion, digestive enzymes act as insurance for proper absorption. Partially or improperly digested foods cause many health issues, such as heartburn, food allergies and constipation.

Digestive enzymes usually include protease, which aids in protein digestion, lipase, which aids in fat digestion and amylase or cellulose which aids in carbohydrate digestion. Some digestive enzymes contain Betaine HCL, which helps with protein digestion. Take it as directed on the package. This supplement is not suited to those with high acidity, intestinal or stomach ulcers.

Ginger

Ginger is a root that has been used for centuries for digestion and a poor appetite. It acts as an anti spasmodic and stimulates the gastrointestinal tract. Ginger is thought to have a mild antibiotic effect against various bacteria. It also has some anti inflammatory properties. Ginger is not well tolerated by those with a sensitive stomach as it is a hot herb. Typical dosage is 500 mgs two to three times a day or taken fresh with hot water.

Probiotics

Every person has billions of bacteria in their intestinal tract. Most bacteria are beneficial and maintain health. A small percentage of bacteria in our intestines are harmful if they spread. Those who have gastroparesis tend to have more bad bacteria because the food sits and ferments in the stomach. These bad bacteria overgrow and cause immune dysfunction, infections, constipation and/or diarrhea.

Good flora helps to maintain the immune system and displace the bad bacteria in the gut. It also helps to sustain normal arrangement and function of the intestine's cells. The most popular beneficial bacteria are lactobacillus acidophilus and Bifidobacteria. The lactobacilli can be found in fermented foods such as yogurt, miso, tempeh and kefir. However, the number of bacteria is not standardized. The bacteria may not be an active culture if they are not stored properly.

It is best to use a standardized capsule of probiotics. It should be stored in the refrigerator which helps ensure that it is a live culture. Follow the directions on the package. Typical dosage for a probiotic supplement is one to 10 billion cells per capsule. One to three capsules can be taken daily. There are no known side effects from probiotics.

HOMEOPATHIC REMEDIES FOR GASTROPARESIS

There are many homeopathic remedies for gastroparesis. Some of the more common remedies are listed with their symptoms here. For more information on how to self prescribe a homeopathic remedy, go to Chapter Two. If you cannot find a remedy suited to you, or find you are not improving or your symptoms get worse, seek the help of a professional homeopath or your medical doctor.

EUPATORIUM PERFOLIATUM

Common indications include:
- bitter or tasteless belching
- sensation of an obstruction
- **great thirst for cold drinks**
- vomiting or purging of bile
- hiccoughs
- weakness even to faint
- soreness in the region of the liver
- **tendency to bone pains**
- abdomen is full and distended
- restlessness with great desire to move

NATRUM CARBONICUM

Common indications include:
- very weak digestion
- sleepy after meals
- **dyspepsia**
- **food allergies**
- watery, sour burping and much flatulence
- diarrhea from milk products
- these types can be sluggish physically and mentally and sensitive to heat
- these types catch many colds
- **these types are gentle and refined, sensitive to music**
- **aggravated by milk**, vegetables, cold drinks and starches

NUX VOMICA
Common indications include:
- **stomach is very sensitive to pressure**
- food sits heavily in the stomach for many hours after eating
- **cramping and sharp pains**
- **constipation with ineffectual urging**
- bloating under the ribs with pressure as of a stone
- these types crave stimulants, fats, tobacco or coffee
- **these types tend to have constipation and reverse peristalsis (where the muscles of the throat, stomach and intestines may not contract in a sequence)**
- passing only small quantities of stool with much urging
- **craving for alcohol, spices and fats**
- **aggravated by overindulgence, morning**, after eating, in cold weather
- improved in the evening while resting, after a bowel movement

NUX MOSCHATA
Common indications include:
- **mouth is very dry and saliva is like cotton**
- **dry eyes**
- **tongue is dry and adheres to the roof of the mouth**
- after eating they are soon full
- pain in the stomach shortly after eating
- abdomen is very distended after each meal
- **stubborn constipation, must remove the stool with one's finger**
- **overwhelming sleepiness and feeling spaced out**
- **forgetful; for example, forgetting why one has come into a room**
- aggravation from cold food and water, after eating or drinking and spirituous liquors
- relieved by wrapping up warmly

OPIUM
Common indications include:

- heaviness in the stomach
- vomiting and pains in the stomach
- slow and weak digestion
- bowels seem to not move at all
- **constipation with no urging**
- **sleep apnea, heavy sleep and/or stupor**
- sensitive and inflated sensation of the stomach
- distended with no powers to eliminate food or stools
- intestines are very sluggish and even the strongest laxatives lose their power
- stools may be hard black balls
- **these types may be dopey or apathetic**
- **aggravated by fright**, stimulants, fear and liquor
- relieved by cold, open air and walking

Globus Hystericus

Globus hystericus is also known as globus sensation, globus pharyngitis or globus. It is a term that means the sensation of having a lump in one's throat. It is the sensation of a remaining lump, object or phlegm. Swallowing is not impeded with this disorder but there may be some inflammation in the larynx. It can be related to other disorders such as reflux or psychological diseases like neurosis, depression or anxiety. This disorder is hard to find natural remedies for. The best way to combat globus is to use homeopathic remedies.

HOMEOPATHIC REMEDIES FOR GLOBUS HYSTERICUS

There are many homeopathic remedies for globus hystericus. Some of the more common remedies are listed with their symptoms here. For more information on how to self prescribe a homeopathic remedy, go to Chapter Two. If you cannot find a remedy suited to you, or find you are not improving or your symptoms get worse, seek the help of a professional homeopath or your medical doctor.

ASAFOETIDA
Common indications include:
- this is a good remedy for hysteria that comes on after suppressing chronic discharges
- **empty or ineffectual belching**
- **sensation of a lump or a plug in the throat** that causes frequent swallowing
- **abdomen very bloated without any passing any flatulence but much burping**
- discharges (for example, a running ulcer, suppressed diarrhea)
- **globus hystericus**
- the bowels, stomach and throat have **reverse peristalsis**, which is a reversal of the natural movement. For example, food goes upward instead of down
- **sensation of a lump or bubble in the stomach rising into the throat**
- spasms and nervous irritability
- **mentally these types may be hysterical**

IGNATIA
Common indications include:
- **moods that may alternate quickly**, for example weeping and laughing
- **these types tend to be suffering from grief, broken heart or humiliation**
- **tendency to sigh and yawn often**
- **choking and constricted feeling**
- **a lump in the throat** that is relieved by belching
- **stitching pain when swallowing**
- spasms in the throat, convulsions and cramps
- **aggravated by grief**, coffee, tobacco, emotions and after eating
- relieved with hard pressure and warmth

MOSCHUS
Common indications include:
- spasm in the throat or glottis
- attacks of fainting or unconsciousness
- pale or blue face
- skin is cold
- spasms of the chest that cause a fear of death
- anxiety with heart palpitations
- **mentally these types are hysterical and have fits of anger**
- **rising sensation of a lump in the throat**
- aggravated by cold, excitement, suppression and eating
- relieved by fresh open air and getting warm

NUX MOSCHATA
Common indications include:
- impaired digestion
- heaviness in the stomach after each meal
- gulps up air which lead to a sensation of a lump in the throat
- lump in throat is relieved by belching
- similar to ignatia with its frequent changing of moods
- thirstless with dry mouth and throat
- **these types are absent-minded and may be spaced out**
- **forgetful of why came to get something**
- **sensation of dry mouth and tongue (cotton mouth)**
- **tongue so dry it adheres to the roof of the mouth**
- **these types are sleepy**
- aggravated by emotions, menstrual periods, pregnancy, cold food and drink, alcoholic drinks and after eating
- relieved by warmth and wrapping up warmly

VALERIAN

Common indications include:

- a warm sensation moves up from stomach into the throat
- sensation of rising lump in the throat
- lump felt whilst sleeping
- nervousness that comes on during menopause or around the menstrual cycle
- sensation of a thread is hanging down deep in the throat which tickles
- slightest pain causes fainting
- sensitive to smells
- these types tend to be anxious, animated and better moving about
- facial nerve pains and sciatica

Halitosis/Bad Breath

Halitosis is a condition that is characterized by foul smelling breath. It can be a persistent and embarrassing problem. It may be worth a visit to the dentist to be sure that an underlying infection or gum disease isn't the cause. There are many causes of bad breath, most of which can be rectified through diet or natural treatments.

What are the causes of bad breath?

- Poor dental hygiene causes bad breath. This would result in mouth bacteria from tooth decay, gum disease or not brushing and flossing properly. Flossing removes decaying food particles from the teeth and prevents gum disease. Both the teeth, gums and tongue need to be brushed on a regular basis. Some dentists recommend a tongue scraper, mouth wash, frequent brushing and periodic check ups to combat this problem.
- Diet that includes eating strong tasting foods, like spices, pepperoni, curry, blue cheese, fish, onions, garlic and excessive protein naturally affects the breath. Fasting can cause bad breath because it may induce ketosis, which is when people break down fats in the liver into usable energy.
- Post nasal drip, sinus, lung and throat disease or infections are linked to foul breath. The odour can be from old mucous and/or bacterial infections.
- Constipation, bad bacteria in the colon and gas affect the mouth flora.
- Bad breath can also be a result of a dry mouth caused by decreased saliva. Saliva rinses the mouth of food particles that cause odour. Certain medications like anti-psychotics or antidepressants may cause dry mouth. Breathing through the mouth may also dry the mouth and throat. Mouth breathing results from blocked nasal passages, polyps or a broken nose.
- Dehydration can cause bad breath. Fluids help to flush out the mouth of bacteria.
- Underlying diseases such as diabetes, kidney and liver disease are linked to halitosis. Liver disease can make breath smell fishy. Urine or breath like mothballs can be related to kidney disease. Fruity breath is linked to diabetes. Diabetics tend to suffer from gum disease more than the general population. This can be another cause of bad breath, as mentioned earlier.

DIETARY MEASURES FOR HALITOSIS

Dietary measures for halitosis include avoiding offending foods that typically cause bad breath. Foods that were mentioned earlier are blue cheese, curry, fish, garlic, onions and excessive protein consumption. Drink lots of water to flush the bad bacteria away from the mouth. It also helps to keep hydrated and saliva flowing. Parsley is an herb that is useful in absorbing bad odours. Chew some from time to time or after eating something with a strong flavor. A healthy diet is one that consists of a wide variety of fruits, vegetables, lean proteins, legumes and whole grains. This diet, along with eating lower glycemic and lower fat foods, helps to keep your body healthy. Lower glycemic foods flip into a sugar less quickly in the blood stream. If you eat foods that turn into sugar quickly in the bloodstream, they feed the bad bacteria that can cause foul breath. For a list of low glycemic foods, see the chart outlined in Chapter Three.

Because diabetics typically suffer from gum disease more often then the general public, be sure to eat wisely. Eat low glycemic, low fat foods and have a lean protein with each meal. This helps to keep blood sugar stable and prevents spikes and lows. Eat healthy snacks between meals, such as nuts, yogurt, low fat cheese or fresh cut vegetables. People with kidney disease are usually asked to avoid salt and reduce animal protein consumption.

Morning Breath Anyone?
Spit is composed of 99% water, a dash of mucous and contains many nifty chemicals to kill bacteria. When you sleep, your saliva glands produce much less saliva and it does not wash out the accumulated bacteria. There are approximately 10 billion bacteria in the mouth that multiply as you slumber. This is the reason that many of us have bad breath in the morning!
Source: *Oh Yuck; The Encyclopedia of Everything Nasty*, by Joy Masaff
(see bibliography)

Some people who have bad breath due to an underlying infection of the sinus, lung or throat may do well by avoiding sugars, refined carbohydrates and dairy products. Sugars and refined carbohydrates feed the bad bacteria. Have you ever noticed how kids get sick after a birthday party with lots of cake and sweets? This is because sugar depresses the immune system temporarily after its consumption. Dairy products tend to be mucous forming and this traps bacteria. Eliminate milk, ice cream, yogurt and cheeses and you will notice you don't produce as much phlegm.

SUPPLEMENTS FOR HALITOSIS

Chlorophyll

Chlorophyll is a substance that is found in green foods like wheat grass, alfalfa and barley greens. It helps to absorb and neutralize bad odours. It freshens the breath and acts as an internal deodourizer. For bad breath, take one teaspoon per day. There are no contraindications with chlorophyll; however, the green pigment is known to stain clothing.

Probiotics

Probiotics such as acidophilus and Bifidobacterium are beneficial bacteria. They help to re-colonize the flora in the GI tract. Everyone always has bad and good bacteria in their gut. Bad breath may result when there an imbalance of good and bad bacteria. Probiotic supplementation may be helpful for halitosis therapy by maintaining a greater ratio of friendly bacteria.

Tea Tree Oil

Tea tree oil is an herb made from the leaves of an Australian tree called melaleuca alternifolia. It is used as an antiseptic, antibacterial and antifungal. It is a component in many natural toothpastes and mouth wash.

Vitamin A

Vitamin A is an excellent supplement to aid in the healing of the mouth and gums. It helps to heal ulcers, skin lesions and aids in vision. It is known as an antioxidant which hinders cellular damage that leads to the aging process. The typical dosage for Vitamin A is 10,000 IU per day. Vitamin A in high doses, such as over 100,000 international units can be toxic. Beta Carotene is a precursor to vitamin A and has no toxic effects if taken in larger doses. The skin may turn an orange tinge, however it is not harmful.

Vitamin C

Vitamin C deficiency is common in mouth and gum disease. A sign of it is bleeding gums and gingivitis. Because it helps with immunity, it helps to control bacterial infections and reduces inflammation. 1,000 to 3,000 mgs of vitamin C can be taken daily.

Zinc

Zinc deficiency is associated with poor healing, immunity and inflammation. Halitosis from oral disease can benefit from zinc supplementation. Typical dosage of zinc is from 15-25mgs per day with meals. Zinc is a mineral that can be toxic in higher doses. Do not take more than 40 mgs per day. A zinc overdose produces dizziness, sweating, headaches, nausea, vomiting and a metallic taste in the mouth.

HOMEOPATHIC REMEDIES FOR HALITOSIS

There are many homeopathic remedies for halitosis. Some of the more common remedies are listed with their symptoms here. For more information on how to self prescribe a homeopathic remedy, go to Chapter Two. If you cannot find a remedy suited to you, or find you are not improving or your symptoms get worse, seek the help of a professional homeopath or your medical doctor.

CARBO VEGETABILIS
Common indications include:
- **offensive breath**
- **breath feels cold**
- **dry mouth**
- tongue is covered with canker sores
- gums are retracted and bleed easily

- **bitter and putrid taste in the mouth**
- boils in the gums and/or loose teeth
- sensation of a lump from tough mucous in the throat
- these types tend to have a lot of flatulence and burping
- **belching which improves the distension of the stomach**
- **short of breath from gas or overeating**
- **these types want to be fanned**
- aggravated by butter, pork and fat
- relieved with belching, being fanned and loosening the clothing

CARBOLIC ACID
Common indications include:
- constipation and **offensive breath**
- ulcerated patches in the mouth and throat
- **redness of the throat**
- pus-like lesions and film covering the mouth
- painful swallowing and burning
- the middle of the tongue is coated with white and yellow fur
- relieved with smoking and drinking strong tea

MERCURIUS SOLUBILIS
Common indications include:
- **saliva is increased** and the tongue is moist
- tongue is swollen and the teeth leave imprints on it
- **gums are swollen, bleed easily** and recede from the teeth
- very foul breath
- **foul, metallic, bitter and/or salty taste in mouth**
- **ulcers in the mouth and throat**
- **teeth have cavities**
- **throat painful with stitching on swallowing**
- tendency to sores and ulcers
- salty metallic taste in the mouth
- these people have a very strong thirst

NUX VOMICA
Common indications include:
- **sour or bitter taste in the mouth**
- **dry mouth** in the morning
- **canker sores** on the tongue
- **bitter, putrid and sour taste**
- these types are often addicted to the use of wine or coffee
- **these types are irritable, fiery, competitive and workaholics**
- **cravings for alcohol, fats, spices, coffee and stimulants**
- **aggravated by overeating and drinking**

RHEUM

Common indications include:

- very sour smell comes from the person, the breath, perspiration and skin
- these types have a tendency to diarrhea
- foul tasting mucous in the mouth
- perspiration from the waist up
- worse after bowel elimination and eating

SULPHUR

Common indications include:

- foul, metallic, **sweet, sour, bitter, slimy taste in the mouth**
- **sour odour and taste in the mouth**, worse after drinking milk
- mouth is dry in the morning
- swollen gums
- tendency to skin symptoms
- very hungry types
- desire for alcohol and sweets
- burning of all mucous membranes
- aggravated by milk, alcohol, suppressed discharges and in the morning
- relieved with open air

Hemorrhoids/Piles

Hemorrhoids or piles are characterized by swelling and inflammation of the veins of the anus or rectum. Similar to varicose veins, the elasticity of the anal veins weaken and form a small pouch where blood collects. They can be external (outside the anus) or internal (inside the anus). Often hemorrhoids simply resolve themselves in a few days. However, some people tend to suffer from them more than others.

Symptoms of Hemorrhoids

Symptoms of hemorrhoids may include bleeding after stools, itching and a swollen lump at the anal opening. Blood may be present on the stool, in the bowl or on wiping. There may be pain in the rectum during and after stools and on sitting.

What Conditions are Linked to Hemorrhoids?

Conditions that contribute to this problem are constipation, sitting for prolonged periods of time, pregnancy and aging.

- Constipation with urging for stools puts pressure on the lower pelvic floor.
- Heavy lifting can cause a hemorrhoid strain.
- Pushing during childbirth and/or heavy lifting also adds strain on that area.
- Pregnancy naturally puts a lot of pressure in the veins of the pelvic area. They have more blood flow and baby weight. People who are expecting also tend to have constipation more than others. If you are expecting be sure to eat a lot of fibre filled foods like whole grains, beans, fruits and vegetables.
- Extra body weight contributes to hemorrhoid development.

- Sitting for long periods of time creates a lot of pressure in the rectal area. Blood flow is less likely to become stagnant if one exercises. The capillaries push the blood flow all around the body. It is enhanced when one exercises and moves around. As people age, the vessels in the anal area may weaken.

Medical Treatments for Hemorrhoids

- Sitz baths are recommended to those who have had surgery in the area of the rectum or to ease the pain of hemorrhoids. This is a bath that can be placed on the toilet and is filled with warm or cold water. Some people put salt in the water to help dry out a wound. Warm water is best for soothing the pain of hemorrhoids.
- Surgery may be required in some cases. A rubber band ligation is a procedure where the doctor puts a tiny rubber band around the bottom of the hemorrhoid. This cuts off the circulation and it then just falls off. This is a simple procedure done in the doctor's office. Sclerotherapy is a process where the doctor injects a chemical solution to quell the blood supply through the vessel. This shrinks the hemorrhoid. There are a few other procedures such as stapling or a full surgery. The surgery is used if the other treatments were not successful or if you have large hemorrhoids. A local anesthetic or general anesthetic is used and the hemorrhoid is cut out.
- Topical analgesics, compresses or pads are used to dull the pain and sooth the hemorrhoid. Witch hazel pads or cortisone cream may be recommended.

DIETARY MEASURES FOR HEMORRHOIDS

Diet is crucial for health and proper digestion. Drink eight to 10 glasses of water per day. Coffee and tea do not count, as they have a dehydrating effect on the tissues. Water is perfect and has no calories. Water keeps you hydrated and prevents constipation. The typical recommended dosage of water is eight glasses per day.

Diet is crucial in preventing and healing hemorrhoids. Eat a high fibre diet that includes lots of fruits, vegetables and whole grains. Read Chapter Three on healthy eating. Consume low glycemic and healthy fats, found in primarily in column one of the chart in chapter three. These foods are higher in fibre and decrease the prevalence of many other diseases such as heart disease, diabetes, cancer and hormone imbalances.

When you are filling your plate, visualize it like a pie. Grains should represent only a quarter of your plate. Another quarter should be a lean protein or legumes. The other half should be fruits and vegetables. Eat a wide variety of colours of fruits and vegetables to ensure that you are getting optimum nutrition from your food. For example, orange vegetables are high in beta carotene and dark leafy vegetables contain folic acid. Try to consume mostly raw fruits and vegetables because they have more nutrients than cooked.

Foods to limit and/or avoid:

Sugar, alcohol and refined carbohydrates feed bad bacteria in the gut that cause constipation. These foods do not contain fibre. Animal protein and fat can make your system more acidic. An acidic condition can lead to inflammatory conditions such as arthritis, gout, heart disease, irritable bowel and muscle pains.

Foods that are beneficial for constipation:

Foods that are high fibre help with constipation. Increase your fibre slowly every day. Some people experience cramps or diarrhea if they have a steep increase in fibre at once. Examples of high fibre foods are brussels sprouts, kale, cabbage, cooked legumes, ground flaxseed and whole grains. Whole grains that are high in fibre are brown rice, bulgur, millet, oat bran, slow cooked oatmeal, quinoa, whole wheat and wheat bran.

SUPPLEMENTS FOR HEMORRHOIDS

Horse Chestnut

Horse chestnut is an herb made from a tree that grows fruits that are brown, small and prickly. The parts used are bark, flowers, leaves and seeds. It has medicinal value in helping to strengthen the veins and circulation. It helps to decrease the swelling in the veins and causes constriction of the veins and reduces the permeability of the veins.

Typical dosage for horse chestnut is 300 mgs twice per day. Side effects from horse chestnut may include dizziness, nausea and headaches. However, it is usually well tolerated. This herb is not suitable during pregnancy and in those with liver damage, latex allergy or kidney disease.

Psyllium Fibre

Any fibre source is beneficial for hemorrhoids, because it prevents the straining of constipation which aggravates the veins in the rectal area. Psyllium is a type of bulking agent that is useful in those who tend to become constipated. If you do not drink enough water, do not bother taking psyllium as it needs water to expand. If you become dehydrated, it will sit and cause more constipation. However, it expands with water and gently scrubs along the intestinal walls to clean out the bowels.

Vitamin C and E

Vitamin C is useful for healing and strengthening the blood vessels. Another vitamin, namely vitamin E, is excellent for that as well. Take 1,000 to 2,000 mgs of vitamin C daily. Take 400 IU of vitamin E per day.

HOMEOPATHIC REMEDIES FOR HEMORRHOIDS

There are many good homeopathic remedies that help hemorrhoids. Some of the more common remedies are listed with their symptoms here. For more information on how to self prescribe a homeopathic remedy, go to Chapter Two. If you cannot find a remedy suited to you, or find you are not improving or your symptoms get worse, seek the help of a professional homeopath or your medical doctor. An external application made of the mother tincture of Aesculus, Hamamelis, Phytolacca and olive oil helps to soothe and shrink piles. The rest of these remedies are taken orally.

AESCULUS
Common indications include:
- purple **hemorrhoids** with or without a backache
- **pain as if full of sticks**
- **rectal pains are sharp, sticking, burning, sore and/or with urging**

- stool may be stuck and ulceration of the veins may happen
- sensation of fullness in the anus
- **sharp pains that radiate upwards from the rectum into the back**
- intense rectal pain for hours after a bowel movement
- **itching of the rectum**
- **hemorrhoids associated with back pain or sciatica**
- constipation with difficulty passing stools
- **worse after passing stool, moving, walking** and after washing
- relieved by warmth

COLLINSONIA
Common indications include:
- stubborn hemorrhoids that bleed continually
- itching of the anus
- **bleeding hemorrhoids**
- **pain during stools**
- congestion of the veins in the lower pelvic area
- painful and bleeding piles
- sensation of sticks, sand or gravel in the rectum
- **constipation with ineffectual urging**, hard stools, alternates with diarrhea
- hemorrhoids during pregnancy especially in the later months
- worse with suppression of hemorrhoids (such as after surgery other symptoms appear), during pregnancy and from emotions
- relieved by warmth

HAMAMELIS
Common indications include:
- hemorrhoids that bleed very profusely
- sore, heavy and burning sensation in the rectum
- anus feels as if it is raw and chapped
- **bleeding hemorrhoids, especially after stool**
- **external hemorrhoids**
- blood may be profuse and very dark
- aggravated by pressure, riding in a car and touch
- relief from resting and lying

NUX VOMICA
Common indications include:
- **bleeding hemorrhoids**
- **irritability with hemorrhoids**
- **constipation from sedentary habits**
- **constipation with ineffectual urging**
- **cutting pains after stools**
- hemorrhoids come on after overeating, alcohol, spices and stimulants

- **painful constriction of the rectum**
- **sticking, stinging and pressing pains**
- itchy piles that may prevent the sleep
- sensation as if part of the stool is still in the rectum
- **mentally these types tend to be competitive, workaholics and irritable**
- **aggravated by overeating, spices, stimulants, alcohol** and prolonged sedentary lifestyle
- relief from rest, warmth and passing stools

PAEONIA

Common indications include:

- **burning and cutting pains after stool, lasts for hours**
- itching and swelling of the anus
- these types may suffer from pasty sudden stools
- **rectal pains**
- chills felt after stools
- constipation or diarrhea
- extreme pain after stool
- person may have to lie for a time with buttocks separate to prevent touching the painful area
- **aggravated by touch of the rectum**

Picture this….

A young man aged 21complained that he could not sit down. He had long-lasting rectal pains after a bowel movement. His rectum was itching and burning. He was not eating properly and had very frequent soft bowel movements. They were dark and bloody.

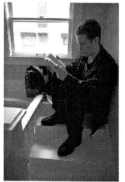

He had been suffering from heartburn. He smoked cigarettes and drank alcohol quite often. He was college age when kids are in the "party mode" when drinking and late night parties are the fashion. His mother was interested in natural remedies and sent him to a Homeopath she had read about in a magazine.

His symptoms were related to over indulgence. Nux Vomica 30 CH, probiotics, fish oil and B12 with folic acid were taken. His diet was adjusted to include more fruits and vegetables, and to avoid deep fried and rich foods. Within one month he said that he felt a lot better. He only got pain occasionally. His bowel movements improved and he had no blood or dark stools. His heartburn had improved and he was feeling well.

Hiatal Hernia

A hiatal hernia is characterized by a protrusion of the stomach above the diaphragm. It is quite common and people may not suffer from any symptoms. Detection of this disorder is commonly seen via an X-ray or gastroscopy. A hiatus hernia allows the stomach contents to move into the esophagus because the muscles that move food along are not in the correct location.

Hiatus hernia does not necessarily cause any symptoms. Symptoms can include heartburn, difficulty swallowing, chest pains and burping. Heartburn may occur when bending over or lying down. Eating may be a trigger for symptoms. If this condition is left a long time, the acid can destroy the esophagus, cause scarring, ulcers and cancer.

Causes of Hiatus Hernia are usually unknown but may be related to a congenital abnormality, trauma or overeating. There is no specific medical treatment for a hiatus hernia, other than not eating large meals before bed or sleeping with the head of the bed elevated. In rare cases surgery may be necessary. For treatment see Acid Reflux/Heartburn, Barrett's Esophagus and Dysphagia for treatments.

Hiccoughs

A hiccough is an involuntary spasm of the diaphragm. It may be a repetitive occurrence, every few minutes. Air travels quickly into the lungs and causes the epiglottis (a flap in the throat) to close. This makes this noise "hic". Usually hiccoughs are temporary and resolve on their own. However, they may be long-lasting and require treatment. Certain conditions can bring on hiccoughs such as:

- drinking a cold drink while eating a hot meal
- eating hot or highly spiced foods
- eating too quickly
- coughing
- consuming alcoholic beverages in excess
- smoking
- crying
- pregnancy
- certain prescription drugs such as chemotherapy
- tumours or kidney disease
- electrolyte imbalances like hypokalemia or hyponatremia

Hiccoughs are said to help dislodge food particles that are stuck in the throat. When a large piece of food is swallowed and our natural swallowing reflex is taxed, pressure is put on the phrenic nerve which stimulates the hiccough. The diaphragm contracts and creates suction in the thoracic cavity. This makes a region of high pressure where the food is closest to the mouth. This pressure aids in normal swallowing by helping the muscles of the throat to contract in an orderly manner.

Many cures focus on controlled breathing via holding the breath, breathing shallow, deep or into a paper bag. These methods may provide short term relief. Breathing into a paper bag creates respiratory acidosis. This increases the amount of carbon dioxide inhaled. Increased levels of CO_2 levels in the blood lower the pH which causes depression of the nervous system and increased blood flow to the muscles. Some people may find this makes them dizzy and can have potentially harmful side effects such as passing out and injury. Swallowing sometimes helps hiccoughs, especially drinking water alone or with one's nose plugged. Psychological intervention such as distracting someone from their hiccoughs by concentrating on another task, such as counting backwards, may be helpful. Trying to scare someone's hiccoughs away is an old remedy. My brother and I would try this as kids and it never worked for us!

Using homeopathic remedies is an easy way to effectively treat hiccoughs. Usually they resolve on their own, but can become painful if they are left for a long period of time. Remedies such as peppermint oil, lemon juice or baking soda revolve around relieving gas and may help with hiccoughs.

COMMON HOMEOPATHIC REMEDIES FOR HICCOUGHS

There are many homeopathic remedies for hiccoughs. Some of the more common remedies are listed with their symptoms here. For more information on how to self prescribe a homeopathic remedy, go to Chapter Two. If you cannot find a remedy suited to you, or find you are not improving or your symptoms get worse, seek the help of a professional homeopath or your medical doctor.

CICUTA
Common indications include:
- loud **hiccoughs**
- spasms and belching
- heartburn and flatulence
- nausea in the morning when eating
- violent vomiting with headache
- **aversion to company**
- **mentally can be childish**
- **craving for inedible things**
- thirst and dryness of throat

CYCLAMEN
Common indications include:
- coated tongue
- nausea and a fluid filled mouth
- violent hiccoughs while eating or before
- **hiccoughs**
- worse whilst pregnant
- burning in the esophagus
- **thirst in the evening**
- **food tastes salty**
- aching in the stomach that extends through the back
- **aggravated by fat, pork**, during pregnancy and while resting
- relieved with motion

IGNATIA
Common indications include:
- worse after eating or drinking and in the evening
- warm food aggravates
- **constriction of the throat or lump sensation**
- hiccoughs from strong emotions, feeling restless and weepy in the evening

- **ailments from grief, lost love and anger**
- **aggravated by tobacco** and coffee

NUX VOMICA
Common indications include:
- **hiccoughs from smoking and alcoholism**
- **worse from cold drinks**
- frequently comes before dinner
- used most often in hiccoughs with great success
- **eructations bitter, sour and rancid**
- hiccoughs from overeating
- **ineffectual urging for stools and belching**
- **chronic constipation**
- **mentally these types are workaholics, competitive and irrtible**
- **ailments from overendulgance**

SULPHUR
Common indications include:
- hiccoughs in the morning, evening or **when fasting**
- worse lying in bed
- **indigestion and burning pains**
- belching of air
- hiccoughs with pain in the back of the palate
- fullness of the stomach that bring on hiccoughs that last 15 minutes
- **tendency to skin problems**
- **cravings for sweets, spices, fat and alcohol**
- **mentally these types tend to be messy, lazy and intellectual**

Indigestion
See Dyspepsia

Irritable Bowel Disease

Irritable bowel disease (IBS) is a disorder that is more of a term then an actual disease. Many people are labeled with irritable bowel disease when they have undergone a gamut of tests and nothing is detected. Many people are tested for parasites, bacteria, ulcerative colitis, Crohn's disease, lactose intolerance, celiac and many other things. These medical tests show nothing out of the ordinary, although the person is still suffering with irregular bowel movements. This disorder affects more women than men and occurs more frequently between the ages of 20 to 30. IBS responds very favourably to natural remedies and dietary changes.

What are the Symptoms of IBS?
- frequent bowel movements
- constipation alternating with diarrhea

- lower abdominal pains
- spastic pains in the bowels
- flatulence and bloating
- belching and acid reflux
- food sensitivities to one food or many
- poor appetite
- vomiting
- headaches
- mucous in the stools
- pains caused by eating food or one particular food
- pain may be relieved after bowel movements
- joint pains

What Causes IBS?

- Stress affects the nervous system. The nervous system and the bowels are tightly connected. When we are stressed we release hormones that put our nervous system on high alert. We all know someone who has a nervous stomach or gets diarrhea during times of stress.
- Stimulants such as tobacco, coffee and tea all stimulate the bowels. Smokers have a higher than normal occurrence of intestinal disorders such as Crohn's disease.
- Other diseases that may not be diagnosed are related to IBS. They are diseases such as bacterial, parasitic or fungal infections, malabsorption, pancreatic insufficiency, Crohn's disease, diverticulitis, food poisoning, ulcerative colitis, lactose intolerance, colon cancer and/or celiac disease. There are many other disorders that cause symptoms of IBS.
- Drugs such as antibiotics, antacids and laxatives may cause symptoms of irritable bowel syndrome. If you suspect your medication may be causing your problems ask your pharmacist for a report on your medications and their side effects. If you have any inkling that your drug is causing the troubles, talk to your doctor about adjusting your prescription.
- Food sensitivities are a major factor in IBS. Go to Chapter Three for more information about food sensitivities. It will help you detect your triggers.
- Low fibre diets contribute to irritable bowel syndrome. Refined flours such as white flour and sugars are high glycemic, which means they flip into a sugar quickly in the blood stream. They also feed bad bacteria in the gut. Constipation may cause some residual build up of stool along the intestinal canal. Stools actually are passed between this debris and are not properly absorbed. They may be loose and contain food particles.

Diagnostic tools

Medical doctors use a number of tests to determine the cause of irritable bowel syndrome. They use a barium enema, colonoscopy, sigmoidoscopy and stool exam to detect blood, bacteria or parasites. Often these tests reveal nothing and the term irritable bowel syndrome labels this disorder. A syndrome is a compilation of symptoms rather than a specific disease they can diagnose. The diagnosis of irritable bowel is very vague.

Although the terminology is vague, the good news is that natural remedies actually work better than most medications.

DIETARY MEASURES FOR IRRITABLE BOWEL SYNDROME

If you suffer from IBS, eat a bland diet. Drink plenty of water to replace any fluids lost. Do not use a lot of hot spices, acids and citrus fruits. Steer clear of deep fried or fatty foods, caffeine, sugar and alcohol. Dairy products may cause further diarrhea in some, so avoid them until your symptoms improve. Eat smaller meals with fresh fruits and vegetables, lean meat, fish and whole grains. If you have chronic diarrhea, you may do better on cooked vegetables and fruits. However, if you can tolerate fresh fruits and vegetables, they have more enzymes and beneficial properties than cooked.

Read Chapter Three about healthy eating. Eat foods mostly from column one and some from column two found in the chart in that chapter. Foods that are lower fat and low glycemic help to keep you healthy overall. Plus any food that flips into a sugar quickly, such as high glycemic foods, feeds bad bacteria in the gut. So if you have any bacterial, fungal, viral or parasitic infections, these critters will be happy to have lots of sugar. Reduce these foods to keep your bowel flora in balance.

Commit to avoiding any food sensitivities that you may have. As mentioned earlier, go to Chapter Three to find out more about it.

SUPPLEMENTS FOR IRRITABLE BOWEL SYNDROME

B12 and Folic Acid

B12 and folic acid is useful to improve energy in those with bowel disorders. B12 and folic acid may not be properly digested and absorbed. It aids in proper absorption of foods, protein synthesis, metabolism of carbohydrates and fat, improves mood and prevents anemia. Use this supplement in a sublingual form. Typical dosage is 1,000 mcgs of B12 and 400 mcgs of folic acid per day.

Essential Fatty Acids (EFAs)

Essential fatty acids – mainly flax and fish oil – are good for pain, allergies, inflammation, dry skin, gas, bloating, gastrointestinal function and secretion and immune system deficiency. These can also help with other problems such as depression, concentration problems, joint pains, inflammation, skin eruptions and cardiovascular disease. Be sure to keep your EFAs in the fridge to prevent rancidity. Do not use your EFA liquid for cooking. Once it is heated it releases free radicals.

Eicosapentaenoic acid (EPA) found in fish oil is most beneficial for inflammatory bowel disease and diarrhea. EPA can be found in cold water fish such as herring, trout, salmon and mackerel. It increases a type of prostaglandin that actually decreases inflammatory proteins. Take about 1,000 mgs of EPA per day. An enteric coated fish oil capsule is advantageous because it releases in the intestinal tract not the stomach. This would ensure that you would be getting the maximum EPA into the intestinal tract.

Probiotics

Every person has billions of bacteria in their intestinal tract. Most bacteria are beneficial and maintain health. A small percentage of bacteria in our intestines are harmful if they spread. If these bad bacteria overgrow, it may have negative health consequences such as immune dysfunction, infections, constipation and/or diarrhea.

Good flora helps to maintain the immune system and displace the bad bacteria in the gut. They also help to sustain normal arrangement and function of the intestine's cells. The most popular beneficial bacteria are lactobacillus acidophilus and Bifidobacteria. The lactobacilli can be found in fermented foods such as yogurt, miso, tempeh and kefir. However, the number of bacteria is not standardized and some people who have IBS are lactose intolerant. The bacteria may not be an active culture if they are not stored properly.

It is best to use a standardized capsule of probiotics. It should be stored in the refrigerator which helps ensure that it is a live culture. Follow the directions on the package. Typical dosage for a probiotic supplement is one to 10 billion cells per capsule. One to three capsules can be taken daily. There are no known side effects from probiotics.

Digestive Enzymes

If you suffer from undigested food in the stool and your diarrhea is a result of poor digestion, digestive enzymes may be an answer. Digestive aids that contain pancreatic enzymes (protease, lipase and amylase) aid in digestion and help the body to absorb nutrients from food. Protease helps one to digest protein, lipase helps with fats and amylase with carbohydrates. Supplementing with enzymes is particularly helpful for diarrhea caused by food allergy and nutritional malabsorption disorders. If you have ulcers, do not take enzymes with hydrochloric acid in them. Take as directed on the label.

L-Glutamine

L-glutamine is a supplement that provides metabolic fuel for the intestinal cells. It helps to sustain the villi and absorptive surfaces of the intestinal tract lining. Vitamin C and B complex help to enhance the absorption of L-glutamine. Recommended dosage for adults is two to six grams per day with meals. There are no known side effects of L-glutamine.

Peppermint Oil

Enteric coated peppermint oil capsules are helpful in relieving gas, fullness and spasms of the intestinal tract. The oil is also considered to be anti-bacterial. Typical dosage is 200 mgs to 400 mgs per day. Those with a very sensitive stomach may be bothered by this herb. This herb is not suited to those with gallbladder or liver disease.

HOMEOPATHIC REMEDIES FOR IRRITABLE BOWEL SYNDROME

There are many homeopathic remedies for irritable bowel syndrome. Some of the more common remedies are listed with their symptoms here. For more information on how to self prescribe a homeopathic remedy, go to Chapter Two. If you cannot find a remedy suited to you, or find you are not improving or your symptoms get worse, seek the help of a professional homeopath or your medical doctor.

ALOE SOCOTRINA
Common indications include:
- distended abdomen after drinking water
- rumbling and gurgling gas
- urgent diarrhea after eating
- **jelly-like stools that contain mucous** and/or blood
- anus is burning with itching hemorrhoids
- weakness of the anal sphincter
- **involuntary stool while urinating or passing gas**
- **urgent stools at 5:00 a.m.**
- suited to beer drinkers who lead a sedentary life
- mental and physical work causes fatigue
- **lumpy stool mixed with liquid**
- **early morning diarrhea that drives one out of bed**
- pain felt in the stomach when walking and making a misstep
- pain radiates to the back and upwards with every belch
- **hemorrhoids that are congested like grapes are relieved by cold bathing**
- aggravated by eating, heat, after eating
- relieved by passing gas with distension, drinking cold water, bending forward

ARSENICUM ALBUM
Common indications include:
- abdominal distension with a **burning sensation**
- may have both vomiting and diarrhea
- painful glands in the groin or inguinal (abdominal wall) area
- burning rectum with stools and intense cutting pain
- watery, painful diarrhea
- useful for traveler's diarrhea
- **anxiety, restlessness with exhaustion**
- **chilly with the feeling they can never get warm enough**
- **desires hot drinks and applications despite burning sensation**
- **great thirst yet only takes small sips of water**
- nausea after meals
- **worse after midnight**, after eating, cold, during rest
- **relieved by hot drinks, warmth, motion** and exercise

NUX VOMICA
Common indications include:
- said to treat dysentery effectively
- constipation and diarrhea with painful urging
- **spasmodic cramps** and flatulence
- errors in diet aggravate these types
- enlarged liver and gallstone colic

- pain felt two or three hours after eating
- **stomach pains worse from anger and tight clothes**
- sour, watery, bitter heartburn after meals
- painful ulcers in the mouth and throat
- bleeding piles with urging for stools
- nausea and vomiting in the morning or after meals
- **mentally these types are irritable, ambitious and impatient**
- suited to sedentary types who do a lot of mental work
- **chilly types who seek the warmth**
- **cravings for alcohol, spices, coffee and fat**
- **aggravated by overindulgence, alcohol,** in the morning, mental overwork, coffee, overeating and drugs
- **relieved by warmth,** rest, and during damp weather

PHOSPHORUS
Common indications include:
- watery stools preceded by great rumbling noises and expelled like a hose
- stools may be involuntary, watery, green, mucous-filled, bloody
- anus feels like it is wide open, stool easily escapes
- loss of appetite and hunger soon after eating
- **tendency to hemorrhages**
- distended, painful abdomen worse after dinner
- tearing and burning pain in the stomach, worse in morning
- sour and burning belching
- **these types may suffer from lung problems such as asthma or bronchitis**
- enlarged and/or cirrhosis of the liver
- desires cold food and drinks
- **cold drinks vomited after they warm up in the stomach**
- **cravings for cold food, spices, salt, milk, wine and chocolate**
- **mentally these types are open, anxious and like company**
- **relieved by eating, cold drinks or food**
- **aggravated by spices, warm food and fat**

PODOPHYLLUM
Common indications include:
- this remedy acts on the liver and digestive tract, especially the duodenum and rectum
- **rumbling and gurgling in the abdomen before a stool**
- **stools are sputtering and mixed with air**
- green sour stools in the mornings
- diarrhea typically in the morning and better in the evening
- exhaustion from stools
- **explosive diarrhea**
- **profuse watery and offensive-smelling stool,** pours out like a hydrant

- undigested food in stool, jelly-like, green and watery
- **stool can be yellow, pasty, mucous-filled or bloody**
- liver area in right side under rib feels swollen and sensitive
- thirsty for large quantities of cold water
- desires sour foods
- **anxious sinking sensation after a bowel movement**
- **worse from morning at 5:00 a.m.**, hot weather, whilst teething, during stools and from motion
- relieved by bending double, external warmth, lying on the stomach and rubbing the liver

SULPHUR

Common indications include:

- diarrhea with stools that contain undigested food
- **sour smelling diarrhea that lingers on the person**
- **stool drives him out of bed in the morning (5:00 a.m.)**
- parts around the anus becomes red and excoriated
- pulsation in the anus after a stool
- feeling hot and sweaty
- **redness of the margins of the skin (lips, anus and eyes)**
- burning sensation anywhere in the body
- **skin eruptions are common in these types**
- **itching and burning of the rectum**
- **hemorrhoids**
- feels very weak with the diarrhea, hates standing
- **craving for sweets, fat, spices, beer or whiskey**
- **aversion to eggs**
- **these types tend to be messy, lazy and intellectual**
- **aggravated by warmth of bed, whilst standing, at 11a.m., suppressed discharges**, change of weather, milk products or alcoholic beverages
- relieved by lying down on the right side and in open air

Picture this…

You are a young woman who owns a small business. Over the past four years, you have had stomach problems. Whenever you traveled for work, you would have to stop to

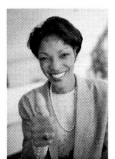

have a bowel movement. Your bowels were moving three to four times a day. Although you had no cramps, you did have a foul odour to your stool. You had been feeling a lot of stress with work and also about your digestive issues because they were embarrassing. You had to plot your travels along with known pit stops that had a washroom.

You decide to check in with a local Homeopath. You cut back on sugars, white bread and fried foods. You take 1,000 mgs of fish oil, acidophilus and a homeopathic complex for detoxification of the intestinal tract. After one month you are still having trouble with loose stools. You have a fear to pass gas or whether you could make it to the washroom. Your

Homeopath adds Aloe 30 CH. After another month you have no diarrhea and are surprised at how well you feel. Your energy is good and you feel less stress due to your improved digestion.

Lactose Intolerance

Lactose intolerance is a disorder which results in the inability to digest lactose which is milk sugar. This is usually due to a deficiency or a defect in the enzyme lactase. This enzyme is produced in the lining of the small intestine and breaks down lactose in dairy products. When someone consumes milk products and is lactose intolerant, the food will go through the intestinal tract undigested. The lactose collects water, ferments and results in many unpleasant digestive symptoms up to two hours after its ingestion. Oddly some people's degree of lactose intolerance varies. It may be worse at certain times, such as during pregnancy, stress or when the person feels physically run down. Lactose intolerance is not the same as a milk allergy. An allergy is an immune system reaction where it mounts a response to the milk and it can cause swelling of the mouth, throat and digestive tract.

What are the Symptoms of Lactose Intolerance?
Symptoms may occur immediately or up to two hours after ingestion of lactose containing foods. Symptoms are bloating, gas, nausea, diarrhea, vomiting and abdominal cramps. The stools may smell like curdled milk, be frothy and/or yellow in colour. Symptoms in children may include diaper rash or delayed weight gain.

What Causes Lactose Intolerance?
1. In countries where people do not regularly consume dairy products, lactose intolerance is commonplace. This is because people lose the enzyme to digest milk when they do not use it. Some genetic changes occur and the enzyme lactase is lost. Certain cultures have almost 100 percent lactose intolerance, such as Africa, Asia and South America. This disorder is so prevalent that it is not considered an abnormal occurrence.
2. Infections caused by certain microbes such as viruses, bacteria and parasites can cause lactose intolerance. Some common bugs that are culprits are giardia, the Norwalk virus and rotavirus.
3. Those who suffer with celiac disease, Crohn's disease, irritable bowel syndrome or gastroenteritis may all have difficulty digesting milk products. Any disease that affects the border of the small intestine may lead to lactose intolerance.
4. Some people are born without the ability to digest milk. It is a genetic disorder.

How is Lactose Intolerance Diagnosed?
1. One method is to ingest more lactose than what one is used to. Symptoms may be observed half an hour to two hours after ingestion.
2. Doctors may do a "Hydrogen Breath Test" where one consumes 50 grams of lactose. Then, over the course of six hours, hydrogen levels are measured from the breath. Hydrogen is a byproduct of undigested lactose that is fermented from lack of absorption in the intestinal tract.
3. An intestinal biopsy is done in some cases. However, it is not usually performed or necessary.

4. Food elimination testing is the easiest method of detecting lactose intolerance. If you have a hunch you are sensitive to dairy products, you can do an allergy elimination test to see just how sensitive you are. If you are fully lactose intolerant, you should see symptoms a few hours after consuming milk products. If you are just sensitive to milk in general, you may see other symptoms, such as rashes, headaches, sinus pressure etc., up to 72 hours after its ingestion. See Chapter Three for the Allergy Sensitivity Survey where you can note your symptoms before and after consuming dairy products.

To do a milk challenge test, eliminate the following foods for three weeks: all milk products, dried, evaporated and skimmed milk, butter, calcium caseinate, casein, caseinates, cheese of any kind, cream, creamy sauces and soups, curds, dried milk solids, lactose, lactoalbumin, margarine (some may contain milk products), mayonnaise (some may contain milk products), puddings, whey and yogurt. Packaged foods such as muffin, pancake and cake mixes may contain dried milk. When you re-introduce these foods into your diet, you will notice symptoms shortly after their consumption. Keep in mind some people can tolerate a small amount of lactose and may require a higher dose of it to elicit symptoms.

DIETARY REGIMES FOR LACTOSE INTOLERANCE

Re-habituation
Some authorities recommend consuming small portions of dairy products a few times a day to get the intestinal tract accustomed to milk products. This may work in some people who have a reduced ability to digest lactose. This process is called "re-habituation." If one has complete lactose intolerance, it likely would not be a good idea to challenge the digestive tract further. If your symptoms are worse with dairy products in any form, re-habituation is not for you.

Avoid These Foods
Check labels for binding agents, brown sugar flavouring, butter, butter fat, buttermilk, butter oil, butter solids, calcium caseinate, casein, cheese, cow milk products, cream, cream sauces and soups, curds, custard, dried milk solids, evaporated milk, frozen yogurt, ghee, hydrolysates, hydrolyzed casein, ice cream, lactate, lactulose, lactose, lactoalbumin, margarine, milk, natural butter flavor, potassium caseinate, pudding, sour cream, whey, whey powder, whey protein concentrate, whey protein hydrolysate and yogurt. Become a detective and read all labels!

Eat Alternative Sources of Calcium
Foods that contain calcium are almonds, apricots, asparagus, blackstrap molasses, bok choi, broccoli, cabbage, clams, collard greens, dandelion greens, dried figs, filberts, kale, kelp, calcium fortified orange juice, oats, okra, prunes, rhubarb, sardines, salmon with the bones, spinach, tofu, dark green leafy vegetables, soybeans, sesame seeds, parsley, turnip greens, white beans, rainbow trout, sweet potatoes, soya milk, rice milk and almond milk.

Alternative Lactose-Free Foods
Milk alternatives are: lactose free milk, almond beverage, amazake, cashew nut beverage, hazelnut beverage, rice milk and soymilk.

Ice cream alternatives are: fresh fruit sorbet, fruit smoothies, juice popsicles, juice ice cubes, tofutti products, soy delicious and rice dream

Mayonnaise alternatives are: avocado, mustard, nut butter, soya yogurt, and tofu sour cream.

Cheese alternatives are: ground nut butter, tofu and soya cheese.

Butter alternatives are: non-hydrogenated margarine (check label for dairy free), flax oil and olive oil.

SUPPLEMENTS FOR LACTOSE INTOLERANCE

Probiotics

Every person has billions of bacteria in their intestinal tract. Most bacteria are beneficial and maintain health. A small percentage of bacteria in our intestines are harmful if they spread. If they overgrow it may have negative health consequences such as immune dysfunction, infections, constipation and/or diarrhea.

Good flora helps to maintain the immune system and displace the bad bacteria in the gut. They also help to sustain normal arrangement and function of the cells in the intestinal lining. The most popular beneficial bacteria are lactobacillus acidophilus and Bifidobacteria. The latter, bifidobacteria is said to aid in the digestion of milk products. The lactobacilli can be found in fermented foods such as yogurt, miso, tempeh and kefir. Yogurt and kefir are dairy products. They may not be a good choice for those with lactose intolerance. Also in foods, the number of bacteria is not standardized. The bacteria may not be an active culture if they are not stored properly.

It is best to use a standardized capsule of probiotics. It should be stored in the refrigerator which helps ensure that it is a live culture. Follow the directions on the package. Typical dosage for a probiotic supplement is one to 10 billion cells per capsule. One to three capsules can be taken daily. There are no known side effects from probiotics.

Calcium, Magnesium and Vitamin D

Bone loss is not caused by a lack of cow's milk, but other factors, such as acidity, digestion, lack of sunlight and a sedentary lifestyle. Minerals such as boron, calcium, magnesium, strontium and vitamin D are useful for bone building. They can be found in cow milk and other foods, such as almonds, broccoli and salmon with the bones. Cow milk is for baby cows and human milk is for baby humans.

Take a 2:1 ratio of calcium to magnesium. Typical daily dosage would be 800 to 1200 mgs of calcium and 400 to 600 mgs of magnesium. It is best to split this into two or three doses throughout the day. Calcium citrate or hydroxyapatite is a better form of calcium for bone building.

Enzymes for Lactose Digestion

Enzymatic lactase supplementation may help those with lactose intolerance. It replaces the enzyme that is lacking. Take a pill right when you sit down to eat a meal that contains dairy products. See the directions on the individual package.

HOMEOPATHIC REMEDIES FOR LACTOSE INTOLERANCE

There are many homeopathic remedies for lactose intolerance. Some of the more common remedies are listed with their symptoms here. For more information on how to self prescribe a homeopathic remedy, go to Chapter Two. If you cannot find a remedy suited to you, or find you are not improving or your symptoms get worse, seek the help of a professional homeopath or your medical doctor.

AETHUSIA
Common indications include:
- teething babies with gastrointestinal problems
- **vomiting of mucous, curdled milk and** cheesy appearance
- **milk products cause violent vomiting**
- falls asleep or becomes drowsy immediately after drinking milk
- **vomiting and diarrhea of newborns**
- **may see eruptions at the tip of the nose**
- poor ability to focus attention or think
- **mentally these types love animals and have many pets**
- **difficulty studying or concentrating**
- **aggravated by milk, after eating**, hot weather and from teething
- relieved by covering up and resting

CALCAREA CARBONICA
Common indications include:
- this remedy is also suited to teething children
- **vomiting of cold milk**
- **flatulence and rumbling**
- **heavy set people**
- milk upsets the person's stomach; they vomit sour curds
- acidity with sour belching, vomiting and stool
- chronic diarrhea with clay like stools
- **hearty appetite**
- **nausea after milk**
- **heartburn, indigestion with sour belching**
- **perspiration on the head**
- **sensitive to cold and damp air**
- diarrhea may be green, watery and contain undigested foods
- **cravings for eggs**
- aggravated by milk, evening and during a full moon
- relieved by resting

CARBO VEGETABILIS
Common indications include:
- excessive formation of gas
- **passing gas helps relieve discomfort**
- milk causes a lot of gas

- **foul smelling gas**
- weak digestion
- simple foods aggravate
- **frequent belching which helps the stomach**
- belching and flatulence with colicky pains
- **tremendous bloating and indigestion**
- unceasing passing of flatus
- **heartburn, belching and flatulence**
- **shortness of breath from gas or overeating**
- cannot bear anything around the waist
- **bloating and gas felt under the ribs**
- **abdominal pains may extend to the legs**
- **desire to be fanned or have open air**
- weak and tired people with slow thinking
- aggravated by butter, warmth and tight clothes
- **relieved by belching, being fanned** and loosening the clothing

CHINA
Common indications include:
- **debilitated and exhausted from diarrhea**
- weight felt after eating a small amount of food
- pain comes on alternating days
- **pains that are sensitive to light touch but better by hard pressure**
- **distension and flatulence a long time after eating**
- eating at night causes food not to digest at all
- **cutting pains**
- diarrhea can be watery and containing undigested food
- involuntary stool with fruits
- loosens the belt after eating
- **craving for sweets**
- **relieved with** hard pressure on the abdomen, bending double
- **aggravated by loss of bodily fluids (perspiration, diarrhea, urination or blood), light touch** and eating late
- aggravated from eating fruits, diarrhea, milk, night, fish, tea

LAC DEFLORATUM
Common indications include:
- intense pounding headaches with nausea and vomiting
- **aggravated by and an aversion to milk**
- sour vomiting
- profuse clear urine
- constipation with great urging
- stools are dry, large and cause pain and tears the anus
- these types are very chilly

- aggravation from drafts, in the morning, from noise and light, motion and during the menstrual flow
- **relieved by** urinating, resting, bandaging and warm covers

MAGNESIA CARBONICA
Common indications include:
- good for people with an irritable and nervous disposition
- tongue is coated yellow
- colicky pains that cause one to bend double and are better after a bowel movement
- bloating and flatulence after milk
- painful mouth ulcers that prevent eating
- the person's whole body is sour smelling
- **heartburn, sour belching and taste in the mouth**
- stools are green, frothy and sour
- abnormal cravings for meat
- **worse before bowel movements**, evenings, night, rest, around the menses, every three weeks, milk, temperature changes and whilst pregnant
- **relieved by** passing stools, warm air and walking outdoors

NATRUM CARBONICUM
Common indications include:
- very weak digestion
- sleepy after meals
- **dyspepsia**
- **food allergies** (such as dairy products)
- stools are emitted quickly with noise
- watery, sour burping and much flatulence
- diarrhea like orange pulp from milk products
- these types can be sluggish physically and mentally and is sensitive to heat
- these types catch many colds
- **these types are gentle and refined, sensitive to music**
- **aggravated by milk**, vegetables, cold drinks and starches
- aggravated by mental exertion, thunderstorms, music and the sun
- **relieved by** motion, rubbing and after eating

SULPHUR
Common indications include:
- diarrhea with stools that contain undigested food
- **sour smelling diarrhea that lingers on the person**
- **stool drives one out of bed in the morning (5:00 a.m.)**
- parts around the anus becomes red and excoriated
- pulsation in the anus after a stool
- feeling hot and sweaty

- **redness of the margins of the skin (lips, anus and eyes)**
- burning sensation anywhere in the body
- **skin eruptions are common in these types**
- **itching and burning of the rectum**
- **hemorrhoids**
- feels very weak with the diarrhea, hates standing
- **craving for sweets, fat, spices, beer or whiskey**
- **aversion to eggs**
- **these types tend to be messy, lazy and intellectual**
- **aggravated by warmth of bed, whilst standing, at 11a.m., suppressed discharges**, change of weather, milk products or alcoholic beverages
- **relieved by** lying down on the right side and in open air

TUBERCULINUM

Common indications include:

- these types are sensitive to dairy products, cats and dogs
- they tend to be fair skinned, freckled and very skinny despite eating well
- these types like open air and catch many colds
- **painless diarrhea**
- **offensive smelling stool**
- tendency to lung troubles, such as pneumonia, bronchitis and asthma
- they love to move about and travel
- diarrhea that occurs early in the morning and is sudden
- diarrhea may be dark, brown, watery and foul smelling
- diarrhea is discharged with great force
- night sweats and weakness
- **cravings for smoked meat**
- aggravated by milk, cold weather, dampness, morning, whilst sleeping and before a storm
- **relieved by** open air, moving and in the mountains

Picture this….

This is a case of a 60-year-old woman who had various digestive difficulties with vertigo. She suffered from irritable bowel syndrome, lactose intolerance and hypertension. This case was a difficult one due to the number of prescription medications she was taking. She wisely decided to seek the help of a professional Homeopath. Her symptoms included diarrhea alternating with constipation. She suffered from diarrhea and stomach cramps from shrimp and milk products. She also had nightly sweats on the scalp area. She already took probiotics, fish oil and a multi-vitamin. The two remedies that made the most impact on her health were Calcarea carbonica200 CH and Carbo Vegetablis 3 CH. She reports much less diarrhea, bloating and gas and only occasionally does she have the sweating.

Pancreatitis

Pancreatitis is an acute or chronic inflammatory condition of the pancreas and can be a serious condition. This large gland is located behind the stomach and excretes digestive enzymes into the small intestine via the pancreatic duct. These enzymes are amylase (for digestion of fats), protease (for digestion of proteins) and lipase (for digestion of fats). The pancreas also plays a role in blood sugar stability.

Acute Pancreatitis

Acute pancreatitis occurs more often in men than women. It is often caused by alcohol abuse and gallstones. Diagnostic tests for pancreatitis include an ultrasound, CAT scan or a blood test to see if there are elevated pancreatic enzymes such as amylase and lipase in the blood. These high levels return to normal when the pancreas is not inflamed. Typical medical treatment varies from fasting, medication to surgery. Often acute pancreatitis resolves on its own. However, it is important to seek medical help because pancreatitis can be life-threatening in some cases.

Chronic Pancreatitis

The pancreas' own enzymes can attack and destroy itself. These enzymes digest foods. Enzymes that are released inappropriately lead to inflammation, pain and scarring of the affected tissues. Often, chronic pancreatitis is linked to alcoholism, smoking, autoimmune diseases, medications, cystic fibrosis or blocked ducts. In some occasions its cause is unknown. In severe cases, diabetes may be a result of the damage to the pancreas.

Symptoms of Pancreatitis
- swollen and tender abdomen
- pain worse after eating
- pain in upper left abdomen
- pain on lying down
- pain in the left shoulder blade
- nausea and vomiting
- weight loss
- foul smelling stools
- fatty stools
- high fever
- rapid heartbeat
- diabetes in chronic stages
- back pain
- dehydration

DIETARY REGIMES FOR PANCREATITIS

While in the hospital, some people are advised to fast while they are sick with pancreatitis. This gives the pancreas a break from producing digestive enzymes. Treatment depends on your doctor's choice of treatment and the severity of your case.

Proper digestion starts in the mouth, so be sure to chew your food well. Our saliva contains digestive enzymes that help with starch digestion. Chewing your food into small particles makes it easier to digest and break down in the intestinal tract.

Diet is crucial for health and proper digestion. Eat a high fibre diet that includes lots of fruits, vegetables and whole grains. Consume low glycemic and low fat foods, found in column one of the diet guidelines outlined in the chart in Chapter Three. These foods are higher in fibre and decrease the prevalence of many other diseases such as heart disease, diabetes, cancer and hormone imbalances.

When you are filling your plate, visualize it like a pie. Grains should represent only a quarter of your plate. Another quarter should be a lean protein or legumes. The other half should be vegetables. Eat fruit alone because it is a simple carbohydrate. It is quickly digested and, when thrown in with other foods may lead to gas and bloating.

Eat a wide variety of colours of fruits and vegetables to ensure that you are getting optimum nutrition from your food. For example, orange vegetables are high in beta carotene and dark leafy vegetables contain folic acid. Try to consume some raw fruits and vegetables because they have more nutrients than cooked.

Foods to limit and/or avoid
Sugar, fried foods, fat, alcohol and refined carbohydrates contribute to ill health and may aggravate pancreatitis.

SUPPLEMENTS FOR PANCREATITIS

B Complex
B vitamins such as B3 and B5 assist in the production of enzymes that help to digest carbohydrates and fat. B3 or niacin is thought to help prevent the development of diabetes by helping the pancreatic cells with insulin sensitivity. B5 or pantothenic acid help to lower blood lipid levels. Typical dosage of B complex is 50 to 100 mgs per day. However, B5 and B3 can be taken in higher potencies for better results.

Chromium
Chromium is a mineral that is useful for keeping blood sugar stable. This is beneficial for those who have diabetes. It helps to reduce sugar cravings, aids in weight loss and lowers blood glucose levels. It also improves muscle mass in those who do strenuous exercise. Typical dosage of chromium is 200 to 400 mcgs per day with meals. Do not exceed the recommended dose as chromium can be toxic in high doses.

N-Acetylcysteine (NAC) and Vitamin C
NAC is a sulphur containing amino acid and antioxidant that is useful in reducing inflammation in acute pancreatitis. It helps the liver to detoxify alcohol, tobacco and other environmental pollutants. It slows cellular damage involved in aging. Typical dosage is 200 to 500 mgs per day. If you are taking NAC, you should take a 1,000 mgs of vitamin C with it because it aids in its antioxidant properties. NAC may not be appropriate for those with diabetes because it interferes with insulin.
Do not exceed the recommended dose because it causes toxic side effects.

Pancreatic Enzymes

The use of pancreatin as a digestive enzyme is said to be useful in reducing pain in chronic pancreatitis. High potency pancreatin increases the level of the enzymes in the small intestine. This decreases the amount of destructive enzymes produced by the pancreas and improves digestion. Pancreatin includes lipase, amylase and protease. Follow the directions on the individual package.

HOMEOPATHIC REMEDIES FOR PANCREATITIS

There are many homeopathic remedies for pancreatitis. Some of the more common remedies are listed with their symptoms here. For more information on how to self prescribe a homeopathic remedy, go to Chapter Two. If you cannot find a remedy suited to you, or find you are not improving or your symptoms get worse, seek the help of a professional homeopath or your medical doctor.

ARSENICUM ALBUM
Common indications include:
- **burning pains**
- difficulty swallowing
- **great thirst for hot drinks but only takes sips**
- **nausea and vomiting**
- vomiting of green mucous, bile, black matter
- stomach very easily irritated
- swollen abdomen
- bowel movements cause great burning
- **chilly people who cannot get warm enough**
- hates the sight and smell of food
- **very exhausted**
- **great anxiety, restlessness and fears about health**
- **aggravated by cold and** wet weather
- **relieved by heat and warm drinks**

BELLADONNA
Common indications include:
- **high fevers with hallucinations**
- **intense heat felt**
- **pains are cramping, burning, cutting and/or come and go quickly**
- **retching and vomiting**
- **dilated pupils and light sensitivity**
- pain in the right hand side worse with slight touch
- colicky pains that come and go as fast as they appeared
- pains lessened by bending over or backward
- **cold hands and feet but face is hot**
- **constipation**
- **cramping across the transverse colon**
- **fear of dogs**

- **thirstless**
- **craving for lemons and lemonade**
- **worse at 3:00 p.m., being jarred, motion, around menstrual period, right side**, slight touch, night, swallowing liquids, draughts of air, looking at bright objects, summer sun
- amelioration from rest, bending forward or back and a warm room

COLOCYNTHIS
Common indications include:
- **colicky, cutting and knife-like pains**
- **pains compel the person to bend double**
- **distended abdomen**
- **constriction sensation**
- **stitching pains in the sides and/or around the belly button**
- **chills during pains**
- **vomiting and diarrhea**
- **anger and irritability**
- **restless during the pains**
- **aggravated by anger, indignation**, night time, eating after, at rest and with movement
- **relieved by bending double, hard pressure, lying on the abdomen**, heat and coffee

CONIUM
Common indications include:
- acute pancreatitis
- **band like constriction felt under the ribs**
- **cutting and stitching pains**
- **swollen glands**
- nausea, burning heartburn and belching
- painful spot of above the sternum
- sensitive stomach with sharp pains and a bruised sensation
- heat and burning after bowel movements
- weakness after every stool
- irritable and restless
- **mental dullness, anxiety and indifference**
- **emotionally flat or hard people**
- **relieved by passing stool**, immediately after eating and fasting
- **aggravated by suppressed sexual desires**
- worse a few hours after meals

IODUM
Common indications include:
- abdomen enlarged

- **ravenous hunger and thirst that must be appeased**
- **excessively thin and emaciated despite eating**
- **much saliva**
- cutting pains in the abdomen
- constipation and diarrhea
- bloody stools
- **mentally these types are anxious**
- **better with eating, walking and open air**
- **aggravated by fasting, lying in bed, from physical exertion/labour but better for exercise**
- aggravated by quiet, warm room and hunger

IRIS
Common indications include:
- **nauseating headaches with gastric complaints**
- **vomiting from nauseating headache offers no relief**
- copious saliva
- **sour belching**
- **burning sensation from the mouth to the anus**
- poor appetite
- **nausea and vomiting**
- **right sided headaches, in the temple, above or below the eye**
- **headaches with blurred vision**
- nightly watery diarrhea
- cutting pains
- worse in the evening, night and at rest
- better with movement

PHOSPHORUS
Common indications include:
- burning heat between the shoulders and up the back
- watery chronic diarrhea
- undigested foods in the stool
- **nausea and vomiting**
- **vomits when consumed cold water warms up in the stomach**
- **ravenous appetite**
- sensation as if the rectum remains open
- stools are thin and long
- desires cold drinks and food such as ice
- vomiting and nausea of drinks when they warm up in the stomach
- **mentally these types are sympathetic, fearful and enjoy company**
- **cravings for chocolate, ice cream, salt, spices, milk and wine**
- **worse with fasting, lying on the left side**, change of weather, thunderstorms, morning and evening, after eating and drinking

- **relieved by cold food and drinks, sleep, being massaged** and lying on the right side

Picture this….

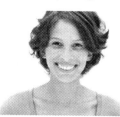

You are a young woman diagnosed with acute pancreatitis and are told that you have gallstone sludge. This means that there is a mash of thick bile formed and residing in the gallbladder and bile ducts. You hate the thought of surgery so you opt to try a homeopathic approach. Your Homeopath warns you that you may require medical intervention if the pancreatitis doesn't improve because it can be serious. Your symptoms are pain in the back and between the shoulder blades, nausea and fever. You started a low fat and low glycemic diet. You take a fibre supplement and 1,000 mgs of vitamin C per day. Once a day for two weeks you take Phosphorus 30 CH. You also take digestive enzymes containing Pancreatin with each meal. After one month your symptoms have not returned. You follow this regime over a period of six months and have no further aggravation from the pancreas or symptoms of gallstones.

Polyps, Intestinal

Intestinal polyps are an overgrowth of tissue of the mucous membranes in the small or large intestine. A polyp results from an abnormal overgrowth of cells that line the intestines. They are single or multiple and come in a variety of shapes. In most cases, polyps are benign without symptoms and have limited growth. The tendency to form polyps occurs as people age. It is thought that up to 30% of all people have polyps. Occasionally they can grow quite large and become cancerous.

Symptoms of polyps
- rarely causes abdomen pain and cramps
- painless bleeding
- rectal bleeding
- bloody stools
- anemia and fatigue
- bowel obstruction in severe cases
- nausea and vomiting in severe cases
- change in bowel habits

What are the risk factors for developing polyps?
- men tend to suffer from polyps more than women do
- a parent or sibling with polyps
- smoking
- drinking excessive amounts of alcohol
- being over age 40
- high fat and low fibre diets
- a sedentary lifestyle
- genetic abnormalities

Genetic disorders related to intestinal polyps:

- **Familial adenomatous polyposis** is a disorder that results in hundreds to thousands of polyps. It can cause severe bleeding and anemia. This is a genetic disorder that is also linked to cancer of the duodenum and stomach. Jaw cysts, sebaceous cysts and bone tumours are all related to familial polyposis. This disorder typically leads to colon cancer before the age of 40. Medical treatments usually include surgical removal of the affected portion of the intestinal tract.

- **Gardner's syndrome** is a syndrome that has multiple polyps in the colon, skull, thyroid and skin. Often people who have impacted supernumerary teeth have Gardner's syndrome. Supernumerary teeth are extra teeth that do not surface past the surface of the gums. Cancerous malignancies are common in this disorder. Gardner's syndrome is considered to be a variant of familial polyposis.

- **Lynch's syndrome** is a genetic disorder that is characterized by an increased risk of colourectal, ovarian, liver, brain, urinary tract and skin cancer. Genetic testing is required for a diagnosis of Lynch's syndrome.

- **Turcot syndrome** is a disorder that is related to intestinal and central nervous system tumours. The link between Turcot syndrome and genes are unclear. Some believe it is another variant of familial polyposis.

- **Peutz-jeghers syndrome (PJS)** is a disorder that is characterized by intestinal polyps. Infants tend to have freckles or abnormal pigmentation around the mouth, gums and surrounding mucous membranes. This disorder is linked to other types of polyps and cancer, such as ovarian, breast, lung, uterus and colon.

Medical Screening for Polyps

There are many medical tests for polyps. It is typically recommended that everyone over age 50 have a colonoscopy to screen for intestinal cancers and polyps early. With early detection comes a high survival rate (90%) for cancerous lesions. The screening methods used by the medical profession are as follows:

1. A fecal occult blood test simply checks a stool sample for blood. If blood is present other factors need to be ruled out such as hemorrhoids, polyps or other conditions.

2. A sigmoidoscopy is a diagnostic tool that looks at the last two feet of the colon. It is a flexible lighted tube.

3. A colonoscopy is the test of choice for most doctors. It is more accurate at detecting polyps than other tests. The colonoscope is a long tube that has a video camera attached to it, for your doctor to see inside the intestinal tract. He/she then will likely remove any polyps that are found and biopsy them.

4. A barium enema allows for your doctor to view your large intestine with an X-ray. Barium is a dye that coats the lining of the bowel. This helps contrast the edges of the intestine for viewing with the X ray.

5. Genetic testing may be recommended to rule out any ominous disorders that may lead to cancer or other tumour growth.

7. A simple digital rectal exam may be performed. Your doctor will check the first few inches of the rectum with a gloved finger. They will check for lumps or tumours. It is safe and painless but it also may miss small polyps and the rest of the bowel.

DIETARY REGIME FOR INTESTINAL POLYPS

Intestinal polyps that are not genetic can be prevented with a healthy diet. Those who have had polyps removed or a family history of polyps should follow a low glycemic diet outlined in the chart in Chapter Three. Eating a high fibre diet also helps to remove waste from the bowel. This decreases the amount of time the stool is in contact with the lining of the intestinal tract. Stool contains toxins and waste that can aggravate the lining of the intestinal tract. Foods that contain antioxidants like berries, dark green leafy vegetables and orange vegetables are helpful to prevent free radical damage that may signal for uncontrolled cell growth of the mucous membrane cells.

SUPPLEMENTS FOR INTESTINAL POLYPS

Probiotics

Every person has billions of bacteria in their intestinal tract. Most bacteria are beneficial and maintain health. A small percentage of bacteria in our intestines are harmful if they spread. If they overgrow it may have negative health consequences such as immune dysfunction, infections, constipation and/or diarrhea.

Good flora helps to maintain the immune system and displace the bad bacteria in the gut. It also helps to sustain normal arrangement and function of the cells in the intestinal lining. Most of the body's immune defenses are found in the intestinal tract. The gut associated lymph tissue is in the intestines is one of our powerhouses for the immune system. If we keep our gut flora balanced, we can inadvertently support our immune system. When our immune system works well, it can recognize abnormal cell growth and eradicate it.

The most popular beneficial bacteria are lactobacillus acidophilus and bifidobacteria. The latter, bifidobacteria is said to aid in the digestion of milk products. Use a standardized capsule of probiotics. It should be stored in the refrigerator which helps ensure that it is a live culture. Follow the directions on the package. Typical dosage for a probiotic supplement is one to 10 billion cells per capsule. One to three capsules can be taken daily. There are no known side effects from probiotics.

Calcium and Vitamin D

Recents studies show that a lack of calcium and vitamin D are linked to colon cancer. According to Life Extension Foundation (www.lef.org), calcium is protective against advanced polyps that cause cancer. A study group of 930 patients found that those who had cancerous polyps removed and took 1200 mgs of calcium per day had 18% less risk of hyperplastic polyps and a 35% reduction of cancerous lesions. This calcium protective effect is most pronounced in those with a high fibre diet.

Take a 2:1 ratio of calcium to magnesium. Typical daily dosage would be 800 to 1200 mgs of calcium and 400 to 600 mgs of magnesium. It is best to split this into two or three doses throughout the day. Calcium carbonate is thought to be best for the colon because it is not well absorbed. This mineral then goes through the intestinal tract and absorbs toxins. Calcium citrate is a better absorbed form of calcium for those who need it for bone building and easier digestion.

Vitamin D and calcium have a synergistic effect in cancer prevention. Those with higher levels of vitamin D are said to have less incidence of cancer. Vitamin D3, cholecalferol, taken as 1,000 to 2,000 IU per day is recommended.

Resveratrol

Resveratrol is an antioxidant found in red wine. It is considered to be an excellent cancer preventative. It is thought to help those with inflammatory bowel disease and prevent oxidative damage caused by the disease. Typical dosage is 100 to 250 mgs per day. This supplement may contraindicate prescription drugs such as cyclosporine, anticoagulants, drugs for erectile dysfunction and calcium channel blockers.

Curcumin

Curcumin is the yellow pigment from tumeric. It is an anti-inflammatory and anti-cancer remedy. By keeping inflammation down, it aids in preventing undifferentiated cell growth and tumours of the intestinal lining. Typical dosage is 300 mgs three times a day. This herb may enhance the effects of anti-coagulant drugs.

Selenium

Selenium is a mineral that is said to prevent tumour formation. People who have a tendency to colon adenomas have low selenium levels (www.lef.org). Selenium works well with vitamin E to reduce free radicals. Foods that contain selenium are brazil nuts, sunflower seeds, crabs, liver and oysters for example. Typical dosage for selenium is 50 to 200 mcgs. High doses of selenium can be toxic.

HOMEOPATHIC REMEDIES FOR INTESTINAL POLYPS

There are many homeopathic remedies for intestinal polyps. Some of the more common remedies are listed with their symptoms here. For more information on how to self prescribe a homeopathic remedy, go to Chapter Two. If you cannot find a remedy suited to you, or find you are not improving or your symptoms get worse, seek the help of a professional homeopath or your medical doctor.

CALCAREA CARBONICA
Common symptoms include:
- **bleeding and itching of the rectum**
- **constipation without urge for stool**
- **sour, watery belching and heartburn**
- stubborn constipation or diarrhea
- polyps that tend to bleed easily
- **abdomen bloated**, hard and sensitive to pressure
- milk and eggs upset the digestion
- **these types tend to be heavy set**
- **head and neck tends to perspire**
- **cravings for eggs and sweets**
- **aggravated by cold damp weather**, eggs and milk
- better in a dry climate

CALCAREA PHOSPHORICA
Common indications include:

- burning around the navel
- gas, bloating and heartburn
- bleeding during bowel movements
- headaches from mental exertion, school work and stress
- anal fistulas, hemorrhoids and polyps
- anal problems come on after suppressed chest symptoms (asthma and bronchitis)
- bone pains are common
- **cravings for bacon, ham and smoked meats**
- **mentally these types can be peevish, complaining, bored, have a desire to travel**
- **aggravated by cold, drafts**, dampness, changeable weather and mental work
- better in a warm and dry climate

NITRIC ACID
Common indications include:

- anal fissures, fistulas, hemorrhoids and polyps
- tearing pains in the anus after stools
- bowels tend towards constipation
- **cutting pains from trapped gas**
- **constipation alternating with diarrhea**
- **constriction and spasm of the rectum during stool**
- easy bleeding from the rectum
- **stitching or splinter-like pains (especially in the rectum)**
- **mentally these types are angry, unmoved by apology and anxious about health**
- **cravings for fat and salt**
- aggravated by hot and cold weather and in the evening
- improved by riding or driving

PHOSPHORUS
Common indications include:

- **easy and profuse bleeding** of polyps and hemorrhoids
- **stools are thin and narrow**
- **ravenous appetite**
- **thirsty for cold drinks**
- sensation that the rectum remains open
- **typically these types are very open, sympathetic, friendly and enjoy company**
- **cravings for chocolate, cold drinks and food, salt, spices, milk and wine**
- aggravated by thunderstorms, touch, physical or mental exertion
- **relieved by cold applications, eating or fasting, cold food and drink** and open air

SILICEA
Common indications include:

- painful spasms of the rectum
- fissures, hemorrhoids and polyps
- **difficult stools that come down and seem to recede again**
- sensation that feces remain in the rectum
- fatigue of the mind and body
- **sour perspiration**
- **these types may be clammy and chilly**
- **promotes expelling of foreign bodies (slivers)**
- **mentally these types lack self-confidence, are timid and anxious**
- **aggravated by drafts, suppressed foot sweat**, milk, washing, dampness, cold and lying down
- relieved by wrapping up, warmth, summer and humidity

THUJA OCCIDENTALIS
Common indications include:

- **suitable for spongy tumours, polyps, warts and growths**
- bleeding and moist growths
- anal fissures and polyps that bleed easily
- stomach is rumbling as if something moving in the abdomen
- **cravings or aversion to onions and garlic**
- **history of vaccinations** (ill effects from shots)
- **mentally these types may feel unattractive, have low self esteem or are secretive**
- aggravated by onions, coffee, fat, night, bedtime and after vaccinations
- **better during a cold**, from lying on the left side

Picture this….

Your husband, age 55, was concerned after a routine colonoscopy. Polyps were detected and he had them surgically removed. The doctor advised that he should be

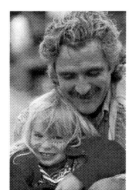

rechecked yearly for the next five years. He was also told he had some inflamed patches in the intestinal tract. He had a history of upset stomach, diarrhea and heartburn. He ate all foods and the only trigger he could pinpoint was onions. He suffered from heartburn at other times as well. You had always felt he ate the wrong foods, such as high sugar and starchy foods, like white bread and pasta. He always said that this was the way he grew up and the way his family ate.

You recommended he seek the help of a local Homeopath and get some nutritional counsel. Surprisingly, he took your advice without a fight! The Homeopath recommended that he adhere to a low

glycemic diet and eat lots of fruits and vegetables. He was to steer clear of deep fried foods. He took a fibre supplement, 1,200 mgs of calcium and magnesium and four pellets of Thuja occidentalis 30CH once a week.

After a few months his digestion had greatly improved and he lost ten pounds. You notice he has a lot more energy and is not complaining of heartburn and diarrhea. At his yearly colonoscopy, his doctor noted his intestinal tract was clear and the inflamed patches were healed.

Rectal Itching

Rectal itching can be an aggravating problem that lingers. It is usually not related to a serious disease. It can be caused by several factors such as poor wiping, eczema and an acid pH. Medications that may cause candida or diarrhea tend to cause rectal itching. Using strong soaps, scented products and harsh toilet paper may all strip the natural oils from the skin of the rectal area. This leaves one open to irritation from stools or urination. Infection and allergic reactions can sometimes affect the rectal area. Infections would include pinworms, candida, scabies or genital warts. Treatment for rectal itching depends on the cause. Some people who have hemorrhoids have rectal itching. See the Hemorrhoid section for the proper treatment. Try to eliminate as many possible irritants. Go to the individual headings to research your cause such as hemorrhoids, candidiasis, parasites or allergies.

Tips for Reducing Itching

- Wipe yourself until you are clean. If you find that even after a few wipes, the paper is not clean, wet the paper and then wipe. It is gentler on the skin and helps clean the area.
- Make sure you keep dry. Just like when babies are wet, adults tend to get rashes when damp. Damp and hot areas tend to breed bacteria such as yeast. If you tend to sweat, try to use cornstarch and clothes made of natural fibres like cotton that breathe.
- Use unscented and gentle bath products. Sometimes artificial scents in soaps, bubble bath and even toilet paper can cause allergic reactions.
- If you tend to enjoy coffee, chocolate or tomatoes, these may be a trigger for rectal itching. Eliminate them one at a time and keep track of your itching. To determine if you have food allergies go to Chapter Three for extensive information on how to detect hidden allergies.

TOPICAL TREATMENTS FOR RECTAL ITCHING

Aloe Vera Gel

Aloe vera is a cactus that makes an incredible healing gel within its leaves. One can drink it or apply directly to irritated skin. It also has soothing and healing properties. It can be applied as needed to the affected area.

Lavender Oil

Lavender oil has many beneficial properties. Lavender has soothing, antiseptic, pain relieving and anti-inflammatory properties. It can be diluted with carrier oil, such as mineral or olive oil, and applied to the affected area.

Rose Oil

Rose oil is a substance that also has many useful properties. It is calming, antiseptic, anti-bacterial and anti-viral. It also helps to soften scar tissue. Rose oil can be diluted with carrier oil and applied to the affected area.

Vitamin A and E ointment

Vitamin A and E ointments have beneficial healing properties, plus they act as a barrier cream. This means that any irritants such as clothing, wiping and feminine hygiene products do not directly contact the skin and further irritate it.

Witch Hazel

Witch hazel is an excellent remedy for itching caused by hemorrhoids. It is an effective pain killer and reduces inflammation and swelling of hemorrhoids. You can use witch hazel on a cotton pad or buy pre-packaged compresses.

SUPPLEMENTS FOR RECTAL ITCHING

Essential Fatty Acids (EFAs)

Essential fatty acids, mainly flax and fish oil, are good for symptoms such as pain, inflammation, dry skin, gas, bloating, gastrointestinal function and secretion, and immune system deficiency. EFAs can also help with other problems such as depression, concentration, joint pains, inflammation, skin eruptions and cardiovascular disease.

Eicosapentaenoic acid (EPA) found in fish oil is most beneficial for its anti-inflammatory properties. EPA can be found in cold water fish such as herring, trout, salmon and mackerel. It increases a type of prostaglandin that actually decreases inflammatory proteins. Take about 1,000 mgs of EPA per day. An enteric coated Fish Oil capsule is advantageous because it releases in the intestinal tract not the stomach. This would ensure that you would be getting the maximum EPA into the intestinal tract which is where its anti-inflammatory properties are needed. Be sure to keep your EFAs in the fridge to prevent them from spoiling. Do not use your EFA liquid for cooking. Once it is heated, it releases free radicals that cause damage to cells.

Probiotics

Every person has billions of bacteria in their intestinal tract. Most bacteria are beneficial and maintain health. A small percentage of bacteria in our intestines are harmful if they spread. If they overgrow it may have negative health consequences such as immune dysfunction, infections, constipation and/or diarrhea. The bad bacteria may also cause rectal itching. Good flora helps to maintain the immune system and displace the bad bacteria in the gut.

It is best to use a standardized capsule of probiotics. It should be stored in the refrigerator which helps ensure that it is a live culture. Follow the directions on the package. Typical dosage for a probiotic supplement is one to 10 billion cells per capsule. One to three capsules can be taken daily. There are no known side effects from probiotics.

Vitamin A

Vitamin A is an excellent supplement to aid in the healing of the epithelial cells of the skin. It helps to heal ulcers, skin lesions and aids in vision. It is known as an antioxidant which hinders cellular damage that leads to the aging process. The typical dosage for Vitamin A is 10,000 IU per day. Vitamin A in high doses, such as over 100,000 international units can be toxic. Beta carotene is a precursor to vitamin A and has no toxic effects if taken in larger doses. The skin may turn an orange tinge, however it is not harmful.

Vitamin E

Vitamin E is a fat soluble vitamin that acts as an anti-oxidant. It improves circulation and is necessary for tissue repair. It can reduce scarring from lesions and aids in healing the skin. Typical dosage of vitamin E ranges from 200 to 400 international units per day.

HOMEOPATHIC REMEDIES FOR RECTAL ITCHING

There are many homeopathic remedies for rectal itching. Some of the more common remedies are listed with their symptoms here. For more information on how to self prescribe a homeopathic remedy, go to Chapter Two. If you cannot find a remedy suited to you, or find you are not improving or your symptoms get worse, seek the help of a professional homeopath or your medical doctor.

CINA
Common indications include:
- itching of the anus
- worms and parasites
- **spasms/convulsions from worms**
- **emaciation despite ravenous appetite**
- white balls of mucous with bowel movements
- loose and involuntary stools
- irritable and restless at night causing a poor sleep
- cutting and pinching pain in the abdomen
- **miserable whilst suffering from worms**
- **mentally these types are irritable and indifferent to caresses**
- **cannot be consoled**
- **children who shriek at night and may hit or strike out**
- **desires cold drinks and food**
- **appetite is unpredictable**
- worse at night, summertime and from worms

GRAPHITES
Common indications include:
- these types tend to be solid people, heavy set working types
- sore and itching anus
- **fissure, hemorrhoids that are worse after wiping**
- **rectal pains that sore, stitching, burning and raw**

- burning, painful and swollen skin
- **rectum is moist and sticky**
- **excoriation of the rectum, must itch it until it raw**
- **constipation with sensation of stool remaining in the rectum**
- cracks or sores may ooze a yellow serum or pus
- stools may be hard with mucous or loose
- **mentally these types are simple, earthy folks who may have poor concentration**
- **weeping from music**
- worse at night, when warm or surrounding menstruation
- better in the dark and wrapping up

IGNATIA
Common indications include:
- itching and stitching in the rectal area
- itching as if from a nettle rash
- **rectal spasms**
- **hemorrhoids internal**
- burning or chapped sensation of the rectal opening
- stools may pass with difficulty and the rectum may feel constricted
- **mentally these types can be moody, tearful and have ailments from grief and romantic disappointments**
- **aggravated by sweets**, mornings, coffee, after meals and warmth
- relieved by changing position

SULPHUR
Common indications include:
- **itching rectum**
- **itching worse from the heat of the bed**
- **itch makes one want to scratch which doesn't help**
- **burning pain whilst sitting** and itching around the anus
- **diarrhea drives one out of bed in the morning**
- **redness of the anus**
- **voluptuous itching**
- skin may form vesicles or pustules
- the more one scratches, the more it is itchy
- **tendency to skin problems**
- skin may be rough or coarse
- hemorrhoids with dark blood
- constipation or diarrhea
- **mentally these types can be lazy, messy and/or intellectual**
- **worse at 11:00 a.m.**, in the evening or early morning, in a warm bed, **bathing**, after milk or alcoholic beverages
- relieved by walking and in open air

TEUCRIUM MARUM VERUM
Common indications include:

- this is a remedy for worms where there is immense itching of the anus
- creeping sensation in the rectum that is worse at night in bed
- itching after stools, in the evening and in bed
- these types can suffer from unusual hunger
- violent and jerking hiccoughs
- sensation of something crawling in the nostrils
- aggravation night, from the warmth of the bed and after nursing
- amelioration in the open air

Picture this....

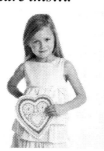

Your sister was telling you about your niece, age 7, having terrible sleep with fits and restlessness. On questioning, she reported having an itchy anus. Her mother said that when she was five, she had a bad case of pinworms which had been treated successfully by her doctor. However, her sleep was never the same. For the last two years your niece has been a terrible sleeper. She has no signs of diarrhea or constipation. You have knowledge of homeopathic remedies and recommended she try Cina 4CH, four pellets twice a day for a few days. To your sister's surprise, her daughter started to sleep well and stopped itching.

Ulcerative Colitis

Autoimmune conditions are becoming more and more prevalent today. These are illnesses characterized by the body's immune system marking a particular organ as the enemy and attacking it. Many alternative health practitioners believe that autoimmune diseases are related to an event(s) that happened before age seven, even in utero. Many types of autoimmune diseases exist, such as lupus, rheumatoid arthritis, Hashimoto's thyroiditis, ulcerative colitis and multiple sclerosis. Despite the different symptoms, there is often a common thread in all of these disorders. The immune system becomes abnormally reactive to a particular organ in the body. Autoimmune sufferers have had a series of toxic insults to their system, whether they are subtle or obvious. Some of these include physical injuries, psychological stress, food sensitivities, parasites, viruses, fungi, vaccinations and heavy metal toxicity.

What is Ulcerative Colitis?

Although ulcerative colitis is considered a separate disorder from Crohn's disease, its treatment is very similar. Ulcerative colitis typically occurs between the ages of 15 and 30. It affects both sexes equally and has a hereditary component. Caucasians and Jewish people tend to be more affected by this disease.

Ulcerative colitis is an autoimmune inflammatory bowel disease. Like most autoimmune diseases, it has active periods followed by remission. It is characterized by inflammation that can affect the lining of the rectum and the colon.

It causes inflammation and ulcerous lesions. Inflammation caused by this disorder attacks the membrane lining of the colon and ulcerous sores result. This inflammation also causes bloody diarrhea. Lesions can be superficial or cause scarring that result in thickening of the intestinal wall. This disorder is often confused with Crohn's disease because the process of destruction to the intestinal wall is similar. However, ulcerative colitis affects the lower portion of the intestines and Crohn's disease affects any portion from the mouth to the rectum.

What are the Symptoms of Ulcerative Colitis?
- abdominal pain
- bloody stools
- diarrhea
- anemia
- fatigue
- weight loss
- loss of appetite
- fever
- rectal bleeding
- dehydration
- nausea
- malnutrition
- skin lesions
- joint pain
- osteoporosis
- growth failure in children

Diagnosis and Medical Treatment
Medical diagnosis is done using several blood tests to determine an elevated white blood cell count, elevated sedimentation rate and C-reactive protein. A barium X-ray, colonoscopy, biopsy and upper GI series are useful to detect lesions associated with ulcerative colitis. Often a Medical Doctor will then differentiate ulcerative colitis from Crohn's disease, enterocolitis and cancer.

Typical medical treatment includes the use of corticosteroid drugs, immunosuppressive drugs, salfasalazine and broad spectrum antibiotics. Surgery may be recommended by your doctor. Immunosupressive drugs may be necessary,but they leave a person open to more infections. Sulfasalazine decreases folic acid and iron stores. Steroids such as prednisone expend more vitamin C, calcium and magnesium. Antibiotics kill the beneficial bacteria in the gut. Supplementation may be necessary to counteract the effects of the medication and to aid in vitamin deficiencies.

Seek Professional Help for Autoimmune Diseases
Autoimmune conditions are difficult to treat and there is no overnight cure. An autoimmune condition can take upwards of six months to halt the condition and another six to heal. For this reason, you have to have confidence in your practitioner and their method of healing. Steer clear of any overnight success claims. Seek the help of a professional when taking any remedies. There can be interactions between prescription medications and natural supplements. Medications can cause other health problems.

Immune suppressants, anti-inflammatories, steroids and prednisone all have side effects. For example, immune suppressants can leave the body open to serious infections and cancer. Steroids can weaken bone strength, skin integrity and eyesight. They can also sap the energy from the adrenal glands.

What Causes Ulcerative Colitis?

There is no known single cause of ulcerative colitis. There are many factors that may contribute to the development of a faulty immune system that turns on itself. Some of the main factors that contribute to autoimmune conditions are imbalanced intestinal flora, dysbiosis, leaky gut syndrome, improper diet, hygiene hypothesis and external toxic insults.

1) Imbalanced Intestinal Flora

The intestinal flora is comprised of delicately balanced healthy and non-healthy bacteria. It is said that 60% of our immune system comes from our intestinal tract. This is our gut associated lymphoid tissue (GALT). If our natural flora is compromised our GALT may not be as effective at maintaining proper health.

There are immune system cells throughout the gut that influence the body's capability to fight off invaders. It is important to note that the gastrointestinal tract is in contact with the outside world. It is an open passage for food, toxins and the like to enter our system. Without a healthy gut flora, we can fall prey to outside offenders such as parasites, viruses, fungi and environmental toxins (such as pesticides, heavy metals and pollution).

In utero, children acquire their intestinal flora from their mother. Neonates also acquire part of their healthy gastrointestinal flora from breastfeeding. Often newborns or breast-feeding mothers are required to take antibiotics that strip the healthy flora of the gastrointestinal system. This creates an imbalance of the good and bad bacteria in the gut if not properly replenished with probiotics. A person's natural flora is usually set in the first few years of life. Thus, if a child is exposed to a variety of toxic insults or the mother's flora was imbalanced, the child may have more of a chance of developing other disorders later in life. These disorders can be allergies, immune dysfunction, ADHD, intestinal problems and the like.

2) Dysbiosis and Leaky Gut Syndrome

A few hypotheses for the cause of autoimmune disorders are leaky gut syndrome and dysbiosis. Leaky gut syndrome is characterized by the gut lining of the intestinal tract as having small perforations or opening in the tight junctions of the cells, allowing waste and food particles into the bloodstream. Due to the nature of the body's immune system, it mounts an inflammatory attack on these particles. Particles circulated in the blood may also be deposited into unsuspecting organs, such as the liver, kidneys or joints. This inflammatory reaction causes the body to unknowingly mount an attack on itself.

Dysbiosis is characterized by an imbalance of the gut flora as discussed. Dysbiosis can lead to leaky gut syndrome. It also creates dysfunction by not properly protecting the gastrointestinal lining that provides a safe barrier between the environment and your internal organs. This is a very basic explanation of the complexities of autoimmune disorders. Nevertheless, it provides basic information for those to understand and heal autoimmune problems.

3) The Hygiene Hypothesis

Another theory, about the prevalence of food sensitivities, allergies and autoimmune disease, is the "hygiene hypothesis". Studies have shown that kids who grew up in a sterile clean environment have more immune reactions and allergies then ones who live with a dog or a mother who wasn't the best housekeeper. Research has also shown that kids who have been exposed to certain parasites actually show less allergy and asthma. We overuse antibiotics which kill all good and bad bacteria in the gut. In children, an early introduction of antibiotics prevents the development of a healthy immune system. It depletes both good and bad bacteria in the gastrointestinal (GI) tract. If our GI tract has an aseptic environment, without both good and bad bacteria, our immune system becomes deranged. It is thought that bad bacteria in balance with the good, actually trains the immune system to properly function. If it doesn't function normally, it recognizes harmless things as potential allergens and organizes an inflammatory attack. We need a balance of both good and bad bacteria to be healthy.

4) Improper Diet

Many types of foods actually increase inflammation and dysbiosis in the body. These two factors are the root cause of many diseases like inflammatory bowel disease, hypertension, arthritis and even cancer. Inflammation causes a chain of cellular events that release inflammatory proteins in the body. These proteins cause immune system reactions which include the destruction of healthy cells called oxidation. Both high fat and high glycemic foods increase inflammatory reactions and feed the bad bacteria which cause dysbiosis.

The term "high glycemic" means the food such as refined carbohydrates like white bread, white rice and sugar quickly converts into a sugar in the bloodstream. For a list of low, medium and high glycemic and fat foods see the chart in Chapter Two. Fats that cause inflammation are saturated, hydrogenated fats or those high in arachadonic acid (A.A.). A.A. is said to be one of the major players in inflammatory responses and is found in animal products such as organ meats, red meats, pork, animal fat and skin. Oils that are re-used for cooking become rancid and cause oxidation which also damages the cells. Stimulants such as caffeine, nicotine and alcohol affect the nervous system. The nervous system and the gut are tightly connected. When it is stimulated, it can cause a chain reaction of gastrointestinal upset, gas, bloating, constipation and diarrhea.

Food sensitivities may play a role in autoimmune conditions. If you have a reaction to certain foods, you may inadvertently be causing an inflammatory reaction in your body. Take care to avoid certain foods that are triggers for your condition.

5) External Insults

External insults from our environment such as stress, vaccines and heavy metal toxicity can weaken our immune system. The nervous system and the gastrointestinal tract are tightly connected. Stress hormones can cause bowel disruptions such as constipation or diarrhea. Heavy metal toxins such as lead, mercury, aluminum, arsenic and barium can cause intestinal and immune system abnormalities. Detection of heavy metals can be done using a hair mineral analysis. Some Medical Doctors use a chelating drug to bind heavy metals and then test the urine for their excretion. Vaccinations are thought to prime our immune system to recognize a virus so that we will not succumb to it. This is a good theory and has prevented many merciless diseases. However, some vaccines still contain toxic ingredients such as mercury and formaldehyde. What happens with those toxins when we are injected with them? How can we excrete something injected right into our blood without it being deposited into some of our tissues? Obviously we cannot.

DIETARY MEASURES FOR ULCERATIVE COLITIS

Ulcerative colitis like Crohn's disease is a condition that has a great deal of individuality. Some may have a severe case and others may have a very mild one. Food restrictions are very individual as well. Follow the diet outlined in Chapter Three because it reduces inflammation, dysbiosis and prevents many other diseases. Any food on this list that has a "#" sign beside it should be avoided. These foods contribute to intestinal dysbiosis, which is an inappropriate balance of bad and good bacteria in the intestinal tract.

Food sensitivities are a factor in most ulcerative colitis cases. Try the food challenge test as outlined in chapter three or be tested by a professional for food sensitivities. With either method, you will have more knowledge to control your symptoms. Typical offenders are wheat, dairy, citrus, gluten, peanuts, corn, soya or sugar. In practice, wheat and dairy are the top two culprits because people tend to overeat them which creates sensitivity. For more information about food sensitivities see Chapter Three.

A book that contains beneficial dietary information for inflammatory bowel disease (IBD) is called *Breaking the Vicious Cycle* by Elaine Gottschall (see bibliography). It covers inflammatory bowel conditions such as Crohn's, colitis, irritable bowel syndrome and celiac disease. Although the diet outlined in this book is very restrictive, it helps most people with IBD. Some of the foods mentioned to avoid in this book are all canned foods, processed meats, sugar and grains like barley, corn, rye, oats, rice, buckwheat, millet, triticale, bulgur and spelt. Potatoes, yams, parsnips, okra, chickpeas, bean sprouts, turnips, soy, mung, fava and garbanzo beans are not acceptable. No milk products, yogurt, soya milk or coffee substitutes can be used. The list of foods to avoid is longer than mentioned here. However, it is a good option for those who do not have the resources to see a Homeopath to do the home food challenge test.

GENERAL SUPPLEMENTS FOR TREATING ULCERATIVE COLITIS

With serious illness, often a liquid or powdered variety is more readily absorbed than a tablet form. If a pill is taken, a capsule is preferred to a tablet.

Aloe Vera
Aloe vera juice is very healing to the gastrointestinal tract. It helps to sooth and repair the intestines. Aloe is said to be a tonic, laxative and to stimulate bile flow, eliminate parasites and heal the stomach. Typical dosage is one tablespoon to three ounces, one to three times daily. Start with the lowest dose until you find your comfort zone. If you take too much aloe vera, you may suffer with diarrhea. This supplement is not suited to those who suffer from acute diarrhea, heavy periods, pregnancy and/or kidney disease.

Antioxidants

Antioxidants are useful for ulcerative colitis sufferers because they do not assimilate nutrients well and they have an increased risk for cancer. They prevent oxidative damage which helps slow the cycle of cellular destruction. They also help to heal the gastrointestinal lining.

1. **Vitamin A** helps to heal the lining of the gastrointestinal tract, aids in immunity and helps the lining of the mucous membranes. It is necessary for the maintenance and repair of the mucous membrane lining, thus it heals ulcers. It is needed for new cell growth and is said to slow the aging process. Beta carotene is converted into Vitamin A in the liver. If the liver is not working well, it is best to take Vitamin A. In high doses, beta carotene does not have any side effects, other then turning one's skin orange. Typical dosage is of vitamin A is 10,000 IU per day. Over 100,000 IU has been known to cause liver damage.

2. **Vitamin C** is a powerful antioxidant that helps with tissue growth and repair. It attacks free radicals that can cause cell destruction. This wonder vitamin protects the blood vessels, decreases cholesterol, decreases inflammation and enhances immunity. It is also helps one to absorb iron, L-glutamine and B vitamins. Use an Esterified vitamin C because it is easier on the stomach, not as acidic and is more readily absorbed than a regular vitamin C. Typical dosage for vitamin C is 500 to 3000 mgs per day.

3. **Vitamin E** helps to heal the mucous membrane lining of the gastrointestinal tract and is good for the cardiovascular system and the skin. It helps selenium be absorbed more readily. Typical dosage for vitamin E is 200 to 400 IU per day.

4. **Selenium** is helpful for inflammatory conditions, maintaining proper immune function, protecting the liver, preventing heart disease and cancer. Typical dosage is 200 to 400 mcgs. Do not take selenium in doses higher then 40 mcgs if you are pregnant.

B Vitamins

B complex is useful for people who suffer from autoimmune disease. It aids in toning the muscles of the gastrointestinal tract and acts to combat the effects of emotional stress. Certain medications such as steroids deplete Vitamin B. One can safely take 100 mgs of B complex daily with meals.

B12 and folic acid are useful to better absorb iron and reduce high homocysteine levels. High levels of the amino acid, homocysteine, in the colon and blood may predispose people to both ulcerative colitis and Crohn's disease. It is said to influence other diseases as well, such as Alzheimer's, dementia, depression, ischemic heart disease and stroke, osteoporosis and cancer. Vitamin B6, B12 and folic acid work to decrease homocysteine levels.

Calcium and Magnesium

Calcium and magnesium are useful for people using steroids because they decrease bone mass. It is also one of the more difficult minerals to absorb. However, calcium citrate tends to be better absorbed than carbonate. However, calcium carbonate was studied and is thought to prevent colon cancer. This is likely because it is not absorbed well and binds intestinal toxins and excretes them. One can take up to 1,200 mgs of calcium with 600 mgs of magnesium daily. Check with your doctor for interactions between calcium and your medications.

Essential Fatty Acids (EFAs)

Essential fatty acids, mainly flax and fish oil, are good for pain, inflammation, dry skin, gas, bloating, gastrointestinal function and secretion, and immune system deficiency. They can also help with allergic symptoms. This can also help with other problems such as depression, concentration problems, joint pains, inflammation, skin eruptions and cardiovascular disease. Be sure to keep your EFAs in the fridge to prevent rancidity. Do not use your EFA liquid for cooking. Once it is heated it releases free radicals.

Eicosapentaenoic acid (EPA) found in fish oil is most beneficial for inflammatory bowel disease. Some studies have shown that it may reduce the need for corticosteroids and ensure longer remission. EPA can be found in cold water fish such as herring, trout, salmon and mackerel. It increases a type of prostaglandin that actually decreases inflammatory proteins. EPA improves blood flow and reduces inflammation. Cod liver oil contains EPA but may have too much Vitamin A for some.

One can safely take up to 4,000 mgs of fish oil daily. Ideally you would like to have about 1,000 mgs of EPA per day. An enteric coated fish oil capsule is advantageous because it releases in the intestinal tract not the stomach. This would ensure that you would be getting the maximum EPA into the intestinal tract. The stomach may degrade some of the EPA before it reaches the colon.

L-Glutamine

L-glutamine is a supplement that provides metabolic fuel for the intestinal cells. It helps to sustain the villi and absorptive surfaces of the intestinal tract lining. Vitamin C and B complex help to enhance the absorption of L-glutamine. Recommended dosage for adults is two to six grams per day with meals. There are no known side effects of L-glutamine.

High Potency Multi Vitamin

People who suffer from Crohn's disease are at risk for vitamin and mineral deficiencies. It is wise to take a daily multi vitamin in a liquid or capsule. These are easier to assimilate than a tablet. I usually don't recommend "one a day" types of vitamins because they contain so many vitamins and minerals, they are packed very tightly to enable one to swallow them. If they did not, people would choke on them. If your stomach acid and digestion are not good, you would not be able to properly break down the tablet. Take a liquid form or a multi that you have to take in divided doses throughout the day.

Probiotics

Every person has billions of bacteria in their intestinal tract. Most bacteria are beneficial and maintain health. A small percentage of bacteria in our intestines are harmful if they spread. If these bad bacteria overgrow it may have negative health consequences such as immune dysfunction, infections, constipation and/or diarrhea.

Good flora helps to maintain the immune system and displace the bad bacteria in the gut. They also help to sustain normal arrangement and function of the intestine's cells. The most popular beneficial bacteria are lactobacillus acidophilus and bifidobacteria. The lactobacilli can be found in fermented foods such as yogurt, miso, tempeh and kefir. However, the number of bacteria is not standardized. The bacteria may not be an active culture if they are not stored properly.

It is best to use a standardized capsule of probiotics. It should be stored in the refrigerator which helps ensure that it is a live culture. Follow the directions on the package. Typical dosage for a probiotic supplement is one to 10 billion cells per capsule. One to three capsules can be taken daily. There are no known side effects from probiotics.

Quercitin, Tumeric and Bromelain
These herbs are helpful for a number of reasons:
- they reduce inflammation
- they combat free radicals
- protect the liver against toxins
- decrease allergic reactions
- reduce platelets from sticking to each other which aids in circulation
- decrease cholesterol
- act as an antibiotic, anti-inflammatory and anti-cancer supplement

Take as directed on the individual package; they may come together in one pill.

HOMEOPATHIC REMEDIES FOR ULCERATIVE COLITIS

There are many homeopathic remedies for ulcerative colitis. Some of the more common remedies are listed with their symptoms here. For more information on how to self prescribe a homeopathic remedy, go to Chapter Two. If you cannot find a remedy suited to you, or find you are not improving or your symptoms get worse, seek the help of a professional homeopath or your medical doctor.

ALOE SOCOTRINA
Common indications include:
- distended abdomen after drinking water
- rumbling and gurgling gas
- urgent diarrhea after eating
- **urgent stools at 5:00 a.m.**
- **stools jelly-like that contain lumpy mucous** and blood
- anus is burning with itching hemorrhoids
- weakness of the anal sphincter
- **involuntary stool while urinating or passing gas**
- suited to beer drinkers who lead a sedentary life
- mental and physical work causes fatigue
- **hemorrhoids that are congested like a bunch of grapes, that are better with a cold bath**

- **hot sensation when passing gas**
- **early morning sudden diarrhea that drives one out of bed**
- pain felt in the stomach when walking and making a misstep
- pain radiates to the back and upwards with every belch
- aggravated by from eating, heat, after eating
- relieved by passing gas with distension, drinking cold water, bending forward

---

Did you know?

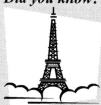

Forty percent of all French Physicians practice homeopathy! A report from 1991 calculated that total costs associated with this type of care per patient was on average 15% less than costs associated with conventional medicine.

Source: Drug Store News, May 17, 1999 "Clinical Study Suggests That Homeopathy Could Save Healthcare Dollars" by Rob Eder
www.findarticles.com

ARSENCIUM ALBUM

Common indications include:

- abdominal distension with a **burning sensation**
- painful inguinal glands
- **burning diarrhea after anxiety, cold drinks and fruits**
- burning rectum with stools and intense cutting pain
- **offensive and putrid discharges**
- fears they may die and it is useless to take medicine
- cold and clammy with the **feeling they can never get warm enough**
- desires hot drinks and applications despite burning sensation
- **great thirst yet only takes small sips of water**
- **tongue is discoloured white**
- canker sores in the mouth
- nausea after meals
- **mentally these types are restless, anxious and fearful of diseases**
- **worse after midnight**, after eating, cold, during rest
- **relieved by hot drinks, warmth**, motion and exercise

BELLADONNA

Common indications include:

- very useful remedy for acute inflammatory flair ups
- **pains comes and goes quickly**
- **high fever with red face**
- **right sided pains**
- bloody diarrhea with great urging
- pains are better when bending or lying the abdomen over a hard chair
- abdomen feels sore and raw
- diarrhea worse during motion
- trembling during stool

- **thirstless during fever**
- flatulent pain with distension felt across the transverse colon
- pain felt in the right groin area
- stomach pain aggravated during a meal
- **cravings for lemons or lemonade**
- aggravation from motion, cold, eating, bright light
- **relieved with pressure**, while bending double or backwards, lying over a hard chair, lying down
- aggravated by jarring, motion or pressure, touch, slightest touch by linens of the bed

CAUSTICUM
Common indications include:
- chilly people who are affected at any change of weather
- burning in the rectum with piles
- **stool is covered with mucous**
- painful swelling of the abdomen
- stool is passed better whilst standing than sitting
- stools seem too slender from rectal cramps
- anxiety is felt after a stool
- colicky pains felt in the morning that extend to the back and chest
- **rectal fissures** and fistulas that are painful whilst walking
- pustules near the anus that discharge blood, pus and serum
- **hoarseness and constant desire to clear the throat**
- **these types tend to have rheumatic complaints**
- **aversion to sweets** and stomach pressure from eating bread
- thirst for cold drinks with a weak appetite
- **cravings for bacon, salt and smoked meats**
- **aggravation from cold**, change of weather, walking, sitting, suppressed skin disease, after eating the least amount of food, tight clothes
- better from standing, bending double

IGNATIA
Common indications include:
- **spasmodic, cramping pains**, painful urging for stool
- stools are pasty, bloody, mucous filled, burning
- sensation of a sharp instrument is in the rectum
- **constriction of the rectum** for one or two hours after a stool
- blind hemorrhoids that are aggravated whilst both sitting and standing
- prolapsed anus
- **these types have a lump sensation in their throat**
- fruit causes diarrhea
- diarrhea alternates with constipation

- **mentally these types are easily offended, have alternating moods and much grief**
- **may sigh or cough often**
- **aggravated by eating sweets, grief, unrequited love** and worries
- aggravated by tobacco, coffee, drug use, fruit, after grief
- relieved by walking

MERCURIUS CORROSIVUS
Common indications include:
- successfully treats dysentery
- bloody frequent motions
- stool are green with mucous, scanty, pure blood, black, pasty, burning, slimy
- burning felt in the anus
- **urging for stools**
- gums may be swollen, purple, spongy
- ulcers are corroding, acid and full of pus
- constriction in the throat with spasms
- **constant urging without remission on passing stools**
- great deal of perspiration and salivation
- complaints in the summer or from May to November
- aggravated by fats, acids, cold, during the summer
- relieved by rest, motion

NITRIC ACID
Common indications include:
- bright red hemorrhage from the bowel after stools
- straining as if stool has been left behind
- pain in the rectum for hours after a bowel movement
- stools are offensive, green and putrid
- breaks into a sweat during stool
- **tendency to rectal warts that bleed easily**
- glands are painful and swollen
- fissures and ulcers of the anus, mouth and throat
- **splinter-like pains, especially in the rectum**
- **these types desire fat and salt**
- raw ulcers that have zigzag edges
- **mentally, these types are anxious, hypochondrical, irritable and hold a grudge**
- aggravated by milk

NUX VOMICA
Common indications include:
- said to treat dysentery
- constipation alternating with diarrhea with painful urging

- **spasmodic sharp cramps and flatulence**
- errors in diet aggravate these types
- enlarged liver and gallstone colic
- **urging to have bowel movement**
- pain felt two or three hours after eating
- **stomach pains worse from anger and tight clothes**
- sour, watery, bitter heartburn after meals
- painful ulcers in the mouth and throat
- bleeding piles with urging for stools
- nausea and vomiting in the morning or after meals
- **cravings for spices, alcohol, fat and coffee**
- suited to sedentary types who do a lot of mental work
- **suited to competitive, impatient, workaholic types who over enduldge**
- **chilly types who seek the warmth**
- worse in the morning, mental overwork, alcohol, coffee, overeating and drugs
- **relieved with warmth**, rest and during damp weather

PHOSPHORUS
Common indications include:

- chronic diarrhea
- watery stools preceded by great rumbling noises
- watery stools expelled like a hose
- **tendency to hemorrhages, nose bleeds etc.**
- stools may be involuntary, watery, green, mucous-filled, bloody
- anus feels like it is wide open, stool easily escapes
- **easily dehydrated and debilitated**
- fistula that secretes a thin, foul smelling pus
- **hunger soon after eating**
- **very thirsty for cold drinks**
- distended, painful abdomen worse after dinner
- tearing and burning pain in the stomach, worse in morning
- sour and burning belching
- enlarged and/or cirrhosis of the liver
- **these types may have lung problems, bronchitis, infections, pneumonia, tickling coughs**
- **desires cold food and drinks, salt, spice, milk and wine**
- cold drinks vomited after they warm up in the stomach
- **emotionally these types are open, anxious, like company and fear thunderstorms or that something bad will happen**
- relieved by cold drinks or food
- **aggravated by fasting, warm foods, salt and spices**

Picture this….

Your son, age 33, is suffering from an acute flair up of ulcerative colitis. He just started with bloody and frequent stools. He had been feeling great prior to this and had been in remission for a few years. However, he has been working hard and eating a lot of fast foods on the run for the past month. He is a single parent on his own and you are worried about his health.

He starts a wheat and dairy-free diet because in the past that had always helped his condition. He feels those foods are his triggers. At your recommendation, he sees your alternative health practitioner who prescribes fish oil, acidophilus and bifidus, plus a herbal combination of quercitin, tumeric and bromelain to be taken daily. After a few weeks, the stools became more solid and his bleeding stops. Like many of us who feel well, pushing the envelope too far can lead to ill health. You know that his condition is very sensitive to being worn down and poor eating habits. Fortunately, his digestion responded quickly because he had taken care of it before it got too bad.

Ulcers

An ulcer is characterized by the eroding of the lining of the stomach (gastric ulcer) or the duodenum of the small intestine (duodenal ulcer). Ulcers occur when the mucus layer that lines the stomach or duodenum loses its integrity. This layer usually provides a slippery protective coating and barrier. Hydrochloric acid made by the stomach for the digestion of food actually comes in contact with the membrane lining when this protective layer is compromised. This condition can be quite painful because this lesion is exposed to corrosive acid. Duodenal ulcers are more common than peptic ulcers. Ulcers are more frequent in men then in women and in people who are blood type O.

Many think there is an emotional or stress component to ulcers. Some metaphysical books attribute the development of ulcers to bitterness that is eating one up inside. It is also related to being defenseless or vulnerable. The body may have a hard time healing if one doesn't have time for forgiveness or is vulnerable. These types of psycho-emotional or spiritual causes are interesting. Nonetheless, they must have meaning to the individual or they are not useful.

What are the Symptoms of Ulcers?
- stomach pain an hour after eating (in gastric ulcers)
- pains before eating (in duodenal ulcers)
- tender abdomen
- bloating
- blood in the stool (via testing)
- black stools
- nausea and vomiting
- heartburn
- fatigue
- belching
- vomiting of blood
- waterbrash

What are the Complications Associated with Ulcers?
Most often proper treatment of an ulcer helps to clear the condition without problems.
- In severe cases an ulcer can erode a blood vessel and cause severe bleeding.
- Perforations may be caused from an ulcer and the stomach or intestinal contents may spill into the abdominal cavity. This can cause a serious condition called peritonitis, which is an inflammation of the inner abdominal cavity.
- Scarring and swelling may cause a narrowing of the duodenum or stomach and block it from expelling its contents.
- Ulcers may penetrate into surrounding organs like the liver and the pancreas.

What Causes Ulcers?
1) Helicobacter pylori
Ulcers used to be thought of as a sign of being stressed. However, researchers have found that most often the culprit is the bacteria called Helicobacter Pylori or H. pylori. This bacteria is found in 50% of people over the age of 50. It is present in 90 to 100% of patients with duodenal ulcers and 70% with gastric ulcers. Doctors test for this bacteria by doing a blood or saliva test to check for antibodies to Helicobacter pylori.

2) Aspirin and NSAIDS
Aspirin and non-steroidal anti-inflammatory drugs (NSAIDS) increase ones risk to having a peptic ulcer. According to the *Encyclopedia of Natural Healing, Second Edition* by Michael Murray and Joseph Pizzorno, (see bibliography), even a low dosage of 75 mgs of aspirin is related to stomach ulcers.

3) Smoking
Smokers tend to have an increased risk, mortality and severity of peptic ulcers.

4) Diet
Foods that may aggravate ulcers and heartburn are fried foods, fat, spices, salt, coffee, tea, sugar, vinegar, carbonated drinks, dried meats, alcoholic beverages, citrus fruits, tomatoes, chocolate and bread. Food allergies are linked to ulcers.

5) Stress
Stress is long thought to be a cause of ulcers. However, the medical literature and studies have not shown that stressful life events cause ulcers. It is not the amount of stress that is the problem, but the person's response to it. Stress can cause increased heartburn symptoms. When we have chronic stress, our blood supply travels to our extremities. This is because we have an evolutionary "fight or flight response." This is to help us run when we are fearful of impending danger. We have no outlet for stress as we cannot ethically or socially attack or run. Thus, the blood supply travels away from the stomach and impacts our digestion. Any worry, stress, shock and anxiety can influence our digestion. Our nervous system is tightly connected to our digestion. For some people any stress manifests in digestive upset.

6) Food Allergies/ Sensitivities

Food allergies can aggravate the stomach lining. In one study 98% of people who suffer with peptic ulcers also have a respiratory allergy. A study of children found that more then half of allergic children had peptic ulcers diagnosed by x-rays. For more information on food sensitivities, go to Chapter Three.

Medical Testing and Treatment for Ulcers

Your medical doctor has a variety of tools to diagnose an ulcer. A barium swallow shows the upper gastrointestinal tract through an x-ray. A scope with a camera can also be put down the throat to look at the stomach and small intestine. Stool samples will be taken to detect blood in them. Blood is checked for anemia. Also Helicobacter pylori can be detected through saliva or blood testing.

Medical doctors use a few medications for ulcers, depending on their symptoms. They are as follows:

- antibiotics for killing the bacteria Helicobacter pylori
- antacids to block excessive acid
- medication for the lining of the stomach and intestines
- bismuth helps to protect the lining and get rid of the bacteria

DIETARY MEASURES

Ulcer sufferers should avoid sugar, tea, pop, spicy foods, coffee, fats, grease, pastries, tomatoes, citrus and alcohol. A variety of fresh fruits, vegetables, lean meat, fish and whole grains are permitted in your diet. Low antioxidant levels are linked to stomach ulcers. By eating a variety of colours of fruits and vegetables you will increase the amount of antioxidants that you ingest. Some juices have healing properties such as raw potato and cabbage juice. They are excellent at healing the lining of the stomach and reducing acid.

Follow the diet guidelines from Chapter Three. Eat foods that are low glycemic which help keep you healthy overall. Avoid foods that trigger your heartburn even if they are in column one.

SUPPLEMENTS FOR ULCERS

Aloe Vera Juice

Aloe vera juice is very healing to the gastrointestinal tract. Aloe is said to be a tonic, laxative, to stimulate bile flow, eliminate parasites and heal the stomach. Typical dosage is one tablespoon to three ounces, one to three times daily. Start with the lowest dose until you find your comfort zone. If you take too much aloe vera, you may suffer with diarrhea. This supplement is not suited to those who suffer from diarrhea, heavy periods, pregnancy and/or kidney disease.

Antioxidants

Antioxidants are useful for ulcers because they help support the healing of the lining of the stomach and small intestine.

1. **Vitamin A** helps to heal the lining of the gastrointestinal tract, aids in immunity and helps the lining of the mucous membranes. It is necessary for the maintenance

and repair of the mucous membrane lining, thus it heals ulcers. It is needed for new cell growth and is said to slow the aging process. Beta carotene is converted into vitamin A in the liver. If the liver is not working well, it is best to take vitamin A. In high doses, beta carotene does not have any side effects, other then turning one's skin orange. Typical dosage is of vitamin A is 10,000 IU per day. Over 100,000 IU has been known to cause liver damage.

2. **Vitamin C** is a powerful antioxidant that helps with tissue growth and repair. It attacks free radicals that can cause cell destruction. This wonder vitamin protects the blood vessels, decreases cholesterol, decreases inflammation and enhances immunity. It is also helps one to absorb iron, L-glutamine and B vitamins. Use an Esterified vitamin C because it is easier on the stomach, not as acidic and is more readily absorbed than a regular vitamin C. Take 500 to 1000 mgs per day.

3. **Vitamin** E helps to heal the mucous membrane lining of the gastrointestinal tract and is good for the cardiovascular system and the skin. Typical dosage for vitamin E is 200 to 400 IU per day.

B Vitamins

B complex is useful for people who suffer from ulcers. It aids in toning the muscles of the gastrointestinal tract, the nerves and acts to combat the effects of emotional stress. Certain medications such as steroids, birth control pills and hormone replacement drugs deplete Vitamin B stores. One can safely take 50 to 100 mgs of B complex daily with meals.

Calcium and Magnesium, 2:1 ratio

Take a 2:1 ratio of calcium to magnesium. It is an alkalinizing mineral that helps to absorb the stomach acid. Take in between meals. Typical daily dosage would be 800 to 1200 mgs of calcium and 400 to 600 mgs of magnesium. It is best to split this into two or three doses throughout the day. Calcium carbonate is a better buffer for acid than calcium citrate or calcium hydroxyapatite.

Deglycyrrhizinated Licorice (DGL)

DGL is an excellent remedy for heartburn and healing the stomach and esophagus. It has been known since ancient Greek and Egyptian times. It is said to help heal ulcers of the gastrointestinal tract. It has anti-inflammatory, antiviral, antimicrobial, mucoprotective and expectorant properties. Typical dosage is 500 mgs half hour before each meal, up to three times a day. Licorice decreases potassium which increases sodium in the body. This is why licorice is not suitable to those who have high blood pressure. Avoid licorice if you have low potassium, during pregnancy, liver disease, kidney disease and heart failure. Avoid licorice if you are taking diuretics or prednisone like drugs.

Garlic

Garlic is a great anti-microbial, which means it is effective in killing yeast, viruses and bacteria. It may be helpful in inhibiting the growth of bacteria that causes ulcers. Garlic is medicinal to the GI tract because it has antimicrobial, anti dyspepsia and beneficial digestive properties.

Note: Avoid garlic if you take blood thinners, prior to surgery and/or have hypoglycemia.

Probiotics

Probiotics such as acidophilus and bifidobacterium are beneficial bacteria. They help re-colonize the beneficial bacteria in the GI tract. You always have bad and good bacteria in your gut. If this bad and good flora become imbalanced, your stomach lining may become irritated. Bifidobacterium has also been shown to suppress Helicobacter pylori, the bacteria responsible for causing peptic ulcers, anemia and gastric cancer. Products that are not refrigerated may be a dead culture, which does not help the beneficial flora to grow. Take as directed on the label.

HOMEOPATHIC REMEDIES FOR ULCERS

There are many homeopathic remedies for ulcers. Some of the more common remedies are listed with their symptoms here. For more information on how to self prescribe a homeopathic remedy, go to Chapter Two. If you cannot find a remedy suited to you, or find you are not improving or your symptoms get worse, seek the help of a professional homeopath or your medical doctor.

ANTIMONIUM CRUDUM
Common indications include:
- **white milky tongue, thick coating on tongue**
- burning in the pit of the stomach
- stomach always feels overloaded
- **overeating causes digestive distress**
- heartburn, nausea, vomiting
- rising of fluid tastes like food that was eaten
- constant
- sensation of something lodged in throat which makes him swallow
- milk becomes curdled in the stomach
- vomits as soon as eats
- **these are warm-blooded types who feel worse from heat**
- **these types tend to be heavy set**
- **people who tend to be irritable, cannot stand to be touched or looked at**
- **cravings for pickles and acids, vinegar, wine**
- aggravated by fats, acids, sweets, vinegar, pork, alcohol
- **aversion to touch**

ARGENTUM NITRICUM
Common indications include:
- heartbeat may be affected by digestion
- **hot blooded with aggravation from heat**
- much flatulence and **loud belching**
- food lodges in the pharynx

- expelling gas relieves symptoms
- pain in the stomach pit with belching
- pain radiates in all directions
- bending double relieves the pains
- pains increase and decrease gradually
- tendency to stomach ulcers
- **craving for sugar which aggravates the stomach**
- ameliorated by warm drinks and alcohol
- aggravated by pressure, any food, **especially sweets**, cold food and drinks
- worse one hour or immediately after eating

Did you know?
Homeopathics help chemotherapy-induced side effects....
Stomatitis is an inflammation of the mouth that causes sores. It can happen with cancer medications. A small study of 15 children taking chemotherapy for bone marrow transplants found that one third of all patients who used a homeopathic preparation called Traumeel S as a mouth rinse did not get stomatitis. Also, 93% of the control patients who received no homeopathic remedy had progressive stomatitis.
Source: Cancer, A Journal of the American Cancer Society (2001; 92:684-90)

ARSENICUM ALBUM
Common indications include:
- water brash
- **burning in the stomach**
- may feel nauseated and low appetite
- **pain feels like a fire**, as if hot coals have are against the affected parts
- chronic digestive disturbance
- irritation of the mucous membrane of the stomach
- red tongue with thin white silvery coating, may have red raised taste buds
- stomach ulcers
- **dry mouth with intense thirst**
- cold water sits in the stomach like a stone
- **suited to chilly, restless and anxious types**
- **improved by drinking small sips of hot drinks despite suffering burning heat**
- aggravated by changing weather, cold and damp, lying with the head low
- **worse with cold drinks, ice**, spoiled meat, alcohol, lobster, salad

CALCAREA CARBONICA
Common indications include:
- **acid, sour risings and loud belching**
- **belching sour, acidic and watery**
- pressure in the pit of the stomach with sensation of a lump
- excessive stomach acid with burning
- rawness with a bitter taste in the throat

- stricture of the esophagus, food will not go down
- throat seems to contract on swallowing
- food tastes sour
- bloated abdomen requires loose clothing around the waist
- **may have sour perspiration, are clammy and perspire a lot on the head**
- **craving for eggs, sweets** and indigestible things like chalk
- **these types may tend to gain weight easily and be heavy set**
- **mentally these types are stubborn, hard working and responsible**
- aggravated by many foods, milk products, beans, sugar, pastries, oil and fats, cold drinks, vegetables and hard and dry foods
- worse during and after eating

HYDRASTIS
Common indications include:
- chronic heartburn
- **stomach feels empty**
- **mucous secretions can be caustic**
- weak digestion with hard bloating in the abdomen
- frequent sour belching
- vomits sour mucous
- struggles to swallow
- regurgitates food by the mouthful
- shortness of breath from digestive disturbance
- all foods turn into gas
- sharp pains in the stomach
- abuse of alkaline and acid mixtures
- tongue large, flabby and has a burnt sensation
- sore and ulcerous mouth
- aggravated by breads, alcohol, vegetables, excess wine and drugs

KALI BICHROMICUM
Common indications include:
- **rheumatism may alternate with stomach problems**
- chronic heartburn
- **increased mucous secretions**
- **ulcers**
- sour or bitter risings with nausea and pain
- dry mouth
- swallowing solids can be difficult, food gets stuck in the throat and may choke whilst eating
- regurgitation of liquids
- a simple diet seems to help most
- raw feeling with burning in the stomach
- may suffer from a stomach or duodenal ulcer

- **chilly people who are worse from cold**
- **mentally these types tend to be gloomy and conventional**
- **desires sweets**, beer and acids, such as vinegar or pickles
- **releived with belching**
- aggravated by attempting to eat or drink
- aggravated by overindulgence in beer, malt liquors and alcohol

MERCURIUS SOLUBILIS
Common indications include:
- **profuse salivation and sweating**
- ulcerations that are deep, bleeding, burning with irregular edges
- **teeth imprints on the tongue**
- moist swollen tongue with great thirst
- sweating severe and may stain the sheets yellow
- **offensive smelling discharges, breath**, urine, stool, sweat
- colic and diarrhea
- **thirsty**
- **worse at night, both hot and cold**, cold weather, warmth of bed and sweating
- better in the morning and whilst scratching

NATRUM PHOSPHORICUM
Common indications include:
- stomach pains, acid stomach and belching
- heartburn, **water brash with sour acid risings**
- trouble swallowing
- **yellow coated tongue**
- regurgitates fluid that is as sour as vinegar
- liquids are not tolerated as well as solid food
- **distension**, fullness after eating very little
- high uric acid in blood
- **cravings for eggs**, beer, fried fish and spices
- worse two hours after eating and with sugar, milk, bitter and fatty foods

NUX VOMICA
Common indications include:
- **bitter, sour and watery belching**
- heartburn and sour taste in the morning before or after eating
- pain in the stomach like a weight or pressure, two or three hours after meals
- bloating and distension
- **sensation of a stone in the stomach after eating**
- putrid bitter taste in the mouth
- **sensitive to clothes around the waist**
- back of tongue is coated brown

- **digestive problems from overeating or overindulging** in alcohol, drugs or excessive spices
- **excessive appetite or aversion to food with hunger**
- reverse peristalsis, spasms from disordered peristalsis, pain when food passes down into the pyloric sphincter
- tightness of the abdomen after eating, must loosen pants
- altered sense of taste for milk, coffee, water and beer
- digestive complaints with accompanying headaches
- **may be suited to zealous, fiery temperaments who overindulge and overwork**
- cravings for fats and tolerates them well
- **cravings for tea, coffee, alcohol and spicy food**
- worse after eating, drug use, tobacco poisoning, **overeating, overindulgence,** alcohol, spices, stimulants, tea and **coffee**

Picture this….

A man age 47 complains of stomach pains before eating. He will eat a bit of food and feel better, but only for an hour. Then his pain returns. He has insatiable cravings for 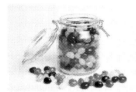 *candies. He will eat them and feel sick. He has a lot of gas and bloating. He is a very anxious person and suffers from heart palpitations. His doctor can't find anything wrong with him and prescribes anti-anxiety medications. He decides not to take them and chooses a natural approach instead. He goes to his local Homeopath. He takes DGL lozenges daily, Argentum Nitricum 30 CH twice daily and probiotics. He finds that after a few weeks his symptoms ease. He feels better without sweets, but he still overdoes it sometimes. His anxiety and heart palpitations stop altogether. His digestion is not an issue. It seems the homeopathic remedy helps him to stop desiring sweets as much.*

Vomiting

Vomiting can be a sign of an underlying problem. Vomiting is the forceful emptying of one's stomach contents through the mouth. The diaphragm contracts downwards and the abdominal muscles simultaneously contract to propel the stomach contents outwards. The feeling that one is about to vomit is called nausea. Signals for vomiting come from a variety of sources such as the brain via the senses, inner ear, the bloodstream or the gastrointestinal tract. Nausea and excessive saliva is often experienced without vomiting.

What are the Causes of Vomiting?
- chemotherapy
- emotional disorders such as bulimia
- food allergies
- food poisoning
- gag reflex that is easily activated
- migraine headaches
- morning sickness
- motion sickness

- overeating
- poisoning from eating non-food items, drug overdose or children getting into their parents' drugs
- viruses, bacteria or parasites

When Should a Doctor be Contacted?
- if you suspect poisoning, over medication, alcohol or drug abuse
- if you suffer from a sore neck or headache
- if you have signs of being dehydrated such as excessive thirst, urine that is infrequent and dark yellow, dry mouth, sunken face and eyes, skin that loses elasticity and doesn't bounce back when it is pinched
- the vomiting lasts more than eight hours
- there is blood or greenish bile in the vomit

Tips for Vomiting
- Drink a lot of water or clear fluids.
- Fast for the day to take the pressure off the stomach.
- If you must eat, consume only bland foods. Avoid spices, fats and solid foods.
- Rest after you eat, so that you do not rile your stomach.
- Do not over consume any food or drinks.
- For morning sickness eat small frequent meals and carry crackers to snack on.
- For motion sickness try to focus on an object in the horizon. Ride in the front seat, not the back.
- If smells bother you, stay out of the kitchen whilst meals are being made or cook odorless food.
- Fresh air may help with nausea. Open a window or go outdoors.

An Anti-Vomit Strategy

Try pressing your thumbs on your wrist, measured about two thumbs' width above the edge of your palm. Putting pressure on this point may help to interrupt the signal to the brain to throw up.

SUPPLEMENTS FOR VOMITING

Ginger
Ginger improves digestion and helps with belching that is associated with nausea and upset stomach. Ginger is usually taken as tea. A fresh piece of ginger can be cut into a small piece and steeped in hot water. There are many commercial packages of ginger tea. It is not useful for those with a sensitive stomach, bleeding conditions, ulcers or inflammatory skin disease. If you are taking Coumadin or Warfarin, do not use ginger. Don't take just prior to surgery.

Peppermint
Peppermint is a digestive aid that helps to relax the muscles of the digestive tract. It has been used since Roman times. It aids in expelling trapped gas, nausea, colic and

dyspepsia. Peppermint is said to help sooth the gut and decrease inflammation. It is useful in reducing colic pains under the diaphragm. It is also useful for nausea and vomiting. Typically, peppermint is bought commercially as a tea. It is available in an oil, which tends to be much stronger then the tea. Typical dosage is two to three grams of fresh leaves, taken as an infusion. Large doses of peppermint may affect male libido by decreasing testosterone. Some people have allergic reactions to peppermint and it may worsen gastroesophageal reflux symptoms.

Probiotics

Probiotics such as acidophilus and bifidobacterium are beneficial bacteria. If these products are not refrigerated, they may be a dead culture, which does not help the beneficial flora to grow. Take as directed on the label. They help re-colonize the beneficial bacteria in the GI tract. You always have bad and good bacteria in your gut. If bad and good flora becomes imbalanced, your stomach may be more easily upset and susceptible to bacterial, viral, parasites or yeast infections. See the Candidiasis or Worms/Parasite section for more information on treatment protocols.

HOMEOPATHIC REMEDIES FOR VOMITING

There are many homeopathic remedies for vomiting. Some of the more common remedies are listed with their symptoms here. For more information on how to self prescribe a homeopathic remedy, go to Chapter Two. If you cannot find a remedy suited to you, or find you are not improving or your symptoms get worse, seek the help of a professional homeopath or your medical doctor.

AETHUSIA
Common indications include:
- teething babies with gastrointestinal problems
- **vomiting of mucous, curdled milk and** cheesy appearance
- **milk products cause violent vomiting**
- falls asleep or becomes drowsy immediately after drinking milk
- **vomiting and diarrhea of newborns**
- **may see eruptions at the tip of the nose**
- poor ability to focus attention or think
- **mentally these types love animals and have many pets**
- **difficulty studying or concentrating**
- **aggravated by milk, after eating,** hot weather and from teething
- improved by covering up and resting

ARSENICUM ALBUM
Common indications include:
- **burning pains with abdominal distension**
- may have both vomiting and diarrhea
- **frequent vomiting of food and after motion and cold drinks or food**
- painful glands in the groin or inguinal area
- burning rectum with stools and intense cutting pain

- watery, painful diarrhea
- **sensitive to the smell of food**
- useful for traveler's diarrhea
- **nausea after a fever**
- **fear of disease**
- cold and clammy with the feeling they can never get warm enough
- **desires to sip hot drinks and warm applications despite burning sensation**
- great thirst yet only **takes small sips of hot water**
- nausea after meals
- **anxiety, restlessness with exhaustion**
- **relieved by hot drinks**, warmth, **motion** and exercise
- **worse after midnight, eating fruits, cold drinks,** after eating, and during rest

COCCULUS
Common indications include:

- this remedy is for those who care for sick people, including being worn down from watching over them at night
- **motion or sea-sickness**
- dizziness with nausea and when rising from bed
- **vertigo with a tendency to fall to the side**
- must lie on the side
- **abdominal distension**
- **vertigo with an intoxicated feeling**
- **faintness on moving**
- **belching and nausea after eating**
- **hates even the sight of food and will not eat**
- sensation of emptiness in the stomach
- thirsty without the desire to drink
- aggravated by noise, least amount of light, lying on the back, smoking, walking, open air, drinking, **being on a boat, riding in car and from night watching**
- improved while in a warm room and by lying quietly

IPECACUANA
Common indications include:

- **constant and continuous nausea**
- **retching, vomiting of blood and bile**
- **incessant inclination to vomit right after retching**
- **tongue is clean and uncoated despite nausea**
- **vomiting from coughing**
- **stitching and cutting pains in the abdomen**
- **stomach feels like it is hanging loose**
- **nausea with hemorrhages, after smoking and coughing**
- **aversion to food**
- vomiting of white mucous

- **aggravated by motion**, overeating, stooping, pork, fats, pastry to candy
- better in open air

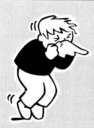
A 1985 study found that patients who took Oscillococcinum, a homeopathic flu remedy, experienced fever reduction in two days, which was much quicker than the placebo group. Also, chills and shivering disappeared on the fourth day. Another study from 1989, printed in the British Journal of Clinical Pharmacology, found that 66% more of the homeopathic group recovered within two days, compared to the placebo group.
Source: www.nationalcenterforhomeopathy.org

NATRUM PHOSPHORICUM
Common indications include:

- stomach pains
- heartburn, water brash
- trouble swallowing
- acid stomach and belching
- vomiting and nausea of pregnancy
- regurgitates fluid that is as sour as vinegar
- **vomiting sour, acid fluids**
- **tongue is coated yellow**
- liquids are not tolerated as well as solid food
- fullness after eating very little
- high uric acid in blood
- **cravings for fried eggs, salt**, beer, fried fish and spices
- worse two hours after eating, sugar, milk, bitter and fatty foods

NUX VOMICA
Common indications include:

- bitter acid and watery belching
- **constant nausea and vomiting with much retching**
- **vomiting from drinking too much**
- **seasickness**
- **nausea from smoking, drugs, alcohol**
- **sensation of a stone in the stomach after eating**
- heartburn may occur before breakfast
- pain in the stomach like a weight or pressure, two or three hours after meals
- bloating and distension
- putrid bitter taste in the mouth
- back of tongue is coated brown
- squeezing stomach aches, tender stomach
- reverse peristalsis, spasms from disordered peristalsis, pain when food passes down into the pyloric sphincter

- acute indigestion of improper foods
- digestive complaints with accompanying headaches
- **may be suited to zealous, fiery temperaments who overindulge and overwork**
- **cravings for fats and tolerates them well**
- **cravings for tea, coffee, alcohol and spicy**
- aversion to food
- **aggravated by anger**, after eating, drug use, tobacco poisoning, **overeating, overindulgence, alcohol, spices, stimulants, tea and coffee**

PHOSPHORUS

Common indications include:
- acute burning sensation
- sour belching and risings
- fullness in throat
- **sour, yellow and/or bitter vomiting of mucous, bile and/or blood**
- **vomit may look like coffee grounds**
- burning in stomach after eating
- **ravenous appetite**
- sharp and cutting pains in stomach after eating
- in some people, stomach feels as if cold as ice
- **great thirst for ice cold drinks and food**
- **vomiting of cold drinks as soon as they warm up in the stomach**
- **may be suited to tall and lean people who are outgoing, sympathetic and have many fears**
- **cravings for ice cream, chocolate, salt, spice, cold drink, milk and alcoholic drinks**
- aversion to warm drinks, coffee, garlic, onions, tomato, tea and boiled milk
- aggravated after every meal and from **warm drinks**

TABACUM

Common indications include:
- dizziness when opening the eyes, looking up or rising
- headache with terrible nausea
- **vomiting before breakfast**
- violent vomiting
- **seasickness**
- **nausea during pregnancy with spitting**
- **desire for tobacco**
- suddenly overcome with nausea, vomiting, weakness and cold perspiration
- **deathly nausea**
- aggravated by noise and light
- **aggravated by motion, a warm room, drinking, opening the eyes**, lying on the left side, riding, evening, room and walking
- relieved by open air, vomiting, vinegar and cold compresses

VERATRUM ALBUM
Common indications include:
- **sudden loss of strength**
- weakness with tremble
- **projectile vomiting**
- cough with vomiting
- cold sensation in the stomach
- **profuse, cold sweat on the forehead**
- violent nausea and vomiting
- watery diarrhea
- **simultaneous vomiting and diarrhea**
- gripping colic pains
- mentally these types are haughty and may have hallucinations when ill
- **craving for sour fruits, lemons, salt and ice**
- **worse during menses**, least motion, drinking, perspiration, pain, from exertion and fright
- relieved by pressure on the head, walking and from stimulants

Picture this….

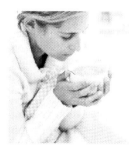

You have had been complaining of a burning feeling in your stomach for the past week. You don't want to eat. You wake up at 1:00 a.m. and throw up. You become overly concerned that you are deathly ill and cannot get back to sleep. You are hot and yet you want to drink hot tea. Your husband is complaining about you pacing the floor at night. Your husband is skilled in homeopathic remedies and sets you straight after three doses of Arsenicum Album 200 CH in one night. Your vomiting clears that night and does not return. Thank goodness both of you can now sleep!

Worms/Parasites

Worms are parasites that inhabit the gastrointestinal tract. The word parasite means that one thing exists by living off another. Parasites are caused by being ingesting or absorbing worms or eggs through eating poorly cook meat, contaminated water, stool and human waste, animals, mosquitoes and poor hygiene. Worm larvae and eggs can enter our body through any opening such as our mouth, anus, nose, genital urinary tract or the pores of our skin.

Worm eggs can bypass the digestive enzymes in our stomach because they have a hard protective layer that is difficult to breakdown. Parasitic infections are thought to be more common in those who travel or live in third world countries. However, we have a considerable number of cases in North America.

The Symptoms of Parasites

Some unknowing people suffer from parasites without symptoms. Those who do suffer with symptoms may experience:

- anemia
- abdominal pain
- anal itching
- bedwetting
- bloody mucous or stools
- breathing difficulties
- bronchitis
- diarrhea
- flatulence
- grinding of the teeth
- insomnia
- itching feet
- joint pains
- poor appetite
- rashes
- restlessness
- urination frequent
- vaginal itching
- vomiting
- weight loss

Types of Parasitic Infections

1. Roundworms are a type of worm that is very common. They include hookworms, pinworms, threadworms and ascarids.

   i. Pinworms are one of the most common parasitic infections in young children. It is frequent in daycare centres, schools and camps. Pinworms are about a third of an inch long, white and thread-like. They are spread by swallowing an egg from a pinworm. Since they lay so many eggs and are moist and resistant to drying, they are easily spread in dirt and dust particles. Children who suck their thumbs and play in sandboxes are good hosts for pinworms. Pinworms can cause severe anal itching which is worse at night and can lead to a restless sleep. Worms tend to come out of the rectum at night to lay their eggs.
   ii. Hookworms can cause itching feet, coughing, fever rash and loss of appetite. Typical hookworms are a half-inch long.
   iii. Threadworms typically cause coughing, bronchitis, gas, itching anus and vagina, stomach pain and loose stools.
   iv. Ascarids are one of the most common roundworm infections. It is common in third world countries, warm climates and rural communities. In some cases, no symptoms are noticed. Lung symptoms may appear such as bronchitis, shortness of breath and wheezing. Other symptoms include nausea, vomiting, bloody diarrhea, weight loss and fatigue.

2. Tapeworms are larger parasites that range from an inch up to 30 feet. These parasites may be seen in the stool; however no symptoms may be felt at all. Some people do feel nausea, fatigue, loss of appetite, pain, diarrhea and weight loss. In severe cases, it can cause cysts outside of the intestines and produce other serious symptoms. Tapeworms typically are passed on through animals (sheep and dogs), contaminated meat (pork, beef and fish), water and soil. These worms can lead to serious complications. Detection is done through a stool sample or blood testing.

Prevention of Parasitic Infections

Some simple tips to prevent a parasitic infection are as follows:

- Wash your hands with soap and water, after using the bathroom and before eating or handling food
- While traveling, wash and cook all foods, including fruits and vegetables with uncontaminated water
- Thoroughly cook meat and fish to kill any parasites or eggs
- Freeze meat or fish for a day to kill any eggs or worms
- Treat your pets or livestock for worms and wash your hands after handling them
- Be sure your water source is uncontaminated
- Cut your fingernails short to prevent eggs being transported
- Avoid nail biting and thumb sucking
- Wear clean underwear every day
- Wash yourself daily and clean around the anal and vaginal opening well to wash any eggs
- Use your own towel and wash cloth
- Vacuum and clean the bed sheets regularly because eggs can adhere to them or linger in dust

DIETARY REGIMES FOR WORM/PARASITIC INFECTIONS

Any bug such as yeast, viruses, bacteria and parasites thrive in an acid environment. It is said that even cancer cells cannot grow in an alkaline environment. They cannot grow in an alkaline intestinal tract. Your pH can shift to be more alkaline through dietary measures. Fifty to 70% of your daily food intake should be alkaline. You can measure your alkaline foods visually by dividing your plate into half or three quarters. The remaining 25 to 50% can be acid forming. Please note, you do still need to consume some acid-forming foods for good health.

Most fruits and vegetables are alkaline-forming. However, citrus fruits tend to aggravate bad bacteria such as candida, so they have some acid properties. On the other hand, millet, almonds and quinoa are very alkaline although they are not a vegetable. Foods that are acid-forming are sugar, animal meats, beans, grains, coffee, tea and alcohol. A percentage of acid forming foods are allowed, however sugar should be avoided because it turns alkaline foods acid. Sugar also tends to feed bad bacteria and help them proliferate. Any food that turns into sugar quickly in the bloodstream can also feed bad bacteria and produce an acid condition of the tissues. Therefore, it is best to eat a low glycemic diet as outlined in Chapter Three. The glycemic index is a measure of how quickly a food turns into a sugar in the bloodstream. The lower the rating on the glycemic index, the less quickly it flips into a sugar in the blood.

Certain foods contain beneficial bacteria that help to displace bad bacteria in the intestinal tract. Fermented products such as plain yogurt, kefir and miso all contain the good bacteria called acidophilus.

SUPPLEMENTS FOR WORM/PARASITIC INFECTIONS

Fibre
Foods that are high fibre help with constipation but also clear bile, cholesterol and toxic debris from the gastrointestinal tract. It is particularly beneficial for sweeping out parasites and debris from the gut. Many parasite cleansing kits contain psyllium, a type of soluble fibre. This is an inexpensive supplement that works well. Drink a large amount of water while you use it to prevent an intestinal blockage. It is healthy to include more fibre in your diet. Examples of high fibre foods are apples, Brussels sprouts, kale, cabbage, cooked legumes, ground flaxseed and whole grains. Whole grains that are high in fibre are brown rice, bulgur, millet, oat bran, slow cooked oatmeal, quinoa, whole wheat and wheat bran.

Garlic
Garlic helps to improve the immune system by stimulating bad bacteria eating cells. It has antibacterial, anti-parasitic, antifungal and antiviral properties and has a good long term effect on those with chronic yeast infections. It is not as strong as antibiotics and has only a modest affect on bacteria. Garlic has been shown effective for cancer, heart disease, immunity, candida, ulcers and parasites.

Typical dosage of garlic is 500 mgs to 1000 mgs per day. Avoid garlic if you take blood thinners or are undergoing surgery.

Oil of Oregano
Oregano oil has a strong anti-microbial effect and acts as an anti-inflammatory, antiseptic and diaphoretic (causes sweating). It comes in oil or capsule form and potency varies, so follow the directions on the individual labels. Side effects may include mild stomach upset and interference with iron absorption. Do not take oregano if you are pregnant or breast feeding, as studies have not confirmed its effect.

Herbal Parasite Formulas
Many health food stores carry a good herbal combination for killing parasites. They usually contain wormwood, male fern root, clove bud, garlic and/or black walnut. These formulas do work well for some people. However, they must be taken with probiotics because they sometimes destroy the good flora along with the bad.

Probiotics
Probiotics such as acidophilus and Bifidobacterium are beneficial bacteria which are found in kefir and yogurt. If you like these products, use an unsweetened variety. These bacteria help to re-colonize the beneficial bacteria in the gut and keep bad bacteria in check. They also help the intestine to metabolize and eliminate toxins.

If these products are not refrigerated, they may be a dead culture which does not help the beneficial flora to grow. They can be purchased in a standardized capsule to ensure the number of live bacteria per capsule. Follow the directions on the package.

Note: Any of these supplements that kill candida should be taken with probiotics to replenish the good bacteria. Like an antibiotic, they may kill some of the good bacteria..

HOMEOPATHIC REMEDIES FOR WORM/PARASITIC INFECTIONS

There are many homeopathic remedies for parasites. Some of the more common remedies are listed with their symptoms here. For more information on how to self prescribe a homeopathic remedy, go to Chapter Two. If you cannot find a remedy suited to you, or find you are not improving or your symptoms get worse, seek the help of a professional homeopath or your medical doctor.

CHENOPODIUM
Common symptoms include:
- suited to hookworm and roundworm
- pains under the breast, right shoulder and scapula
- pain in the head and the eyes
- urination is profuse and foamy

CINA
Common indications include:
- children's **remedy for pinworms**
- **teeth grinding**
- children have an uncontrollable **urge to put their fingers in their nose**
- restless sleep, waking in a frightful state
- **pale or bluish colour around the mouth**
- hungry soon after eating
- **mucous in stool like pieces of popcorn**
- **convulsions associated with worms**
- coughing
- **itching of the anus**
- involuntary diarrhea and urination
- **irritable, striking-out children**
- worse at night, summer, from worms and external pressure
- relieved by motion and laying on the abdomen

FILIX MAS
Common indications include:
- excellent remedy for tapeworms
- worm symptoms with constipation
- inflammation and swelling of the lymph glands
- diarrhea and vomiting

- hiccoughs
- itching of the nose
- weakness and fatigue

IGNATIA
Common indications include:
- itching at anus from pinworms
- hypersensitivity of the nerves
- **changeable mood from laughing to weeping**
- **constriction and spasms of the rectum after passing stool**
- fainting and loss of consciousness
- flatulence and hiccoughs
- diarrhea and a **sharp pain in the rectum**
- **sensation of a lump in the throat** with an inability to swallow
- temporary inability to speak
- **aggravated by grief, smoking**, in the morning, open air, eating and coffee
- relieved by eating and changing positions

SANTONINUM
Common indications include:
- useful for ascarids and threadworms
- itching of the nose
- restless sleep with nightly cough
- laryngitis
- dizziness
- eye symptoms such as pain, pressure and visual disturbances, having the visual hallucination of **things appearing green or having a green haze**
- twitching of the muscles

SPIGELIA
Common indications include:
- itching and crawling of the rectum
- ascarids
- **worms in children**
- ineffectual urging to stool
- pain in the eyes
- **left-sided headaches, especially above the eyes**
- dilated pupils, aversion to light
- fear of sharp things, needles and pins
- **aggravated by smoke**, touch, motion, turning and washing
- relieved by lying on the right side and deep breathing

TEUCRIUM MARUM VERUM
Common indications include:

- this is a remedy for pinworms where there is immense itching of the anus
- creeping sensation in the rectum that is worse at night in bed
- these types can suffer from unusual hunger
- this remedy is good for nasal polyps
- **flatulence**
- violent and jerking hiccoughs
- sensation of crawling in the nostrils
- worse at night, from the warmth of the bed and after nursing
- better in the open air

Picture this….

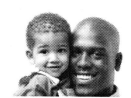

Your two-year-old boy was complaining of an itchy rectum. He had started to have restless sleep and was grinding his teeth. He would cry out in his sleep and thrash about. His stools were loose and he had a runny nose and a slight cough. You called your Homeopath. Based on his symptoms, he was prescribed a remedy called Cina 4 CH, four pellets twice a day for five days and a probiotic powder. After two days, his health returned to normal. His bowel movements were formed, he had no rectal itching and his cough was better.

Bibliography

Allen, H.C. *Keynotes and Characteristics with Comparisons of Some Leading Remedies of the Materia Medica with Bowel Nosodes,* Eighth Edition. Delhi India: B. Jain Publishers Pvt Ltd, 1995.

Anderson, Kenneth, Anderson, Lois and Glanze, Walter Ed. *Mosby's Medical, Nursing and Allied Dictionary, Fourth Edition.* Missouri: Mosby – Yearbook Inc., 1994.

Anderson, Richard. *Cleanse and Purify Thyself, Book 1.5.* California: Triumph, 1998.

Ansorge, R. Metcalf, E, *Allergy Free Naturally: 1,000 Non-drug Solutions for More Than 50 Allergy Related Problems.* USA: Rodale Inc., 2001.

Astor, Stephen. *Hidden Food Allergies: Finding The Foods That Cause You Problems And Removing Them From Your Diet.* New York: Avery Publishing Group, 1997.

Balch, J. and Stengler, M. *Prescription for Natural Cures.* New Jersey: John Wiley and Sons, 2004.

Balch, Phyllis, *Prescription for Herbal Healing.* New York: Avery, 2002.

Balch, P., Balch, J. *Prescription for Dietary Wellness.* Greenfield: Prescription Books for Health Inc., 1992.

Balch, P., Balch, J. *Prescription for Nutritional Healing, Third Edition.* New York: Avery, 2000.

Berkow, Robert ed. *The Merck Manual, Sixteenth Edition.* New Jersey: Merck Research Laboratories, 1992.

Bernard, H., *The Homeopathic Treatment of Constipation.* New Delhi: B. Jain Publishers (P) Ltd., 2004.

Bhanja, K.C. *The Homeopathic Prescriber, Sixth Edition.* Calcutta, N.K. Mitter at the Indian Press Pvt. Ltd., 1989.

Blumenthal, Mark. *The Complete German Commission E Monographs, Therapeutic Guide to Herbal Medicines.* Boston Massachusetts: Integrative Medicine Communications, 1998.

Boger, C.M. *Boenninghausen's Characteristics Materia Medica & Repertory with Word Index.* New Delhi: B. Jain Publishers (P) Ltd., 1996.

Calbom, Cherie, Keane, Maureen. *Juicing for Life; A Guide to the Health Benefits of Fresh Fruit and Vegetable Juicing.* New York: Avery Publishing Group Inc., 1992.

Chilton, Floyd. *Inflammation Nation*. New York: Fireside, 2005.

Clarke, John. H. *Indigestion*. Delhi: Unisons Techno Financial Consultants (P) Ltd. 2002.

Clarke, John. H. *The Prescriber*. Essex: C.W. Daniel Company Ltd, 1992

Gallop, Rick. *The G.I. Diet.* Canada: Random House, 2002.

Gursche, Siegfried and Rona, Zoltan. *Encyclopedia of Natural Healing.* Burnaby B.C., Alive Publishing, Inc. 1997.

Jahr, G.H.G. *Therapeutic Guide; Forty Years' Practice.* New Delhi: B. Jain Publishers PVT. Ltd, 1994.

Joshi, Nish. *Joshi's Holistic Detox, 21 days to a Healthier Slimmer You- For Life.* London: Hodder & Stoughton Ltd, 2006.

Krop, Josef J. *Healing the Planet One Patient at a Time,* Alton Ontario: KOS Publishing Inc, 2008.

Lewith, G., Kenyon, J., Dowson, D. *Allergy and Intolerance: A Complete Guide to Environmental Medicine.* London, Green Print, 1992.

Lilienthal, Samuel. *Homeopathic Therapeutics*. Delhi: B. Jain Publishers (P) Ltd., 1997.

Masoff, Joy. *Oh Yuck; The Encyclopedia of Everything Nasty.* New York. Workman Publishing Company Inc., 2000.

Murray, Michael, Pizzorino, Joseph. *Encyclopedia of Natural Medicine, Revised Second Edition.* California: Prima Health 1998.

Rademacher. *Universal and Organ Remedies.* New Delhi: B.Jain Publishers PVT. Ltd, 2004.

Rivera, R., Deutsch, R. *Your Hidden Food Allergies Are Making You Fat.* California: Prima Publishing, 1998.

Ruddock, E.H. *The Stepping Stone to Homoeopathy & Health.* Thirteenth Edition, New York: Boericke and Tafel.

Schafer, Kristen S. et al. *Chemical Trespass: Pesticides in Our Bodies and Corporate Accountability,* Pesticide Action Network North America, May, 2004. www.panna.org

Shinghal, J.N. *Quick Bedside Prescriber.* New Delhi: B. Jain Publishers Pvt Ltd., 1998.

Thom, Dick. *Coping With Food Intolerance, Fourth Edition.* New York: Sterling Publishing Company Inc., 2002.

Tyler, M.L., *Pointers to the Common Remedies.* New Delhi: B. Jain Publishers Pvt Ltd., 1993.

Ullman, Dana. *The Homeopathic Revolution; Why Famous People and Cultural Heroes Choose Homeopathy.* Berkeley, California: North Atlantic Books, 2007.

Ullman, Robert, Judith, Reichenberg-Ullman. *Homeopathic Self-care: The Quick & Easy Guide For The Whole Family.* Rocklin California: Prima Lifestyles, 1997

Vermeulen, Frans. *Concordant Materia Medica.* Haarlem: Emryss bv Publishers, 1997.

Von Lippe, Adolph. *Keynotes and Redline Symptoms of the Materia Medica.* Delhi: B. Jain Publishers Pvt. Ltd., 1995.

Von Lippe, Adolph. *Textbook of Materia Medica.* Delhi: B. Jain Publishers (P.) Ltd., 2005.

Walker, Richard. *Body; An Amazing Tour of the Human Body.* New York, Dorling Kinderley Ltd., 2005.

Index

<u>About the Author</u>

Since the 1990s, Heather Caruso, B.Sc., DHMS, HD, has been a Homeopath in private practice in Guelph, Ontario, Canada. Her interest in homeopathy grew after a personal 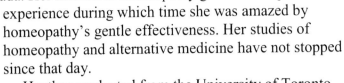 experience during which time she was amazed by homeopathy's gentle effectiveness. Her studies of homeopathy and alternative medicine have not stopped since that day.

Heather graduated from the University of Toronto with a Bachelor of Science. She received her Homeopathic training from the Homeopathic College of Canada. Her post graduate studies included many nutritional courses and teachings with world renowned homeopathic doctors. She has also been trained in various testing methods such electrodermal screening and darkfield microscopy.

Heather believes that education is the key to good health and that everyone has an innate healing ability if they are given the right foundation to express it (i.e. diet, homeopathic remedies and supplements). She has published various informative homeopathic articles in many alternative health magazines and made several television appearances over the years.

In private practice, Heather uses a realistic, natural approach to healthcare that respects the individuality of each client. Her goal is to set each person up to succeed on their healing journey via teaching healthy choices. She believes in a healthy proactive lifestyle through diet, homeopathy and natural supplements. Her conviction is that each person has an innate healing ability that can be expressed if given the correct tools. She uses an alternative health approach but embraces the benefits of both traditional medicine and natural remedies.

For more information on Caruso Homeopathic Clinic, go to
www.carusohomeopathy.com